Computational Intelligence and Applications for Pandemics and Healthcare

Sapna Singh Kshatri
Bharti Vishwavidyalaya, India

Kavita Thakur
Pt. Ravishankar Shukla University, India

Maleika Heenaye Mamode Khan
University of Mauritius, Mauritius

Deepak Singh
NIT, Raipur, India

G. R. Sinha
Myanmar Institute of Information Technology, Mandalay, Myanmar

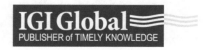

A volume in the Advances in
Medical Technologies and Clinical
Practice (AMTCP) Book Series

Published in the United States of America by
    IGI Global
    Medical Information Science Reference (an imprint of IGI Global)
    701 E. Chocolate Avenue
    Hershey PA, USA 17033
    Tel: 717-533-8845
    Fax: 717-533-8661
    E-mail: cust@igi-global.com
    Web site: http://www.igi-global.com

Library of Congress Cataloging-in-Publication Data

Names: Kshatri, Sapna Singh, 1986- editor. | Thakur, Kavita, 1967- editor.
 | Heenaye-Mamode Khan, Maleika, 1984- editor. | Singh, Deepak, 1986-
 editor. | Sinha, G. R., 1975- editor.
Title: Computational intelligence and applications for pandemics and
 healthcare / Sapna Singh Kshatri, Kavita Thakur, Maleika Heenaye Mamode
 Khan, Deepak Singh, and G.R. Sinha, editors.
Description: Hershey, PA : Engineering Science Reference, an imprint of IGI
 Global, [2022] | Includes bibliographical references and index. |
 Summary: "The primary goal of this book is to introduce the most recent
 technologies and methods for improving the health-care system to take it
 to the next level, discussing the tactics and methods, as well as their
 limitations and performances to grasp the great biomedical potential of
 AI and inspire researchers in relevant areas"-- Provided by publisher.
Identifiers: LCCN 2021054765 (print) | LCCN 2021054766 (ebook) | ISBN
 9781799898313 (h/c) | ISBN 9781799898320 (s/c) | ISBN 9781799898337
 (ebook)
Subjects: LCSH: Medical informatics. | Computational
 intelligence--Industrial applications. | Epidemics. | Organizational
 change.
Classification: LCC R858 .C62397 2022 (print) | LCC R858 (ebook) | DDC
 610.285--dc23/eng/20211215
LC record available at https://lccn.loc.gov/2021054765
LC ebook record available at https://lccn.loc.gov/2021054766

This book is published in the IGI Global book series Advances in Medical Technologies and Clinical Practice (AMTCP) (ISSN: 2327-9354; eISSN: 2327-9370)

British Cataloguing in Publication Data
A Cataloguing in Publication record for this book is available from the British Library.

All work contributed to this book is new, previously-unpublished material.
The views expressed in this book are those of the authors, but not necessarily of the publisher.

For electronic access to this publication, please contact: eresources@igi-global.com.

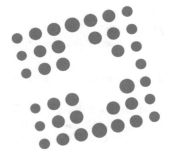

Advances in Medical Technologies and Clinical Practice (AMTCP) Book Series

ISSN:2327-9354
EISSN:2327-9370

Editor-in-Chief: Srikanta Patnaik, SOA University, India, Priti Das, S.C.B. Medical College, India

MISSION

Medical technological innovation continues to provide avenues of research for faster and safer diagnosis and treatments for patients. Practitioners must stay up to date with these latest advancements to provide the best care for nursing and clinical practices.

The **Advances in Medical Technologies and Clinical Practice (AMTCP) Book Series** brings together the most recent research on the latest technology used in areas of nursing informatics, clinical technology, biomedicine, diagnostic technologies, and more. Researchers, students, and practitioners in this field will benefit from this fundamental coverage on the use of technology in clinical practices.

COVERAGE

- Diagnostic Technologies
- Clinical Data Mining
- Biometrics
- Biomedical Applications
- Biomechanics
- Clinical Studies
- Medical Imaging
- Medical Informatics
- E-Health
- Clinical High-Performance Computing

IGI Global is currently accepting manuscripts for publication within this series. To submit a proposal for a volume in this series, please contact our Acquisition Editors at Acquisitions@igi-global.com or visit: http://www.igi-global.com/publish/.

Titles in this Series

For a list of additional titles in this series, please visit:
http://www.igi-global.com/book-series/advances-medical-technologies-clinical-practice/73682

For an entire list of titles in this series, please visit:
http://www.igi-global.com/book-series/advances-medical-technologies-clinical-practice/73682

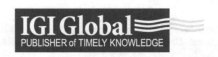

701 East Chocolate Avenue, Hershey, PA 17033, USA
Tel: 717-533-8845 x100 • Fax: 717-533-8661
E-Mail: cust@igi-global.com • www.igi-global.com

Table of Contents

Section 1
From Artificial Intelligence to Good Healthcare: Theory, Framework, and Methods

    Sapna Singh Kshatri, Bharti Vishwavidyalaya, India
    Sameer Sharma, Carl von Ossietzky University Oldenburg, Germany
    G. R. Sinha, Myanmar Institute of Technology, Mandalay, Myanmar

    Simranjit Singh, Bennett University, India
    Mohit Sajwan, Bennett University, India
    Deepak Singh, National Institute of Technology, Raipur, India

    Astha Bhanot, Princess Nourah Bint Abdulrahman University, Saudi
        Arabia
    Naila Iqbal Qureshi, Princess Nourah Bint Abdulrahman University,
        Saudi Arabia

Section 2
From Artificial Intelligence to Good Healthcare: Review, Methods, and Healthcare

Section 3
From Artificial Intelligence to Healthcare: Comparison, IoT, and Cloud

Detailed Table of Contents

Section 1
From Artificial Intelligence to Good Healthcare: Theory, Framework, and Methods

Septic shock, acute respiratory distress syndrome, multi-organ failure are all possible complications of the illness. In this work, machine learning is used to construct and assess mortality risk models that were evaluated (both positive and negative). The authors employed machine learning to gather information about 51,831 individuals (of which 4,769 were confirmed cases of COVID-19). The data collection comprises data from the next week (47,401 tested and 3,624 confirmed COVID-19). It is still uncertain if the SVM classifier ensemble can beat single SVM classifiers regarding the number of positive and negative predictions made in COVID-19. This investigation will investigate the accuracy of ensembled SVM and simple SVM on small and large COVID-19 datasets. The ROC, accuracy, F-measure, classification, and calculation time of SVM and SVM ensembles are evaluated and compared. According to the data, linear-based SVM performs the best when used as a bagging strategy. When dealing with tiny datasets that need feature extraction during pre-processing, bagging and boosting SVM ensembles may benefit.

Simranjit Singh, Bennett University, India
Mohit Sajwan, Bennett University, India
Deepak Singh, National Institute of Technology, Raipur, India

The SARS pandemic has spread throughout the world. Also known as "sporadic" or "spontaneous," the disease is contagious and can spread from someone who is in direct contact with someone else. COVID-19 is most commonly detected through RT-PCR tests, which may take longer than 48 hours. The data obtained from chest x-rays for COVID-19 patients has been found to be very promising for resolving emergencies, urgent care, and overcrowding. Deep learning (DL) methods in artificial intelligence (AI) play a significant role in the identification of the disease COVID using chest x-rays. In this chapter, a novel method for the effective classification of COVID-19 chest x-rays is proposed called XDeep. The developed model is able to achieve high classification accuracy, and the effectiveness is shown by comparing it with state-of-the-art models.

*Astha Bhanot, Princess Nourah Bint Abdulrahman University, Saudi
Arabia*
*Naila Iqbal Qureshi, Princess Nourah Bint Abdulrahman University,
Saudi Arabia*

The COVID-19 pandemic has left the healthcare sector with a slew of problems, including a lack of capacity, supply restrictions, the need for service reform, and financial losses. According to complexity, healthcare delivery organizations are complex adaptive systems that function in extremely complicated and unpredictable situations. Many healthcare organizations suffered ambiguity and inconsistency that was not under control as per requirements. In this chapter, the authors look at an effective management system in the face of COVID-19. In order to tackle the pandemic, Word Health Organization (WHO) is bringing together scientists and health experts from all across the world to speed research and development. The governmental and private sectors in India are viewed as cooperating. Private Indian healthcare organizations stepped up and have been providing everything it requires, including testing, treatment isolation beds, medical professionals, and equipment to the government.

In this chapter, the different dermatological diseases are differentiated using the concept of probabilistic neural networks (PNN). There are different colour transformations for various dermatological diseases. This chapter mainly focuses on the differentiation of psoriasis and dermatitis with the normal one. The colour, shape, and textural features of the patches are studied and analysed for recognising the various dermatological diseases. The colour, texture, mean, median, entropy, standard deviations are considered for feature analysis. The pre-screening system uses the PNN algorithm after the feature extraction. The experimental results define the accuracy and effectiveness of the proposed algorithm, and the system scores sensitivity of 0.91, specificity of 0.94, with an accuracy rate of 96.25%.

This chapter provides a comprehensive explanation of machine learning including an introduction, history, theory and types, problems, and how these problems can be solved. Then it shows some of the most used machine learning algorithms that are used in image classification, ending with the evaluation matrices calculations that are used to assess the performance of the learning models. The open source libraries also mentioned in this chapter facilitate the used codes for building any learning model with the use of machine learning.

Section 2
From Artificial Intelligence to Good Healthcare: Review, Methods, and Healthcare

The internet of things (IoT) and machine learning (ML) are massive technologies that provide enhancement and better resolutions in our daily life, such as in industry, healthcare, space sector, defense, buildings, agriculture, traffic, and so on. The area of IoT has shown a boost over the past decades with the continuous development of the ML tools. The combination of IoT with ML tools has a high impact on medical devices. The application of ML and IoT can provide significant improvements in all parts of healthcare domain from diagnostics to treatment. It is generally believed that ML tools will simplify and boost human work. In this chapter, the authors present the overview of current advance integration IoT and ML application on healthcare care management listed with all benefits and uses. This chapter also supports healthcare professionals to detect and treat disease more efficiently and researchers for their understanding of growth in ML and IoT-based technology.

This chapter is based on a review of heavy metals, high atomic weight, and high-density naturally occurring elements transition elements. In the periodic table, about 80 elements of them are called metals. These metals can be further classified into two categories, those that are essential for survival such as magnesium, potassium, calcium, etc. and those that are nonessential such as lead, mercury, bismuth, and cadmium. These nonessential metals are known as toxic metals. Trace elements such as selenium, zinc, copper, etc. are necessary for maintaining the human body metabolism. These essential elements can be toxic if present at high concentrations. On the other hand, some elements like Hg, Cd, Pb, Bi, Cr, As, etc. are usually toxic to the living organisms when absorbed in small quantities. The source of heavy metals is natural as well as manmade. The toxicity of heavy metals causes carcinogenic effects in human beings related to organ, renal, hepatic, neural, skeletal, and glandular problems.

This work shows the behavioral and heart condition monitoring of the patients during the COVID-19 infection. As the COVID-19 infection spreads very easily through contact, this work introduces a noninvasive technique to monitor such patients. The heart condition monitoring can be done through the analysis of acousticalcardiogram (ACG) as well as the behavioral changes observed through the Formant analysis. The speech of the patient is recorded, digitized, and its analysis is done using the PRAAT software. The required information from the speech samples is extracted and subjected to the analysis. The spectrogram of each utterance is plotted, and its first and second formants are analysed to form the vowel triangle. These vowel triangle provides behavioral monitoring. The monitoring of heart condition can be done using ACG. The Formant analysis of utterance of 12 Hindi consonants provides the assessment technique of the patient heart condition.

This study describes the immediate and long-term effects in behavioral and psychological symptoms due to COVID-19. To handle the situation, the Indian government tried in various levels lockdown, scanning of the patients, social distancing, compulsorily wearing the mask, vaccination, quarantine centers, etc., but in the long-term, all these activities affected social and physiological status. In extreme cases, people suffer from depression, which can be characterized by various factors like tiredness, poor sleep, pessimism, guilt, hopelessness, lack of confidence, low mood, gradual reduction in work output, loss of appetite, feeling helpless, loneliness, etc.

Section 3
From Artificial Intelligence to Healthcare: Comparison, IoT, and Cloud

Chapter 10

Neha Dewangan, Pandit Ravishankar Shukla University, Raipur, India
Prafulla Vyas, Disha College, Raipur, India
Ankita, Pandit Ravishankar Shukla University, Raipur, India
Sunandan Mandal, Pandit Ravishankar Shukla University, Raipur, India

A smart healthcare system is a need of the present world. Artificial intelligence, the internet of things, big data, etc. are essential technologies that build a smart and intelligent healthcare system. Deployment of a smart healthcare system not only serves diagnosis and treatment to more patients but also reduces the workload on health workers. Some patients face difficulties using the technology, which needs to be simplified. The most important issue in a smart healthcare system is cyber security. In smart healthcare systems, wearable devices and hospital management store patient information in digital format, which is available in cloud storage, which can be hacked, and it needs strong cyber security. With the development of technologies, smart healthcare systems can provide more intelligent and convenient applications and services. It can provide better service, self-health management, timely and appropriate medical service that can be accessed whenever needed, personalized medical service, improve the doctor-patient relationship, and reduce the cost of services.

Chapter 11

Manjushree Nayak, National Institute of Science and Technology, India
Anjli Barman, Aadarsh College, Raipur, India

Health is a basic necessity, and access to high-quality healthcare is a human right. Cloud computing provides a base for better reliable and cost-efficient business applications for corporate purposes. Cloud computing provides a good structure and a good cost for the organization with reduced administration. Recent advances in sensor communication, sensor sensing, and microelectronics are focused on monitoring and managing chronic diseases and potential emergencies. Health monitoring can be managed by one or both: the cost of main challenges and citizen-centered care. This likewise permits a specialist to make electronic visits, including no transportation with full correspondence from the specialist to the patient. They can see one another, which permits the specialist to see the wounds. The authors discussed home hospitalization frameworks on the IoT and cloud-based healthcare monitoring systems in this chapter.

    Tanu Rizvi, Shri Shankaracharya Technical Campus, Bhilai, India
    Devanand Bhonsle, Shri Shankaracharya Technical Campus, Bhilai,
        India
    Ruhi Uzma, Anjuman College of Engineering and Technology, India

Behavior of any human is mostly permanent as per their personality, but it gets influenced by a variety of factors originating psychologically and socially. However, some temporary factors such as attitude, surroundings, instant mood, culture, etc. may hamper behavior severely. Researchers have published many articles depending upon human behavior and its approach. This study is aimed to describe the effect of external parameters on human behavior in Indians as well as Europeans due to COVID-19 outbreak globally. This study is a survey made on online platform in Indian premises and studies carried by researchers in four European countries: UK, France, the Netherlands, and Denmark. Comparisons have been done with different levels and parameters between India and European countries. This chapter not only concludes the psychological constraints but also the good habits adopted by peoples during COVID-19 pandemic to have a safer future.

    Arun Kumar, Bhilai Institute of Technology, India
    Padmini Sharma, Chhatrapatishivaji Institute of Technology, India
    Mukesh Kumar Chandrakar, Bhilai Institute of Technology, India

Photoplethysmograph signal carries very useful cardiac information such heart rate, oxygen saturation level, blood pressure, and diabetic condition. Blood pressure is one such cardiac information that can be estimated by extracting features of PPG signal. Cuff-less blood pressure measurement using photoplethysmograph (PPG) signal is one of non-invasive methods. It allows continuous monitoring of blood pressure in simple, rapid, and low-cost mode. This chapter segregates PPG features and re-investigates their effectiveness in terms of BP measurement. Machine learning algorithm based on K-nearest neighbour is applied for classification of samples. MIMIC II multi-parameter database of ECG and finger PPG is applied on the KNN classifiers. Classification accuracy comes to 92%, and correlation between predicted and observed SBP and DSB are 0.89 and 0.85, respectively.

Digitized healthcare technologies provide healthcare enhancements in the field of medical digital technologies and they also provide better accessibility. The research study indicates that digital healthcare is combining or involving more than one academic discipline like biology science, cognitive science, medical science, biochemistry neuroscience, etc. The complete healthcare technologies are based on computational intelligence, artificial intelligence, etc. This chapter gives an overview of the current and future of healthcare technologies and up-to-date research in the area of digital healthcare intelligence. For artificial intelligence or computational intelligence, healthcare is one of the most promising application areas. This review highlights all about applications of artificial intelligence, telemedicine, blockchain technologies, the internet of things, and big data for solving the problems in medical education and healthcare technologies.

Preface

Over the last few decades, lifestyles have shifted dramatically, resulting in many lifestyle-related disorders showing themselves regardless of age or financial bracket. Lack of physical activity and addiction to electronics have increased childhood obesity, emotional insecurity, and various other personality disorders. COVID-19 The pandemic has brought to light a variety of lifestyle-related challenges and refocused lifestyle sustainability and management. Future requirements are a balanced lifestyle that places a premium on automation in wellness and healthcare. Intelligent Systems for Healthcare Management and Delivery discusses relevant and advanced methodological, technological, and scientific approaches to the application of sophisticated AI exploitation, as well as providing insight into technologies and intelligent applications that have gained increasing attention in recent years, such as medical imaging, electronic medical records, and drug development assistance.

Computational Intelligence and Applications for Pandemics and Healthcare is an organized collection of 14 chapters written by renowned authors worldwide that gives a complete look at the use of technology in healthcare, including analytics and visualization. It provides extensive and brief coverage of lifestyle sustainable growth based on artificial intelligence technical developments, emphasizing wellness solutions. The concept of Computational Intelligence's primary goal is to introduce the most recent technologies and methods for improving the healthcare system to the next level. Recently The COVID-19 coronavirus pandemic has been causing a global health crisis. The critical phase in combating COVID-19 is identifying infected patients early and placing them with special treatment. One of the quickest ways to identify patients is to use radiography and radiology images to detect this disease. It is difficult to diagnose a chest infection solely based on chest X-rays. Each chapter begins with an introduction, the need and motivation of the medical modality, and several applications for identifying and improving the healthcare system in every area of biomedical. In this regard, this book helps educate current scientific achievements, comprehend the technology available, grasp the great biomedical potential of AI and inspire researchers in relevant areas, and discusses the tactics and methods and their limitations and performances.

This book discusses theoretical, practical, emotional, and sociological perspectives on life sustainability solutions that incorporate sophisticated technologies such as artificial intelligence, IoT, mental illness, Healthcare Management, Machine Learning, Behavioral Changes, Diagnosis of COVID-19 and Visualization. Can utilize efficiently to advance research and technology in healthcare, precisely wellness solutions in general.

I perceive the compilation of the book as a pragmatic approach in covid 19 and healthcare the use of the 'Artificial intelligence, which is also helpful for a global health crisis. I am pleased to write a foreword for a contemporary subject on "Computational Intelligence and Applications for Pandemics and Healthcare", published by the globally reputed IGI Publishers.

Chapter 1 introduce about machine learning is used to develop and evaluate mortality risk models (both positive and negative). We used machine learning to collect data on 51,831 individuals (in which 4769 were confirmed cases of c0vid 19). The data collection period encompasses the following week (47,401 tested and 3624 confirmed covid 19). It is yet unknown whether the ensemble of SVM classifiers can outperform individual SVM classifiers in terms of the number of positive and negative predictions made in covid 19. This inquiry aims to determine the accuracy of ensembled machine learning techniques using massive covid 19 datasets.

Chapter 2 provide artificial intelligence (AI) algorithms based on deep learning (DL) are critical in identifying the disease Covid utilizing chest X-rays. Also referred to as "sporadic" or "spontaneous," the disease is contagious and can spread through direct touch with another person. COVID-19 is most frequently discovered via RT-PCR testing, which can take up to 48 hours to complete. The data from COVID-19 patients' chest X-rays have been proven to be extremely promising for resolving emergencies, urgent care, and overcrowding.

Chapter 3 manages the Covid-19. The pandemic has created a plethora of complications in the healthcare industry. Healthcare delivery organizations, by definition, are complex adaptive systems that operate in challenging and unpredictable environments. Numerous healthcare organizations encountered uncertainty and inconsistency that did not manage by regulatory requirements. This chapter will examine an effective management strategy in light of the Covid-19. In India, the public and private sectors are considered cooperating. Private Indian healthcare institutions stepped in and provided the government with everything necessary, including diagnostics, treatment isolation beds, medical personnel, and equipment.

Chapter 4 discusses the various dermatological illnesses and how they might be classified using the concept of Probabilistic Neural Networks (PNN). There are other color modifications for a variety of dermatological conditions. This chapter is mainly concerned with differentiating Psoriasis and Dermatitis from typical skin conditions. The patches' color, shape, and textural characteristics are investigated and analyzed to identify various dermatological conditions. Color, texture, mean, median, entropy, and standard deviations are all considered while performing feature analysis. Following feature extraction, the pre-screening system employs the PNN algorithm.

Chapter 5 provides a comprehensive explanation of machine learning, including an introduction to the subject, a history of machine learning, the theory and types of machine learning, machine learning problems, and how we can solve these problems. It then illustrates several of the most commonly used machine learning algorithms for image classification, concluding with the evaluation matrices calculations used to assess the learning models' performance. Additionally, the open-source libraries discussed in this chapter simplify codes for developing any machine learning model.

Chapter 6 presents the current advanced integration IoT and ML application on healthcare care management listed with all benefits and uses. This chapter also supports healthcare professionals to detect and treat disease more efficiently, and researchers for their understanding of growth in ML and IoT based technology. The Internet of Things (IoT) and machine learning (ML) are massive technologies that provide enhancement and better resolutions in our daily lives, such as in industry, healthcare, space sector, defense, buildings, agriculture, traffic, etc.

Chapter 7 reviews heavy metals, high atomic weight, and high density naturally occurring elements. Metals are around 80 elements in the periodic table. These elements, such as magnesium, potassium, calcium, etc., are required for survival. Lead, mercury, bismuth, and cadmium. Toxic metals are non-essential metals. Trace elements like selenium, zinc, copper, etc. are required for metabolism. High concentrations of these necessary components can be harmful. Some elements, such as Hg, Cd, Pb, Bi, Cr, As, etc., are harmful to living creatures even in small amounts. Heavy metals can be natural or man-made. Heavy metal poisoning causes organ damage, including renal, hepatic, neurological, skeletal, and glandular cancer.

Chapter 8 shows the patients' behavioral and heart condition monitoring during the COVID-19 infection. The COVID-19 infection spreads easily through contact, so this work introduces a non-invasive technique to monitor such patients. The heart condition monitoring can be done through the analysis of Acoustical cardiogram (ACG) and the behavioral changes observed through the Formant analysis. The patient's speech is recorded, digitized and its research is done using the PRAAT software. The required information from the speech samples is extracted and subjected to analysis. The spectrogram of each utterance is plotted, and its first and second formants are analyzed to form the vowel triangle. These vowel triangles provide behavioral monitoring. The monitoring of heart condition can be done using ACG. The Formant analysis of utterance of twelve Hindi consonants provides the assessment technique of the patient's heart condition.

Chapter 9 discussed human behaviors related to activities and relationships. In addition, it distinguishes humans from other organisms on the planet. COVID-19 has rapid and long-term behavioral and psychological effects on this study. The government attempted various tactics, including lockdown, patient screening, social segregation, mandatory mask wear, vaccination, and quarantine centers. Chronic weariness, inadequate sleep, pessimism, guilt, hopelessness, and a lack of confidence contribute to depression, as does a progressive decline in work performance, appetite loss, helplessness, and loneliness.

Chapter 10 gives the today's world; smart healthcare is vital. One of the most important components of a smart healthcare system is artificial intelligence. It also reduces the workload of medical personnel. This should be easy for some patients. A smart healthcare system's most essential issue is cybersecurity. Data is stored in a cloud-based format, which is vulnerable to hacking and requires solid cyber protection. Smart healthcare systems will provide more intelligent and convenient apps and services as technology develops. Medical care can be tailored to individual needs, enhancing the doctor-patient relationship and lowering expenses.

Chapter 11 addressed access to high-quality health care as a human right. Cloud computing is a concept that combines computing and networking technologies to create more reliable and cost-effective commercial applications for corporations. Cloud computing reduces administration and provides a good framework. Recent sensor communication, sensing, and microelectronics breakthroughs focus on chronic illness monitoring and emergency detection. Either or both can handle the expense of primary challenges and citizen-centered care. This allows a specialist to conduct electronic visits with patients without travelling. They can see each other, allowing the specialist to see the wounds as the patient intended.

Chapter 12 discovers that various psychological and social factors impact human behaviors. However, transient elements like attitude, environment, mood, culture, etc., can severely affect Behavior. Many papers have been written about human behaviors and its approach. This study describes how the global COVID-19 pandemic affects Indians and Europeans. This study is based on online surveys conducted in India and four other European nations, namely the UK, France, the Netherlands, and Denmark. India and European countries have been compared on several levels and characteristics. This chapter summarizes the COVID-19 pandemic survivors' psychological restrictions and good practices.

Chapter 13 learns that a K-nearest neighbor technique is used to classify samples. They are using the classifiers for better classification. The photoplethysmography signal includes cardiac data like heart rate, oxygen saturation, blood pressure, and diabetes status. The PPG signal can assess cardiac information such as blood pressure. Non-invasive cuff-less photoplethysmography (PPG) blood pressure measuring offers simple, quick, and low-cost continuous blood pressure monitoring. This study attempted to separate PPG features and re-evaluate their BP measuring efficacy.

Chapter 14 discusses using AI, telemedicine, blockchain, IoT, and Big Data to solve medical education and healthcare difficulties. The digitized healthcare technology improves healthcare and accessibility. Research shows that digital healthcare includes academic disciplines like biology, cognitive science, medical science, biochemistry, and neuroscience. The comprehensive healthcare technologies are based on AI and CI. This chapter examines present and future healthcare technologies and current research in digital healthcare intelligence.

Artificial intelligence (AI) transforms every element of human existence, including healthcare and pandemic applications. Numerous intelligent healthcare engineering applications have been developed to address patient healthcare and outcomes, such as disease identification and data collection. AI advancements in healthcare are being pursued to aid in illness identification, health monitoring, and prescription medicine tracking.

This book takes a theoretical, practical, mental, and societal approach to life sustainability solutions that incorporate advanced technologies such as artificial intelligence, the Internet of Things, big data analytics, cloud computing, health management, and covid -19 and healthcare. This book can significantly advance the field of research and technology in the domain of healthcare in particular and wellness solutions in general. The authors of this Handbook come from worldwide. They have significant experience in the artificial intelligence, healthcare-technology, and psychology domains, making this a quality-oriented endeavor to develop healthy and sustainable solutions for a more productive and satisfying living.

TARGET AUDIENCE

The book is designed to serve as a reference for medical students and academics working in this sector. The issues and case studies discussed in this book will aid practitioners in comprehending and disseminating the current state of the art and advancements in artificial intelligence techniques, applications, and healthcare in health care engineering and Big data management to interested readers and researchers.

Sapna Singh Kshatri
Bharti Vishwavidyalaya, India

Acknowledgment

Dr. Sapna Singh expresses sincere thanks to her husband Mr. Yogesh singh Kshatri and son vivant and Viraj, her parents Mr. F. S. Chandel and Mrs. Chandrika Chandel for their wonderful support and encouragement throughout the completion of this important book on Computational Intelligence and Applications for Pandemics and Healthcare with IGI Global Publisher. This book is an outcome of focused and sincere efforts that could be given to the book only due to great support of the family.

Dr Singh is grateful to her teachers who have left no stones unturned in empowering and enlightening him, especially Dr. G. R. Sinha who is like God father for him. Dr Singh also extends his heartily thanks to Dr. Deepak singh Guidance and support.

Dr Singh would like to thank all her friends, well-wishers and all those who keep him motivated in doing more and more; better and better. Dr Singh offers her reverence with folded hands to Swami Vivekananda who has been his source of inspiration for all his work and achievements

The editors would like to express their gratitude to all authors for their contributions. This book is a combined effort of various experts in Artificial Intelligence and Health Engineering and management. Knowledge is not accumulated in a single day. We acknowledge that the chapters contributed by authors are not the output of a single time frame. It results from the various years of their effort in the respective domain. We acknowledge their expertise and the time and effort contributed to this book.

Our sincere thanks to the reviewers who made immensely constructive suggestions and effective efforts to improve the book's chapters' quality, readability, and content. Some of our authors also reviewed others' chapters, and we thank them for their valuable time and efforts. Words cannot express our sincere thanks to all of them without whose timely comments; this book would not have taken its current shape. Last but most important, humble thanks to Team-IGI for great support, necessary help, appreciation and quick responses. Thanks to IGI Global Publisher also for giving me this opportunity to contribute on some relevant topic with reputed publisher.

Acknowledgment

Sapna Singh Kshatri
Bharti Vishwavidyalaya, India

Kavita Thakur
Pt. Ravishankar Shukla University, India

Maleika Heenaye Mamode Khan
University of Mauritius, Mauritius

Deepak Singh
NIT Raipur, India

G. R. Sinha
Myanmar Institute of Information Technology, Mandalay, Myanmar

Introduction

Artificial intelligence (AI) has been developing rapidly in recent years in terms of software algorithms, hardware implementation, and applications in a medical heath care. The goal of this book is to explore the state-of-the-art of computational intelligence approaches in medical data and to classify existing Computational techniques used in medical areas as single or hybrid. The constraints are addressed as difficulties in order to obtain a set of needs for Computational Intelligence Medical Data (CIMD).

The editors have done an excellent job at every stage and have ensured that the chapters are examined by reputable reviewers, as far as I am aware. At the moment, no book exists that tackles this critical collection of public health and health care challenges. The guidebook is intended for researchers, academics, practitioners, policymakers, and postgraduate students working in information technology, health care, technology management, and artificial intelligence.

We explore the most recent developments in AI applications in biomedicine, such as deep learning, artificial neural networks, biomedical information processing, biomedical research, as well as cloud computing, evolutionary computing, and statical technologies. Clinical flow diagram to aid physicians, and laboratory professionals in the management of COVID-19 patients with aspergillosis, candidiasis, mucormycotic, or cryptococcosis as co-morbidities. In addition, we investigate how deep learning models can be used to detect COVID-19 patients in chest radiography images. Early research discovered specific abnormalities in COVID-19, aspergillosis-infected people' chest and body X–ray CT scans.

The Handbook Computational Intelligence and Applications for Pandemics and Healthcare of Research Using machine learning, deep learning, artificial intelligence, big data analytics, and visualization to conduct research on applications for pandemics and healthcare that contribute to the diagnosis, detection, conduct, protection, and technological enhancement, including machine learning, deep learning, artificial intelligence, big data analytics, and visualizations. Additionally, it gives Behavioral Change, which can help enhance lifestyle monitoring and aid in diagnosing mental illness in humans. It is ideal for technologists, students, data scientists, hospital administrators, researchers, academicians, physicians, IT specialists, systems engineers, and technology providers. It covers big data, intelligent medical systems, and cloud-based health technology.

Doctors, clinicians, engineers, and researchers will benefit from the presented approaches in their research and diagnosis. This book is also an excellent guide for undergraduate and postgraduate students and researchers in electrical, computer science, biomedical engineering, and healthcare. This Handbook is an organized compilation of 14 chapters written by renowned authors from across the world that provides a thorough and concise treatment of Lifestyle Sustainability solutions utilizing cutting-edge technical breakthroughs emphasizing well-being.

Sapna Singh Kshatri
Bharti Vishwavidyalaya, India

Section 1
From Artificial Intelligence to Good Healthcare: Theory, Framework, and Methods

Chapter 1
An Investigation of the Coronavirus Disease (COVID–19) Mortality Risk Using Machine Learning

Sapna Singh Kshatri
Bharti Vishwavidyalaya, India

Sameer Sharma
Carl von Ossietzky University Oldenburg, Germany

G. R. Sinha
Myanmar Institute of Technology, Mandalay, Myanmar

ABSTRACT

Septic shock, acute respiratory distress syndrome, multi-organ failure are all possible complications of the illness. In this work, machine learning is used to construct and assess mortality risk models that were evaluated (both positive and negative). The authors employed machine learning to gather information about 51,831 individuals (of which 4,769 were confirmed cases of COVID-19). The data collection comprises data from the next week (47,401 tested and 3,624 confirmed COVID-19). It is still uncertain if the SVM classifier ensemble can beat single SVM classifiers regarding the number of positive and negative predictions made in COVID-19. This investigation will investigate the accuracy of ensembled SVM and simple SVM on small and large COVID-19 datasets. The ROC, accuracy, F-measure, classification, and calculation time of SVM and SVM ensembles are evaluated and compared. According to the data, linear-based SVM performs the best when used as a bagging strategy. When dealing with tiny datasets that need feature extraction during pre-processing, bagging and boosting SVM ensembles may benefit.

DOI: 10.4018/978-1-7998-9831-3.ch001

INTRODUCTION

Today, the world is thinking about coronavirus sickness, which suggests that this pandemic is not unique. Recently, the world has seen remarkable advancements in technology, which plays a vital role in industrialized countries. Nowadays, all aspects of daily life, including education, business, marketing, armies, communications, engineering, and health care, rely on modern technology applications. The health care centre is a necessary profession that relies largely on current technology, from symptom definition to precise diagnosis and computerized patient triage. Healthcare companies urgently need decision-making systems to manage this virus effectively and get appropriate recommendations in real-time to prevent its spread. AI is very adept at simulating human intellect. It may also be critical in comprehending and recommending the creation of a COVID-19 vaccine. This outcome-driven tool is used to evaluate, analyse, forecast, and follow existing and potential future patients. Significant apps are used to keep track of verified, recovered, and wrongful death instances (Vaishya et al., 2020). Strict societal controls, along with current testing, have proved adequate to substantially decrease pandemic numbers, though not to the point of eradicating the virus. Indeed, breakouts are risking a second wave throughout the globe, which was much more destructive in the case of the Spanish flu than the first (Barro et al., 2020). And they often need patients to stay separated for many days until the desired outcome is achieved. In comparison, our AI-based pre-screening technology can check the whole globe daily, if not hourly, for a fraction of the cost. In terms of storage, the everyday rapid diagnostic ability in the US fluctuated between 5 million and 823,000 tests a week times today to July 13, 2020. However, other experts predicted that by June, the demand for 5000,000 tests a day would increase to 20 million per day through July (Tromberg et al., 2020). Our tool's infinite output and actual diagnostic capabilities may aid in intelligently prioritizing who should be examined, particularly in asymptomatic patients. In an assessment of 9 commercially available COVID-19 serology tests, sensitivities ranged between 40% and 86%, and AUCs ranged between 0.88 and 0.97 in the initial stage (7-13 days after the start of illness symptoms) (La Marca et al., 2020). Meanwhile, our technique with an AUC of 0.97 obtains a sensitivity of 98.5 percent.

Records are a significant strategic asset for nations in the digital economy, enhancing governments' abilities to handle social concerns and deliver good public services. Big data technology is used to assist a wide range of health-care operations, disease surveillance, and global health management including the clinical decision support, (Feldman & Martin, 2012). Big data technology, which analyses patient attributes and nursing expenses, has the potential to improve healthcare quality, save lives, and cut health-system expenditures, among other things. The most clinically cost-effective treatment methods may be determined through the use of big data analysis technology to analyse patient files. Through the gathering and analysis of medical procedure data, it is possible to identify individuals who may benefit from preventative care or lifestyle alterations, and the most advantageous patient nursing plans can be developed. In order to forecast epidemics, issue pandemic alerts, monitor and trace sick people, uncover potential pharmaceutical cures, and optimize resource allocation within the health system, significant data technologies are used (Ginsberg et al., 2009).

It has been suggested that effective area daily testing and investigations may serve as a near replacement for area incarceration in terms of containing the virus and avoiding the expenses associated with economic isolation (Marcel, 2020). However, many recent efforts at screening, contact tracing, and isolation, similar to those undertaken by the UK initially, have been a failure (Hunter, 2020). The current focus is continuing testing and survey methods (including contact tracking), network separation strategies, strengthening human services frameworks, and enlightening general society. For populations to comply with mental wellness, physical separation measures must be improved. Physical separations are very costly to society, both financially and socially. De-acceleration is, therefore, a hotly debated topic. Transmission will continue until a population assurance limit is achieved unless contamination levels in a given environment are lowered to a surface level. To put things into perspective for those in India, the 2019–20 coronavirus pandemic began on January 30th, 2020, and it is thought to have originated in China. Since April 14th, 2020, the Ministry of Health and Family Welfare has reported 10,815 cases, 1,190 recoveries, and 353 confirmed fatalities, according to the latest available data. Experts believe that India's low examination rate is to blame for the high sickness count. The illness rate for Covid-19 in India is 1.7, which is lower than the rate in the nations that have been least affected by the virus. Michael Ryan, director of the World Health Organization's health emergency program, stated that India has reached a "colossal breaking point" in terms of dealing with the coronavirus outbreak, and that this will have a big influence on the world's ability to monitor it in the coming days. Another point of emphasis was the economic damage caused by the lockdown, which prohibits transit and market access to casual workers as well as small businesses, farmers, and the self-employed, among others. Per observers, the lockdown has lowered the pandemic's development pace to a point where it is reproducing at regular intervals rather than on a regular timetable, as was the case before the lockdown. India may have had 31,000 cases of the sickness between March 24th and April 14th, according to a study conducted by Shiv Nadar University researchers (Roy, 2020). Developing highly interpretable machine learning-based approaches and performance-enhancing scoring systems for the goal of finding the biomarkers with the highest predictive value for patient death is still a significant unmet need. In order to allocate resources and provide treatment to those who are at heightened danger, it is necessary to identify them and prioritize them. In addition, persons who are at high risk must be identified. Developing advanced interpretable machine learning-based approaches and performance enhances scoring systems for the goal of discovering the most selective predictive indicators of patient death is still a major unsolved challenge. Individuals who are in imminent danger must be identified and given first priority in both resource allocation and medical care, according to the guidelines (Chowdhury et al., 2021).

In addition, higher risk patients should be examined continually during their hospital stay using a validated scoring system, which should be utilized to identify them. Patients with a minimal chance of developing difficulties can self-quarantine more easily, reducing the burden on healthcare institutions. A validated scoring system was utilized to evaluate them on a continuous basis during their hospital stay. Patients with a minimal chance of developing difficulties can self-quarantine more easily, reducing the burden on healthcare institutions.

Coronaviruses were identified in the 1930s, after an outbreak of severe respiratory sickness in chickens that resulted in widespread bronchitis infection (IBV). In the 1940s, two novel coronaviruses were discovered: transmissible gastroenteritis (TGEV) and mouse hepatitis (MHV). The first human coronaviruses were found. The human coronaviruses OC43 and 229E were shown to be the most often discovered in human patients suffering from the common cold virus. There have also been reports of human coronaviruses, with SARS-CoV being discovered in 2003, HKU1 being discovered in 2005, MERS-CoV being discovered in 2012, and SARS-CoV-2 being discovered in 2019. Many of these were related to true respiratory problems. The World Health Organization (WHO) announced on December 31, 2019, the discovery of the new coronavirus strain 2019-nCoV. According to the Intergovernmental Committee on Virus Taxonomy, it was identified as SARS-CoV-2. Since the 1918 influenza pandemic, Covid-19 has been the world's worst public health disaster in history. Because of its genetic resemblance to SARS-CoV and MERS-CoV, this unique Beta-coronavirus is considered to have evolved from a bat-borne coronavirus and been transmitted to humans by an unknown middle-aged, well-evolved creature host, which has not yet been identified.

COVID-19: A MACHINE-LEARNING-BASED PRODUCT

Computer science is the study of artificial intelligence (AI) and machine learning, and it encompasses a diverse range of learning paradigms, including regression, supervised and unsupervised learning, clustering, anomaly detection, and reinforcement learning (RL) (Scarpone et al., 2020). Artificial intelligence (AI) and machine learning are two of the most important topics in computer science. Machine learning models are commonly used in various applications, including classification, dimension reduction, and reward maximization (Gao et al., 2020).

Yan et al. described how They explained how they utilized machine learning to pick three biomarkers (lactic dehydrogenase (LDH), lymphocytes, and high-sensitivity C-reactive protein (hs-CRP)) and then used them to correctly predict individual patient mortality ten days in advance of the event. It has been demonstrated that elevated LDH levels are critical in identifying most persons who require immediate medical attention.1 However, none of the scoring methodologies discussed in this article can assist clinicians in statistically identifying persons who are at risk of developing heart disease. The assertion of an earlier prognosis supports a statistically significant matrix by ten days, which is included in the report. On the other hand, some patients died on the same day they were admitted to the hospital, while others died 32 days after being admitted. As a result, the model's performance on an individual basis will be overstated by this average matrix as a whole. Worldwide, the virus has forced national closures, curfews, and travel prohibitions due to the outbreak. Although COVID-19 infection is usually associated with minor symptoms, it can produce significant and even fatal consequences in certain people. Due to a growing number of COVID-19 cases worldwide, healthcare systems worldwide are being put under strain, even though little is known about the virus. Since the infection with COVID has been the subject of an investigation by scientists from various fields. Machine learning, a subset of artificial intelligence, is concerned with creating systems that can learn from and improve on input samples without the need for explicit programming instructions.

Decision tree, Linear SVM, bagging tree, and Boosted methods are examples of SVM (Support Vector Machine) models. With tenfold cross-validation, the accuracy rate of positive and negative rates is determined. All ROC curve metrics used in this study have been generated and are available in a supplementary excel file. The findings identified which features could produce mortality projections comparable to those produced by the invasive model and on a par with those produced by the linear SVM model. Additionally, features performed better for longer distant expiration intervals, resulting in more accurate near-term mortality projections.

The machine learning algorithm may generate a ground-truth output (continuous or discrete) for each input because it has been thoroughly trained in the SL paradigms on labels data sets. The UL (Anzai, 2012), method, on the other hand, does not give a ground-truth conclusion, and the techniques are typically aimed at uncovering patterns in the data. The goal of the Reinforcement approach is to enhance the cumulative reward for each decision-making activity that is completed (Zhang et al., 2020). As seen in Figure 1, classification is included; regression and unsupervised learning involve clustering methods and dimension reduction; and reinforcement learning (RL), which comprises classification and control, is included.

Figure 1. Types of machine learning algorithms

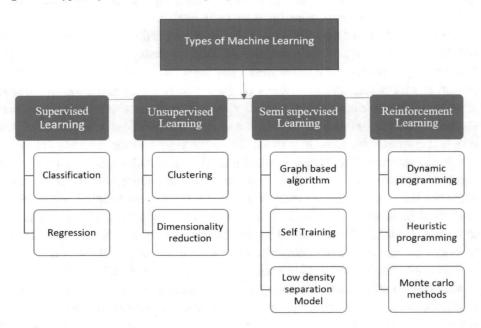

According to O. Dag (Dağ, 2019) the data is sourced from a Portuguese financial institution's direct marketing campaign. The data is classified based on whether or not the customer has a term deposit account. In categorization, standard artificial intelligence approaches such as Support Vector Machines and ANN (Artificial Neural Networks) are used and bagging and boosted algorithms. Statistical outliers and absolute values are excluded from the dataset. It is decided which characteristics will be included in the application using the ReliefF technique, a correlation-based feature selection strategy, and a Chi-Squared attribute evaluation algorithm, among other methods. The data division follows this into five unique training and testing conditions: 10-fold cross-validation, 5-fold cross-validation, 2-fold cross-validation, and an 80% split. In her research, Magorzata (2012) examines the performance of bagging, boosting and fixed fusion strategies compared to one another. This study uses a real-world medical dataset to make a diagnosis of thyroid disease. Both bagging classification trees and boosting classification trees showed the best performance in the experiments, which was determined by the outcomes of those experiments (Yaman & Subasi, 2019). However, there was no significant difference observed between the two approaches.

Numerous review papers have included machine learning in their COVID-19 research. According to Agbehadji et al., big data platforms, artificial intelligence, and nature-inspired algorithms are used to discover and track COVID-19 instances. Bullock et al. (Rajabi Shishvan et al., 2018) highlighted how artificial intelligence is being utilized to address COVID-19 concerns on genetic, clinical, and epidemiological levels. Naudé (Ascent of machine learning in medicine, 2019) explored the application of artificial intelligence in the fight against COVID-19. The following topics are discussed: tracking and predicting, diagnosis, treatment and immunizations, and social control. Albahri et al. (Naudé, 2020) discussed current data mining and machine learning strategies for developing COVID-19 prediction systems. Swapnarekha et al. (Swapnarekha et al., 2020) examined the use of machine learning and deep learning for COVID-19 prediction and screening. They discussed existing machine learning approaches for COVID-19 screening, forecasting, contact monitoring, and medication development. Tayarani-N recently (Tayarani, 2021) expanded their research to cover clinical applications, image processing of COVID-19-related images, and pharmacological and epidemiological studies. The literature has examined deep learning, machine learning, artificial neural networks, and evolutionary algorithms. Wu et al. (Wu et al., 2020) assessed the utilization of advanced big data technologies in China for the covid-19.

Globally, the virus has prompted national closures, lockdowns, and travel restrictions due to its spread. Although COVID-19 infection is frequently linked with very mild symptoms, it can have serious and even deadly implications in certain cases, particularly in children. Despite the virus's relative obscurity, a rise in COVID-19 infections has strained worldwide healthcare systems. Following COVID-19 infection, however, it has been investigated by researchers from a variety of different disciplines. In artificial intelligence, machine learning is a subset concerned with the development of systems that can learn and improve independently without the need for explicit programming (Dargan et al., 2020). Several industries, particularly healthcare informatics, have successfully implemented machine learning techniques. The use of machine learning in COVID-19 is an important area of investigation. A slew of research initiatives is now ongoing to run and develop machine learning algorithms connected to COVID-19. In January 2021, a simple PubMed search yielded 94,609 papers on COVID-19, according to the National Library of Medicine. With the spread of the COVID-19 pandemic, it is vital to allocate resources as efficiently as possible. In either impoverished or developed countries, large-scale RT-PCR testing is not a viable option for diagnosis.

Currently, triage is the only strategy available for screening patients and identifying potential issues as soon as possible. X-rays can replace Real-time PCR testing and CT scans in some cases. The limitations of RT-PCR and CT scans have left us with just CXR pictures to rely on. The use of automated CXR image processing can help in the diagnosis of certain conditions. Large amounts of labeled data are required, which is currently the fundamental restriction of CXR image diagnosis (Dev et al.,

2021). Infection rates of COVID-19 are growing over the world, putting pressure on healthcare systems (Skowronski, 2005). The RT-PCR is the gold standard for identifying viral nucleic acid in the throat and nasopharyngeal swabs. This method takes 4–6 hours and has a modest viral load (Xie et al., 2020), which refers to the amount of virus identified in the sputum after the operation is completed. The availability of test kits, apparatus, and qualified workers is typically constrained in underdeveloped countries due to a scarcity of resources. Because of the limitations mentioned earlier, several countries have been unable to reproduce the procedure.

Figure 2. Detail information about death and newly reported case

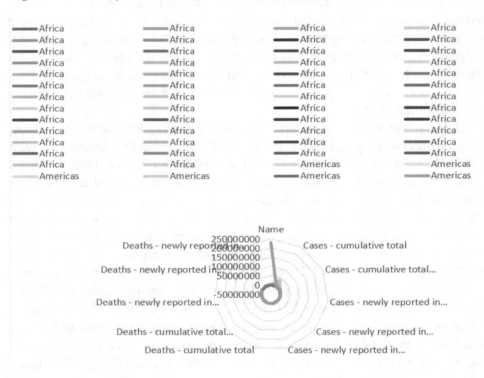

Fig. 2 illustrates the continent-by-continent date of the first verified case. The diameter of the circle varies according to the number of verified cases on the first day. It Displays sample statistics on the number of confirmed cases by region on the first day. In the majority of nations, just one confirmed case was discovered on the first day.

Figure 3. Growth of Covid 19 cases region wise

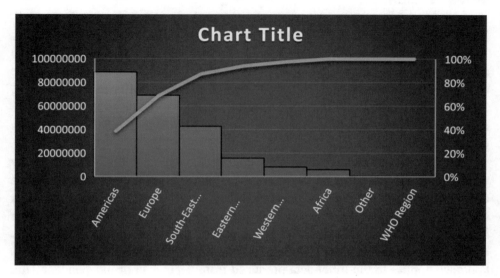

Fig. 3 illustrates the number of instances in each region as a growth. COVID-19 has been recognized for one year. And after a year, these areas continue to be free of infections, with the first cases reported discovered lately. As a result, their crisis management solution may be used as a case study to determine a method for preventing disease of any pandemic. In America, we discovered more instances of covid 19 than in any other European country.

METHODOLOGY

Data Set

The data for this study were taken from the Israeli Ministry of Health's website11. The dataset has been downloaded and is accessible in English at https://github. com/nshomron/covidpred. This dataset provides epidemiological data about the current COVID-19 outbreak. This collection contains the following: We developed a machine learning technique based on 51,831 tested individuals' data (4769 were confirmed to have COVID-19). The test set included data from the next week (47,401 tested people, 3624 tested positive for COVID-19). With a few additional factors, this data may be used to forecast the number of infections at the first day of any pandemic in the future.

Model Evaluation

Model evaluations for covid 19 usage should take the model's purpose into account. The objective of diagnostic models is to classify individuals into their positive and negative rates accurately. However, the goal is more complicated in predictive models. While accurately forecasting if a near-future event will occur is desirable, it is more challenging due to the stochastic character of the occurrence. Accurate risk estimation and categorization into risk strata are frequently the best outcomes possible in this scenario.

The entire area (under the operator operating characteristic ROC) is a frequently used statistic for collecting all the data contained inside the curve. However, when comparing two receiver operating characteristic curves, complications arise when the region of interest does not contain the complete range of false-positive rate (the entire area). The area under a portion of the receiver operating characteristic curve is determined via numerical integration. Variance estimates are derived. The approach applies to binormal data produced from dependent or independent data, regardless of whether the data are continuous or rating scale. The authors provide a case study comparing rating scale data from computerized tomography scans of the head with and without a patient diagnosis. The regions under two receiver operating characteristic curves are investigated throughout an a priori range of false-positive rates and at a specific location.

Model accuracy is multifaceted and frequently defines four model (Namely Bagging boosting Linear SVM, Decision tree) that correspond to the objectives above, namely discriminating and calibration. Discrimination refers to the capacity to discriminate between people with or without disease or between different disease stages. It is the end objective of diagnosis models that attempt to categorize persons. On the other hand, calibration refers to accurately predicting the danger or likelihood of a future event. It quantifies the degree to which projected probabilities, often derived from the model and another algorithm, concur with observed proportions of people getting the disease later in life.

RESULTS

Machine learning technology is a collaborative decision-making system that uses learned classifier predictions to generate new instances. Early research has shown that ensemble classifiers are much more trustworthy than single component classifiers, both experimentally and conceptually. On the data of 51,831 tested individuals, four machine-learning algorithms were employed to train. The data collection includes the next week's (47,401) tested individuals, 3624 of confirmed to have COVID-19.

From the rest of the reviewed data, we randomly selected ten cross-fold negative samples. This approach is successfully used to anticipate sickness in 51,831 tested individuals, and when combined with the 4769 validated datasets, the test set contained a dataset from the next week (47,401).

Envisioned works 10-fold Cross-validation was used to assess the classifier. Cross-validation is a widely used approach for categorizing data sets as testing and training. The data is divided into equal halves according to the required number of folds, and then each split half is used for testing, while the remaining halves are used for training. Cross-validation may be an effective method of resolving the overfitting problem. This indicates that 20% of the whole data set is defined as test data, while the other 80% is labelled as training data. The F1 score, precision, recall, and area under the curve (AUC) evaluate classification performance. For each test dataset, we calculated the number of false-negative (FN), true-negatives (TN), true-positives (TP), and false-positives (FP). Precision and F1 score and recall were calculated using the following formulas:

1. TP rate = correct class/actual class
2. Rate of precision =PT /((TP+FP))
3. F= (2*recall*precision) / ((recall*precision))
4. Recall =PT /((TP+FN))
5. FP = TN/N

Liner SVM

SVMs are a kind of supervised machine learning algorithm. SVM's objective is to find an optimum hyperplane that classifies data covid positive or n. Its purpose is to maximize the margin between the hyperplane and the training samples. This is accomplished by finding two additional parallel hyperplanes that pass through one or more instances, referred to as support vectors, and are positioned optimally relative to the core hyperplane. The unseen sample is then categorized according to the hyperplane side on which they fall.

Linear SVM is extremely efficient in situations involving large amounts of data. While their accuracy on the test set is comparable to that of a non-linear SVM, they train considerably more quickly for such applications. For instance, text categorization applications have a high-dimensional Input Space, and it is unnecessary to add more characteristics to the Input Space since they have little effect on performance (Chauhan et al., 2019).

When developing an SVM classifier, choosing a specific kernel function, such as a polynomial or radial basis function (RBF), is vital as a significant learning parameter. However, there is a shortage of studies evaluating the prediction performance of SVM classifiers constructed using different kernel functions. Additionally, it is widely recognized that grouping several classifiers and ensembles of classifiers, another hot area of pattern classification research, often results in greater performance than single classifiers (Kittler et al., 1998). Experiments demonstrate that a feature ranking algorithm based on linear SVM models achieves acceptable performance even though the train and test data are not uniformly distributed. Comparing the Area Under Curve (AUC) with and without each feature also results in comparable ranks.

Figure 4. Shows the area under the ROC curve of SVM. SVM (linear) obtained the best classification performance with the least error and the greatest accuracy. AUC (Positive 0.74) and AUC (negative=0.79) RT-PCR for COVID 19. positive

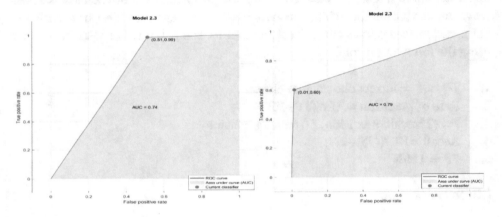

As demonstrated in Table 1, our study reveals that linear SVMs trained on the Causality Challenge data sets are effective. The purpose of this research was to investigate the high sensitivity and specificity of different parameters in identified COVID-19 patients using the ROC curve. The AUC of the present classifier was more than 0.94 in a recent experiment, demonstrating that it is efficient and has a strong predictive value for COVID-19 prediction. Certain blood laboratory indicators seem beneficial in screening persons with a positive reverse transcription-polymerase chain reaction (RT-PCR) for COVID-19.

Table 1. Performance table of Linear SVM classifier based on Covid 19

validation	Accuracy	Sensitivity	Specificity	Precision	F1_score	MCC	Kappa	FPR	Error
Fold - 1	0.954624461	0.947203521	0.984701	0.820618	0.861888	0.854344	0.878999	0.015299	0.045376
Fold - 2	0.967257825	0.944047267	0.987902	0.874253	0.903565	0.892212	0.912688	0.012098	0.032742
Fold - 3	0.956737088	0.944882656	0.981615	0.862291	0.893997	0.879713	0.884632	0.018385	0.043263
Fold - 4	0.964410372	0.941705201	0.98782	0.836183	0.872156	0.866116	0.905094	0.01218	0.03559
Fold - 5	0.942273723	0.945999495	0.981746	0.775339	0.802172	0.805307	0.846063	0.018254	0.057726
Fold - 6	0.94378577	0.943379824	0.979913	0.782035	0.810639	0.81089	0.850095	0.020087	0.056214
Fold - 7	0.949523069	0.94081038	0.983579	0.789564	0.822054	0.823012	0.865395	0.016421	0.050477
Fold - 8	0.936614145	0.940934986	0.977468	0.784926	0.826389	0.816393	0.830971	0.022532	0.063386
Fold- 9	0.943503144	0.944929697	0.981813	0.783864	0.8277	0.821252	0.849342	0.018187	0.056497
Fold- 10	0.940924186	0.941472192	0.978567	0.815388	0.859019	0.843222	0.842464	0.021433	0.059076

Decision Tree

The decision tree is also known as a Classification or Regression Tree. It's indeed capable of resolving both classification and regression problems. Certainly, since forecasting PV power is a regression problem, this chapter will concentrate on the accuracy of COVID-19 regression trees. The process for building regression trees using the least square error norm (0.063) comprises repeatedly building the binary tree by picking the most appropriate features and split points (Wang et al., 2018).

Figure 5. Shows the area under the ROC curve of SVM'. Decision tree obtained the low classification performance with the high error and the lowest accuracy. AUC (Positive 0.86) and AUC (negative=0.79) RT-PCR for Covid 19

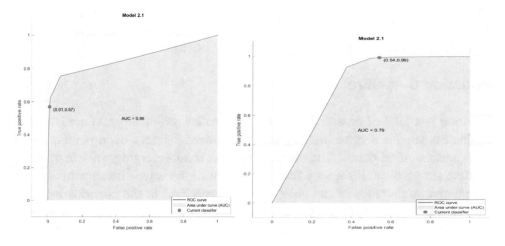

The model was predicted with a 0.79 ROC and 0.92 accuracies for the future test set (Fig. 5). The potential working points are as follows: 0.95 percent sensitivity and 0.95 percent specificity in table 2. show the PPV (positive predictive value) of a COVID-19 classification against positive and negative outcomes with 0.0608 error. All ROC curve measurements used in this research were computed and are available in a dataset (supplementary excel).

Table 2. Performance table of Decision tree classifier with 10 cross validations

Validation	Accuracy	Sensitivity	Specificity	Precision	F1_score	MCC	Kappa	FPR	Error
Fold - 1	0.94367272	0.943471399	0.977652	0.821905	0.864221	0.847055	0.849794	0.022348	0.056327
Fold - 2	0.953903766	0.950861881	0.985169	0.835525	0.880228	0.866404	0.877077	0.014831	0.046096
Fold - 3	0.910125062	0.941636408	0.972848	0.738339	0.788102	0.77534	0.760333	0.027152	0.089875
Fold - 4	0.946060906	0.941138241	0.981906	0.790931	0.833371	0.825629	0.856162	0.018094	0.053939
Fold - 5	0.948498552	0.946386635	0.984331	0.782244	0.819738	0.819402	0.862663	0.015669	0.051501
Fold - 6	0.959690525	0.940521277	0.986291	0.845498	0.880023	0.869781	0.892508	0.013709	0.040309
Fold - 7	0.94582774	0.940354876	0.978399	0.793408	0.823072	0.82067	0.855541	0.021601	0.054172
Fold - 8	0.940952448	0.940262006	0.98214	0.769933	0.802389	0.803086	0.84254	0.01786	0.059048
Fold- 9	0.922935067	0.950850672	0.97766	0.75807	0.777541	0.780222	0.794494	0.02234	0.077065
Fold- 10	0.939108316	0.943501432	0.979238	0.802218	0.84892	0.834377	0.837622	0.020762	0.060892

Ensemble Models

Because of their resistance to uneven class labeling, boosting and bagging classifiers have gained popularity in recent years. They both rely on the ensemble notion to generalize the model and predict previously unknown data; both are used to predict previously unknown data. An unbalanced binary classification dataset is used in this study to test how well a classifier works after it has been bagged and boosted, which is the goal of this research (Singhal et al., 2018).

Boosting Classifire

Boosting is a kind of ensemble learning that makes use of separate models. The incline Boosting is very resilient against imbalanced datasets, owing to the way it treats misclassified points. The boosting process entails merging weak learners to become strong ones. It's a very resilient, owing to the way it iterates, increasing the relative importance of the observable misclassified in the previous iteration with each iteration (Sapna Singh kshatri Verified reviews, 2020). There are several different types of supervised machine learning classifiers. The following are examples

14

of machine learning techniques: naive Bayes, generalized linear models, linear discriminant analysis (LDA) and quadratic discriminant analysis (QDA), stochastic gradient descent, support vector machines (SVM), linear support vector classifiers (Linear SVC), decision trees, neural network models, and nearest neighbours Using ensemble techniques, weak learners' knowledge is pooled in order to develop strong learners. These prediction algorithms are intended to improve the overall accuracy of the predictions. There are two approaches that may be used to achieve this. The use of feature engineering is one method, while the use of boosting techniques is another method of improving performance. In contrast to learning algorithms, boosting algorithms concentrate on training observations that result in inaccurate classifications. The boosting algorithmsCatBoost, AdaBoost, gradient boosting LightGBM, and XGBoost, are the 5 most often used in computer science (Rahman et al., 2020). The true power of Boosting stems out of its reinforcement learning approach. Bootstrap aggregation, commonly known as bagging, is a meta-algorithm for machine learning ensembles that aims to improve the efficiency and consistency of machine learning techniques used in statistics regression and classification. Additionally, it reduces variance and helps minimize over-fitting, which is a frequent problem when decision trees are used to choose features. Bagging is just a subset of the technique's dependability as a measurement model (Sharma et al., 2018).

Figure 6. Shows the area under the ROC curve of boosting. Boosting obtained the good classification performance with the least error and the greatest accuracy. AUC (Positive 0.69) and AUC (negative=0.75) RT-PCR for Covid 19

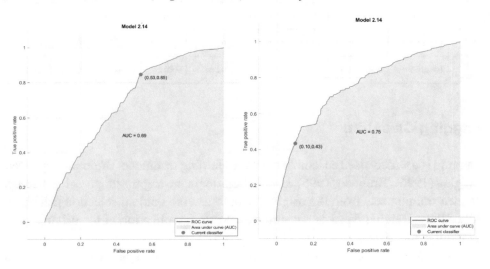

When it came to bagging, the ROC curve revealed that all models obtained an area under the curve more than 0.75, suggesting a high accuracy covid model. Presenting a highly accurate covid model. Numerous prior research utilized the area under the ROC curve's AUC parameters to assess the model's performance (0.53) as in fig 6. The AUC was used to validate the covid mortality models, and the covid negative rate models were deemed legitimate due to their higher AUC values, such as the ensemble model. Cleary table 3 preseant the accuresy rate of bagging is with 10 fold cross valodation is 0.94 but comparative to Linear SVM error rate is higher from 0.05, F1 score 0.86.

Table 3. Performance table of boosting classifier with 10 cross validations

	Accuracy	Sensitivity	Specificity	Precision	F1_score	MCC	Kappa	FPR	Error
Fold - 1	0.969857981	0.945294325	0.987915	0.838282	0.869401	0.868076	0.919621	0.012085	0.030142
Fold - 2	0.964184272	0.957330862	0.988666	0.814565	0.849901	0.853587	0.904491	0.011334	0.035816
Fold - 3	0.945834805	0.94079764	0.981444	0.783676	0.811778	0.813567	0.855559	0.018556	0.054165
Fold - 4	0.946265809	0.942383902	0.982182	0.783052	0.817017	0.81677	0.856709	0.017818	0.053734
Fold - 5	0.942005229	0.940016164	0.976997	0.796841	0.837585	0.825546	0.845347	0.023003	0.057995
Fold - 6	0.956836007	0.941042266	0.98327	0.869689	0.900477	0.883182	0.884896	0.01673	0.043164
Fold - 7	0.953197202	0.93993489	0.982628	0.797433	0.816413	0.823818	0.875193	0.017372	0.046803
Fold - 8	0.971221649	0.949435876	0.991131	0.827461	0.862865	0.864193	0.923258	0.008869	0.028778
Fold- 9	0.953910832	0.940131782	0.985416	0.79327	0.830907	0.828493	0.877096	0.014584	0.046089
Fold- 10	0.949183919	0.943630533	0.983574	0.801107	0.845667	0.83711	0.86449	0.016426	0.050816

Bagging Classifire

Bagging is a widely used ensemble machine learning technique. Breiman suggested bagging (1996) (Breiman, 1996). Every classifier in the bagging approach generates its own training sets from the original data to use the random selection principle. All of these training datasets constitute a bootstrap replication of the original data (Baraldi et al., 2011).

The phases and explanations that follow pertain to the bagging model, which is one of the ensemble algorithms:

Inputs:

D: a d-sample collection k: the model's identifier in a model based on ensembles (e.g., Boosting, neural networks, bagging, random forest, decision tree, etc.).

As a consequence of this procedure, an M *n is generated by the ensemble model.

Figure 7. Shows the area under the ROC curve of bagging. Bagging obtained the lowest classification performance with the hight error and the low accuracy. AUC (Positive 0.91) and AUC (negative=0.84) RT-PCR for Covid 19

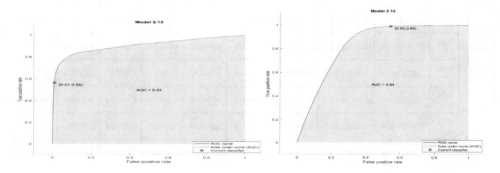

Bagging classifier provides Liner SVM with some competition. Bagging has the same accuracy rate as linear SVM but has a higher error rate. While ensembles offer highly accurate regression models, their practical applicability may be limited by including too many regression models. To be viable and competitive, learning algorithms must run in an acceptable amount of time. The model was predicted with a 0.84 ROC and 0.94 accuracies for the future test set (Fig. 7). The potential working points are as follows: 0.94 percent sensitivity and 0.97 percent specificity in table 4.

Table 4. Performance table of bagging classifier with 10 cross validations

		Accuracy	Sensitivity	Specificity	Precision	F1_score	MCC	Kappa	FPR	Error
Bagged Tree	Fold - 1	0.953246661	0.945669047	0.981009	0.808595	0.843921	0.838584	0.875324	0.018991	0.046753
	Fold - 2	0.938430015	0.952627988	0.981687	0.834717	0.882441	0.862145	0.835813	0.018313	0.06157
	Fold - 3	0.955719635	0.952431015	0.982513	0.834574	0.874447	0.863585	0.881919	0.017487	0.04428
	Fold - 4	0.956150639	0.945757519	0.985412	0.800647	0.839442	0.83635	0.883068	0.014588	0.043849
	Fold - 5	0.9389882	0.946032629	0.978254	0.799893	0.846534	0.83189	0.837302	0.021746	0.061012
	Fold - 6	0.955762029	0.950083555	0.985687	0.797322	0.836578	0.834464	0.882032	0.014313	0.044238
	Fold - 7	0.925839045	0.942194768	0.979477	0.750536	0.780145	0.780012	0.802237	0.020523	0.074161
	Fold - 8	0.913057302	0.94319786	0.973694	0.736217	0.779331	0.770838	0.768153	0.026306	0.086943
	Fold- 9	0.945234226	0.952218623	0.98372	0.799715	0.850849	0.839757	0.853958	0.01628	0.054766
	Fold- 10	0.916017805	0.941520791	0.975827	0.752324	0.770882	0.769938	0.776047	0.024173	0.083982

Mortality Risk Model

It appears that the Random Forest approach has benefited from the current situation since it has fared admirably in terms of f1 score and recall despite just a slight increase in accuracy over the past several years. The low negative f1 score for bagging in this scenario is misleading since it is heavily relying on recollection, which is quite low when compared to a decision tree, and so misleads. To evaluated several classifiers to model all of those above, including Bagging, boosting, Decision tree, and linear SVM. We developed a machine learning technique based on the data of 51,831 persons who were tested for this collection (4769 of whom were confirmed cases of COVID-19 infection). The data set used for the experiment contains information from the next week's data (47,401 tested people, 3624 tested positive for COVID-19). With a few additional factors, this data may be used to forecast the number of infections on the first day of any pandemic in the future. Due to the possibility of bias introduced by random sampling, we selected 4769 negative samples and merged them with the positive dataset to train the classifier. The performance of several classifiers was evaluated using the median value of 1001 outcomes. As indicated in Table 2, we discovered that SVM (linear) performed the best, with accuracy = 0.94, Sensivity = 0.944, Specifity = 0.978, Precision=0.81 F1 = 0.85, and AUC = 0.80. kappa=0.0842, FPR=0.021 shown in fig 8. As a result, it was selected as the final classifier and used in practice. To illustrate the variance induced by sampling, Supplementary Figure S1 shows boxplots of the 1001 training outcomes (precisions, recalls, F1s, and AUCs) with SVM (liner). Accuracy rate of SVM (linear) are shown in Figure. That minimum classifier rate is less than 0.054. with minimum hypothesis rate in optimization result.

Figure 8. Optimization tree of linear SVM algorithm

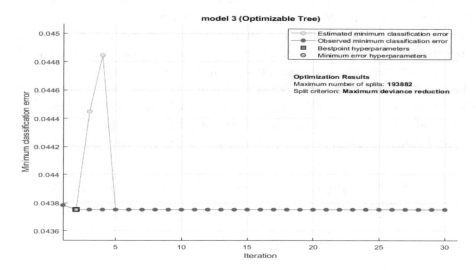

When performance criteria and ROC curves are compared to the results of the algorithms, it is clear that the most successful algorithm. The Linear SVM algorithm, a type of linear regression, is the algorithms under discussion for classifying decisions about subscribing to the term of morality risk of covid based on symptoms. This research determined that linear techniques outperformed ensemble (bagging and boosting) and machine learning algorithms, which are both considered to be conventional artificial intelligence methods.

CONCLUSION

Several researchers have recently investigated whether regression tree and linear regression models are appropriate for use in ensembles (Kotsiantis et al., 2006). Both regression tree and linear regression models are widely used in the machine learning field, and various researchers have recently investigated whether they are appropriate for use in ensembles. Surprise, surprise: In this year's True class labels, the Linear

SVM maintained its lead in the recall component, which is surprising given that recall measures a classifier's ability to generate a small number of false negatives, which is critical when applying machine learning techniques in a production setting. On many occasions, companies place a larger value on recall than on accuracy, precision, and an f1 score as low as feasible for a single false negative, all of which are important. Using an RT-PCR test, we wanted to see how accurate single SVM classifiers and ensemble classifiers constructed using various kernel functions and combination methodologies were in predicting positive SARS-CoV-2 infection. Also included is a comparison of two different scaled datasets. It is also possible to compare the classification accuracy, receiver operating characteristic (ROC), F-measure, and training duration of different classifiers.

To analyse and evaluate linear SVM, decision tree, bagging, and boosting models in fig 9 show the kappa statistics, Root Mean Squared Error (RMSE), area under the Receiver Operating Characteristic curve (ROC), Mean Absolute Error (MAE), and Root Relative Squared Error (RRSE) are all used to find out the conclusion.

Figure 9. Comparison graph of l proposed model (Decision tree, Linear SVM, Bagged tree, Boosted)

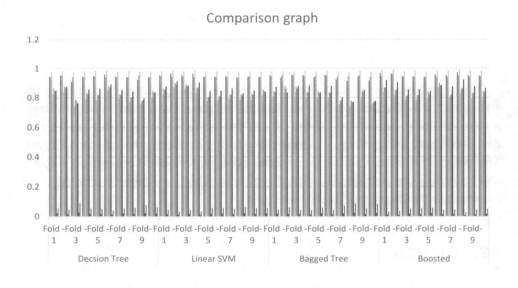

These experimental circumstances have not been shown before. The empirical data help us to get a thorough understanding of SVM and SVM ensemble prediction capabilities and to choose the optimal prediction model(s) for future study.

REFERENCES

Anzai, Y. (2012). *Pattern Recognition and Machine Learning*. Elsevier Science.

Ascent of machine learning in medicine. (2019). *Nature Materials*, *18*(5), 407. doi:10.103841563-019-0360-1 PMID:31000807

Baraldi, P., Razavi-Far, R., & Zio, E. (2011). Bagged ensemble of Fuzzy C-Means classifiers for nuclear transient identification. *Annals of Nuclear Energy*, *38*(5), 1161–1171. doi:10.1016/j.anucene.2010.12.009

Barro, Ursua, & Weng. (2020). The Coronavirus and the Great Influenza Epidemic - Lessons from the 'Spanish Flu' for the Coronavirus's Potential Effects on Mortality and Economic Activity. *SSRN*. doi:10.3386/w26866

Breiman, L. (1996). Bagging predictors. *Machine Learning*, *24*(2), 123–140. doi:10.1007/BF00058655

Chauhan, V. K., Dahiya, K., & Sharma, A. (2019). Problem formulations and solvers in linear SVM: A review. *Artificial Intelligence Review*, *52*(2), 803–855. doi:10.100710462-018-9614-6

Chowdhury, M. E. H., Rahman, T., Khandakar, A., Al-Madeed, S., Zughaier, S. M., Doi, S. A. R., Hassen, H., & Islam, M. T. (2021). An Early Warning Tool for Predicting Mortality Risk of COVID-19 Patients Using Machine Learning. *Cognitive Computation*. Advance online publication. doi:10.100712559-020-09812-7 PMID:33897907

Dağ, Ö. H. N. (2019). Predicting the success of ensemble algorithms in the banking sector. *International Journal of Business Analytics*, *6*(4), 12–31. doi:10.4018/IJBAN.2019100102

Dargan, S., Kumar, M., Ayyagari, M. R., & Kumar, G. (2020). A Survey of Deep Learning and Its Applications: A New Paradigm to Machine Learning. *Archives of Computational Methods in Engineering*, *27*(4), 1071–1092. doi:10.100711831-019-09344-w

Dev, K., Khowaja, S. A., Bist, A. S., Saini, V., & Bhatia, S. (2021). Triage of potential COVID-19 patients from chest X-ray images using hierarchical convolutional networks. *Neural Computing & Applications*. Advance online publication. doi:10.100700521-020-05641-9 PMID:33649695

Feldman & Martin. (2012). *Big Data in Healthcare Hype and Hope*. Academic Press.

Gao, K., Mei, G., Piccialli, F., Cuomo, S., Tu, J., & Huo, Z. (2020). Julia language in machine learning: Algorithms, applications, and open issues. *Computer Science Review*, *37*, 100254. doi:10.1016/j.cosrev.2020.100254

Ginsberg, J., Mohebbi, M. H., Patel, R. S., Brammer, L., Smolinski, M. S., & Brilliant, L. (2009). Detecting influenza epidemics using search engine query data. *Nature*, *457*(7232), 1012–1014. doi:10.1038/nature07634 PMID:19020500

Hunter, D. J. (2020). Covid-19 and the Stiff Upper Lip— The Pandemic Response in the United Kingdom. *The New England Journal of Medicine*, *382*(16), e31. doi:10.1056/NEJMp2005755 PMID:32197002

Kittler, J., Hatef, M., Duin, R. P. W., & Matas, J. (1998). On combining classifiers. *IEEE Transactions on Pattern Analysis and Machine Intelligence*, *20*(3), 226–239. doi:10.1109/34.667881

Kotsiantis, S. B., Kanellopoulos, D., & Zaharakis, I. D. (2006). Bagged averaging of regression models. *IFIP Int. Fed. Inf. Process.*, *204*, 53–60. doi:10.1007/0-387-34224-9_7

La Marca, A., Capuzzo, M., Paglia, T., Roli, L., Trenti, T., & Nelson, S. M. (2020, September). Testing for SARS-CoV-2 (COVID-19): A systematic review and clinical guide to molecular and serological in-vitro diagnostic assays. *Reproductive Biomedicine Online*, *41*(3), 483–499. doi:10.1016/j.rbmo.2020.06.001 PMID:32651106

Marcel, S. (2020). COVID-19 epidemic in Switzerland: On the importance of testing, contact tracing and isolation. *Swiss Medical Weekly*, *150*(11–12), 4–6. doi:10.4414mw.2020.20225 PMID:32191813

Naudé, W. (2020). Artificial intelligence vs COVID-19: Limitations, constraints and pitfalls. *AI & Society*, *35*(3), 761–765. doi:10.100700146-020-00978-0 PMID:32346223

Qiu, H.-J. (2020). Using the internet search data to investigate symptom characteristics of COVID-19: A big data study. *World J. Otorhinolaryngology-Head and Neck Surgery*, *6*, S40–S48. doi:10.1016/j.wjorl.2020.05.003 PMID:32837757

Rahman, S., Irfan, M., Raza, M., Ghori, K. M., Yaqoob, S., & Awais, M. (2020). Performance analysis of boosting classifiers in recognizing activities of daily living. *International Journal of Environmental Research and Public Health*, *17*(3), 1082. Advance online publication. doi:10.3390/ijerph17031082 PMID:32046302

Rajabi Shishvan, O., Zois, D.-S., & Soyata, T. (2018). Machine Intelligence in Healthcare and Medical Cyber Physical Systems: A Survey. *IEEE Access : Practical Innovations, Open Solutions, 6,* 46419–46494. doi:10.1109/ACCESS.2018.2866049

Roy. (2020). *Prediction and Spread Visualization of Covid-19 Pandemic using Machine Learning.* doi: . doi:10.20944/preprints202005.0147.v1

Sapna Singh kshatri Verified reviews. (2020). Academic Press.

Scarpone, C., Brinkmann, S. T., Große, T., Sonnenwald, D., Fuchs, M., & Walker, B. B. (2020). A multimethod approach for county-scale geospatial analysis of emerging infectious diseases: A cross-sectional case study of COVID-19 incidence in Germany. *International Journal of Health Geographics, 19*(1), 1–17. doi:10.118612942-020-00225-1 PMID:32791994

Sharma, S., Srivastava, S., Kumar, A., & Dangi, A. (2018). Multi-Class Sentiment Analysis Comparison Using Support Vector Machine (SVM) and BAGGING Technique-An Ensemble Method. *2018 International Conference on Smart Computing and Electronic Enterprise (ICSCEE),* 1–6. 10.1109/ICSCEE.2018.8538397

Singhal, Y., Jain, A., Batra, S., Varshney, Y., & Rathi, M. (2018). Review of Bagging and Boosting Classification Performance on Unbalanced Binary Classification. *2018 IEEE 8th International Advance Computing Conference (IACC),* 338–343. 10.1109/IADCC.2018.8692138

Skowronski, D. M. (2005). Article. *Annual Review of Medicine, 56*(1), 357–381. doi:10.1146/annurev.med.56.091103.134135 PMID:15660517

Swapnarekha, H., Behera, H. S., Nayak, J., & Naik, B. (2020). Role of intelligent computing in COVID-19 prognosis: A state-of-the-art review. *Chaos, Solitons, and Fractals, 138,* 109947. doi:10.1016/j.chaos.2020.109947 PMID:32836916

Tayarani, N. M.-H. (2021). Applications of artificial intelligence in battling against covid-19: A literature review. Chaos, Solitons, and Fractals, 142, 110338. doi:10.1016/j.chaos.2020.110338 PubMed doi:10.1016/j.chaos.2020.110338 PMID:33041533

Tromberg, B. J., Schwetz, T. A., Pérez-Stable, E. J., Hodes, R. J., Woychik, R. P., Bright, R. A., Fleurence, R. L., & Collins, F. S. (2020). Rapid Scaling Up of Covid-19 Diagnostic Testing in the United States— The NIH RADx Initiative. *The New England Journal of Medicine, 383*(11), 1071–1077. doi:10.1056/NEJMsr2022263 PMID:32706958

Vaishya, R., Javaid, M., Khan, I. H., & Haleem, A. (2020). Artificial Intelligence (AI) applications for COVID-19 pandemic. *Diabetes & Metabolic Syndrome*, *14*(4), 337–339. doi:10.1016/j.dsx.2020.04.012 PMID:32305024

Wang, J., Li, P., Ran, R., Che, Y., & Zhou, Y. (2018). A Short-Term Photovoltaic Power Prediction Model Based on the Gradient Boost Decision Tree. *Applied Sciences (Basel, Switzerland)*, *8*(5), 689. Advance online publication. doi:10.3390/app8050689

Wu, J., Wang, J., Nicholas, S., Maitland, E., & Fan, Q. (2020). Application of big data technology for COVID-19 prevention and control in China: Lessons and recommendations. *Journal of Medical Internet Research*, *22*(10), e21980. Advance online publication. doi:10.2196/21980 PMID:33001836

Xie, X., Zhong, Z., Zhao, W., Zheng, C., Wang, F., & Liu, J. (2020). Chest CT for Typical Coronavirus Disease 2019 (COVID-19) Pneumonia: Relationship to Negative RT-PCR Testing. *Radiology*, *296*(2), E41–E45. doi:10.1148/radiol.2020200343 PMID:32049601

Yaman, E., & Subasi, A. (2019). Comparison of Bagging and Boosting Ensemble Machine Learning Methods for Automated EMG Signal Classification. *BioMed Research International*, *2019*, 9152506. doi:10.1155/2019/9152506 PMID:31828145

Zhang, Y., Xin, J., Li, X., & Huang, S. (2020). Overview on routing and resource allocation based machine learning in optical networks. *Optical Fiber Technology*, *60*, 102355. doi:10.1016/j.yofte.2020.102355

Chapter 2
COVID-19 Chest X-Rays Classification Using Deep Learning

Simranjit Singh
Bennett University, India

Mohit Sajwan
Bennett University, India

Deepak Singh
National Institute of Technology, Raipur, India

ABSTRACT

The SARS pandemic has spread throughout the world. Also known as "sporadic" or "spontaneous," the disease is contagious and can spread from someone who is in direct contact with someone else. COVID-19 is most commonly detected through RT-PCR tests, which may take longer than 48 hours. The data obtained from chest x-rays for COVID-19 patients has been found to be very promising for resolving emergencies, urgent care, and overcrowding. Deep learning (DL) methods in artificial intelligence (AI) play a significant role in the identification of the disease COVID using chest x-rays. In this chapter, a novel method for the effective classification of COVID-19 chest x-rays is proposed called XDeep. The developed model is able to achieve high classification accuracy, and the effectiveness is shown by comparing it with state-of-the-art models.

DOI: 10.4018/978-1-7998-9831-3.ch002

INTRODUCTION

The COVID-19 pandemic officially started on 31st December 2019, when in China (a city name Wuhan), a patient was afflicted with an unidentified type of pneumonia (WHO, 2020; Huang et. al., 2020; Wu et. al., 2020). The WHO (World Health Organization) later renamed the SARS-CoV-2 from COVID-19, a nomenclature that has been used previously (WHO). After that, from Wuhan to other cities and provinces in China, this new virus spread in just 30 days. A global health emergency of global concern was first proclaimed on 30th January 2020, by the WHO (World Health Organization) (Apostolopoulos et. al., 2020). Up to November 15th, 2021, there will be 254,186,130 confirmed cases of C0VID-19, of which 19,226,194 are active, resulting in 5,118,347 deaths (www.worldometers.info/coronavirus).

On January 20, 2020, United States of America (USA) recorded its initial seven cases of the disease. And On 21st July 2020, 39,63,376 cases of COVID-19 and 1,43,889 deaths were registered in the country (Apostolopoulos et. al., 2020). However, even though covid-19 result of its zoonotic origin, this virus was able to be transmitted from wild animals to humans, where it was then spread by direct person-to-person contact. Two coronavirus families have existed in the past., notably SARS-CoV and MERS-CoV, triggered serious respiratory illnesses and mortality in humans (Huang et. al., 2020). The genome of COVID-19 has undergone numerous mutations during its existence.

COVID-19 virus-caused coronavirus illness, In the year 2019, SARS-CoV-2 pandemic presents enormous problems to healthcare systems around the world and puts clinicians under extreme time constraints to make quick clinical decisions. After months of exhausting medical teams, hospitals are again working with new waves of patients who seek medical assistance, many of whom need life-saving treatment. Some individuals come to the hospitals with respiratory symptoms, while others are asymptomatic but have tested positive for COVID-19 for a variety of reasons (Kanne et. al., 2020).

Among the most symptoms and common signs of SARS-CoV-2 are fatigue, headache, sore throat, sneezing, fever, coughing, throat swelling, malaise, shortness of breath (Singhal et. al., 2020), and in most cases, covid 19 makes a huge impact on the lungs. Where, RTPCR, known as Real-time reverse transcription-polymerase chain reaction, most employed COVID-19 technique for identification, even though numerous nations offer immunological tests. Also, the RTPCR test is a time-consuming test and as has a low sensitivity of 60%–70%. In a solution for the RTPCR test, the detection of COVID-19's in their early stages, can be used by harmful consequences can be achieved by evaluating images of x-ray having lungs of the patients. (Singhal et. al., 2020; Kanne et. al., 2020). For COVID-19 pneumonia,

X-ray is a more sensitive approach and can be used in conjunction with RTPCR as an additional screening tool.

According to one study, survivors of COVID-19 pneumonia, lung illness caused by this virus is among the most dangerous. After ten days of experiencing symptoms, their X-ray began to show anomalies that were not there before (Pan et. al., 2020). With the lack of resources for RTPCR tests, many doctors are urged to make choices only on the basis of chest X-ray findings. X-ray pictures are extensively employed in areas where there is a lack of testing kits for COVID-19 detection. According to researchers, detection at an early stage of COVID-19 is critical and may be improved by the combination of clinical imaging aspects and laboratory results. In most studies, for COVID-19 patients, it has been noticed in the changes of X-ray images (Pan et. al., 2020; Zhao et. al., 2020; Shi et. al., 2020). Also, shown that image of COVID-19 X-ray showed signs of disease progression even before the onset of clinical symptoms (Chan et. al., 2020).

Deep learning models have demonstrated remarkable ability in image-related tasks, covering a variety of radiologic situations (MacLean, et. al., 2020). Despite their immense potential, they require a lot of training data before being used in COVID-19 management. While there should be no differences among images from different classes while training neural networks for image classification; consequently, all images acquired from the same machines should be important. As a result, the network would be able to discern these distinctions. Hence in this chapter, various models of deep learning applied on images of X-ray were employed, studied, and evaluated to distinguish the covid 19 patients from others.

In recent years, LSTM (Liu et. al., 2017) and CNN (Albawi et. al.,2017) has become a number of the most often used AI techniques. Ultrasonography (Liu et. al., 2017), X-ray (Liu et. al., 2018), MRI (Zou et. al., 2017), CT scans (Zhao et. al., 2018), etc., have all been successfully used with CNN and LSTM in medical image analysis. Computer vision (CV), Speech recognition (SRC), Natural language processing (NLP), and audio recognition (AR) are all areas where CNN, LSTM and other deep learning models have performed well. There are several algorithms that can recognize relationships in a dataset using a process that bears a striking resemblance to the human brain. Pattern recognition and image processing can benefit greatly from this algorithm. As input, it receives images and creates a model that performs image processing so that they can be used for feature extraction of images (Chen et. al., 2015) and recognizes a pattern (Chen et. al., 2016). By employing the pattern as a guide, deep learning models like LSTM, and CNN, are able to identify the similarities between fresh inputs as accurately as feasible.

Hence, COVID-19 detection using the different models of deep learning have become a widely used research method since the pandemic has spread worldwide. CNN, LSTM, and other deep learning models-based research efforts using X-ray image, aids to identify and classify COVID-19 have been proven to be outstanding. Even while deep learning-based approaches have shown impressive results, they are still not a substitute for actual testing procedures.

While many researchers are working in establishing the deep learning models against covid -19, wherein most of the approach's researchers have castoff together the x-ray and CT scan images. After which deep learning approaches is built by the researchers used clinical pictures which helps them for the identification of COVID-19, X-rays of the chest in order to combat the COVID-19 outbreak. An overview of newly created systems, where they have employed deep learning approaches which can helps us for the detection of COVID-19 is presented in this paper. In VGG19 was proposed by (Apostolopoulos et. al.,2020) to categorize COVID- 19 negative, COVID-19 positive, and normal patients using X-ray and CT scans, and reached an accuracy of 93.48%. After which, the COVID-Net model, developed by Wang and Wong (Wang et. al.., 2020) for similar 3-class categorization, had a 92.4% of accuracy when applied to images of X-ray only. (Hemdan et. al., 2020) suggested a COVIDX-net model for two-class classification that reached a 90.0 percent accuracy. (Ahsan et al., 2020) employed X-ray image and developed a model called as DarkCovidNet, which obtained a high level of precision of 98.08 percent for two-class classification and 87.02 percent for three-class based classification using the model. In another study, (Narin et al., 2020) found that their model named as Deep CNN ResNet-50 have used two-class based classification was extremely accurate, with an accuracy of 98 percent. While to address the restricted data available for forecasting approaches, according to (Apostolopoulos et al., 2020), they developed a transfer learning technique involving CNN that was capable of autonomously diagnosing the cases of COVID-19 by collecting critical characteristics from the X-rays of chest. To categorise COVID-19 photos, the system used the 5 CNN versions, Inception, VGG19, MobileNet, Inception-ResNetV2, Xception, and as well as the Inception-ResNetV2 to categorise. Each patient in the study was photographed in 224 photographs of COVID-19 disease, 700 photographs of pneumonia disease, and 504 photographs of regular disease. Where data set was divided based on the notion having cross-validation of 10-fold for the objectives of training the model and testing the model. The VGG19 deep learning approach was chosen as the primary deep learning model in the designed application because of its accuracy, specificity and sensitivity were 93.48 percent, 92.85 percent, and 98.75 percent respectively. According to (Sethy et al.,), proposed a deep architecture for COVID-19 detection based that makes use of X-ray photos has been proposed and demonstrated using the images of X-ray. Photographs of COVID-19 patients were included in the data collection, as were images of pneumonias (4290 images) and 1583 photographs of normal cases (76 photos). It was found that the method had a 98.3 percent accuracy for the COVID-19 cases. Later, due to data restrictions, (Horry et al., 30) conducted a case study of deep learning using a combination of composite fuzzy rule induction and Monte-Carlo (CMC). A deep learning algorithm was developed by (Sethy et al., 2020) to categorize COVID-19-infected persons based on the image's chest X-rays, and the technique was validated., which they used to their findings. For feature extraction, the system made use of 9 pre-trained models, and for classification, it made use of SVM. The two data sets had a number of 158 X-ray scans of individuals who were mutually COVID-19 and non-COVID-19. The coupled of SVM model and ResNet50 outperformed all the other methods in F1-score and high accuracy, with the value of 95.52% and 95.38% respectively. In (Hemdan et. al., 2020), COVID-19 detection system developed by Horry et. al., for detecting COVID-19 from X-rays images of chest that was based on pre-trained models. The system was named after the COVID-19 virus. For categorization, the proposed system made use of the Xception, VGG, ResNet, and Inception algorithms. It contains 115 photographs of COVID-19 patients, while pneumonias are depicted in 322 images., and 60361 images of normal subjects, which together make up the dataset used by the system. The recall and precision of the VGG19 and VGG16 classifiers were approximately same (i.e., both were having 80% precision). In the article (Belchior et. al., 2021), authors have developed a strategy of transfer learning by incorporating three phase technique that helps to identify the symptoms of COVID-19, which they called the "transfer learning approach." To locate the abnormalities in the CT scans, the enhanced pictures were employed to various models (i.e., models which were already pretrained), and the ResNet18 architecture achieved an accuracy of 99.4 percent when examined on real-world data.

The objective of this work is to demonstrate how a set of X-ray medical lung images was used to train a LSTM that can identify between, non-COVID-19 and COVID-19 infection. In this paper, we proposed a framework named XDeep, which employed LSTM to effectively classify the x-rays of chest in non-covid and covid class. The dataset is converted into 1D image vectors, which are provided as input to the LSTMs for effective learning as LSTM will interpret these vectors as sequences that form the robust neural connection. Other deep learning models like CNN takes a 2D image for classification. The prepared model is then contrasted with some of the other models of deep learning (i.e., 2D CNN, 1D CNN and GRU) to show the effectiveness of the proposed framework.

The following sections comprise the paper: Section 2 is a background of current scholarly papers pertinent to this research. Section 3 provides a detailed explanation of the present scheme, comprising data collecting and preparation procedures. Section 4 depicts the results of the experiments and a comparison of the suggested deep learning system's performance with other systems. At the end Section 5 covers the conclusion.

BACKGROUND

Dataset

The dataset is developed by DarwinAI Corp (Narin et. al., 2020), it has a total of 55 x-ray images of the chest. The images have 3 (RGB) bands. The corresponding metadata file is also added for more information. There are three classes are that are defined in the metadata. Three classes are- Covid positive, Covid negative and No finding. We pre-processed the data and removed the no finding class. The covid images are shown in figure 1.

Figure 1. Sample images from the Covid chest x-rays dataset

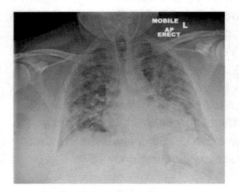 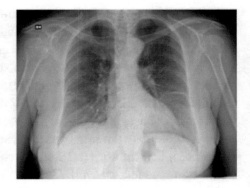

LSTM

LSTM as shown in figure 1 is a category of recurrent neural network (Rumelhart et. al., 1986) which is able to perform exceptional in case of the sequential input (Hochreiter et. al., 1997). The recurrent neural networks have a problem of vanishing gradient which is solved by LSTM (Hochreiter et. al., 1998). That is why we have employed LSTM rather than vanilla RNNs. LSTMs are able to sequential problems like Time series, stock market prediction effectively as it can forget irrelevant information with the help of foreget gate which is not present in vanilla RNN. We have employed these technique for building a robust classification model. The training process of LSTM is defined below:

I. Input gates

$$
\begin{aligned}
net_i &= W_i \cdot \left[O_{it-1}, x_{it} + b_i \right] \\
i_t &= \sigma\left(net_i \right) \\
net_{c_t} &= W_c \cdot \left[O_{it-1}, x_{it} + b_c \right] \\
\hat{c} &= \sigma\left(net_c \right),
\end{aligned}
\tag{2.1}
$$

Where σ is the sigmoid activation function.

II. Forget gates

$$
\begin{aligned}
net_{f_t} &= W_f \cdot \left[O_{it-1}, x_{it} + b_f \right] \\
f_t &= \sigma\left(net_f \right)
\end{aligned}
\tag{2.2}
$$

III. Cell States

$$
c_t = i_t \circ \hat{c} + f_t \circ c_{t-1},
\tag{2.3}
$$

Where ∘ denotes the hadamard product and t is the present time.

IV. Output gate

$$
\begin{aligned}
net_{o_t} &= W_o \cdot \left[O_{it-1}, x_{it} + b_o \right] \\
m_t &= \sigma\left(net_o \right)
\end{aligned}
\tag{2.4}
$$

V. Next hidden state

$$
o_{it} = m_t \times tan(c_t),
\tag{2.5}
$$

Where *tanh* is the tangent hyperbolic activation function.
Afterwards, the hidden value is obtained at the end, which is utilised to find the perdicted value:

$$
p = w_p \cdot o_{it} + b_p,
\tag{2.6}
$$

Where b denotes the bias.

The error is given as:

$$E = \frac{1}{2} \times (a - p)^2, \qquad\qquad (2.7)$$

Where a is the actual and p is the predicted output.

Equations 2.1 to 2.7 show the forward pass of LSTM. These process is performed over and over until the error value is minimal.

Figure 2. Long short-term memory network

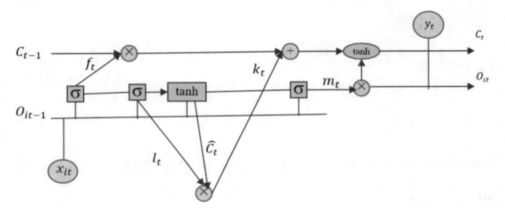

PROPOSED FRAMEWORK

We have proposed a framework in this section for the effective classification of chest X-rays using deep learning called Xdeep, as shown in Figure 2. The image dataset of X-ray (https://github.com/agchung/Figure1-COVID-chestxray-dataset) taken developed using the standard procedure. The images have three bands which are converted to one band image for decreasing the size of the dataset. The converted images are then preprocessed and converted the images into 1D vectors, which are then divided into training and testing. Training images are passed to Long Short Term Memory networks, a sequence-based deep learning model for effective supervised learning of the model. The model is then given the remaining testing images into a trained model that predicts whether the patient has covid based on the X-ray. The predicted data are compared with ground truth values for the model evaluation. As the data is converted into 1D vectors, LSTM is able to perform effective training as it interprets the data sequentially.

Figure 3. Proposed framework XDeep

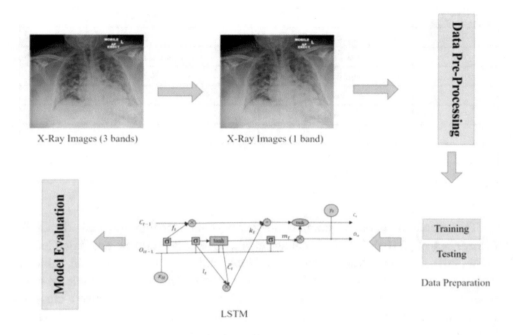

X-Ray Images (3 bands)   X-Ray Images (1 band)

LSTM

EXPERIMENTAL ANALYSIS AND DISCUSSIONS

Experiments are conducted on real chest X-rays. The X-ray set contains 3 classes-Covid, Not Covid, No finding. We have eliminated the No finding class in order to convert this problem into a binary classification problem. The dataset has a total of 55 images, and after elimination, the image count becomes 38. Every image is of different dimension which is then resized to 28 ×28 and then it is converted to 1×784 to form the 1D image. The pre-processed images are divided into training (75%) and testing (25%). 75% of the images are employed for effectively training the LSTM. The obtained trained model is given the remaining 25% of the images as input for prediction. The predicted values are compared against the truth values for evaluating the robustness of the model. The prepared model used total of 1024 neurons with a loss function set as Categorical Cross entropy (Zhang et. al., 2018). The Model also uses a SoftMax activation (Martins et. al., 2016) function with 2 dense layers. Table 1 depicts the parameters we have used for our experiments.

Table 1. Parameter set in LSTM

Sr. No	Parameters	Values
1	No of Neurons	1024
2	Loss Function	Categorical Crossentropy
3	Activation	SoftMax
4	Epochs	50
5	batch size	10
6	Dense Layer	2
7	Training	75%
8	Testing	25%

The prepared model is compared against other learning models- 2D CNN (Martins et. al., 2016), 1D CNN (Albawi et. al., 2017), Gated Recurrent Unit (Chung et. al., 2014), Support Vector Machines (Noble et. al., 2006), as shown in Table 1. The majority of the models are deep learning-based. The proposed model is able to outperform the remaining models and perform the best. GRU is also a class of recurrent neural networks, which is why it is able to perform well. Like LSTM, GRU also do not have the vanishing gradient problem. The parameter of GRU is set similar to LSTM.

Table 2. Parameter set in 2D CNN

Sr. No	Type	Filters	Kernel Size
1	Convolutional	32	(3,3)
2	Convolutional	64	(3,3)
3	Maxpooling	--	(2,2)
4	Fully Connected	128	--
5	Fully Connected	2	--

Table 3. Parameter set in 1D CNN

Sr. No	Type	Filters	Kernel Size
1	Convolutional	128	3
2	Maxpooling	--	2
3	Convolutional	64	3
4	Convolutional	32	3
5	Maxpooling	--	2
6	Fully Connected	256	--
7	Fully Connected	128	--
8	Fully Connected	64	--
9	Fully Connected	32	--
10	Fully Connected	2	--

The parameter employed in 2D CNN and 1D CNN is shown in Table 2 and 3 respectively. There are 2 Convolutional layers that are set in 2D CNN with 1 maxpooling and 2 fully connected layer. Similarly, 3 Convolutional layers are set in 1D CNN with 5 fully connected layers and 2 max pooling. SVM is the popular classification method which is able to attain high classification accuracy in many problems. The kernel SVM is employed with radial basis function with epsilon value of 0.1 and cache size of 200.

Table 4. Comparison of XDeep with other models

Sr. No.	Models	Accuracy
1	2-D CNN	0.91
2	1-D CNN	0.90
3	XDeep	0.99
4	GRU	0.98
5	SVM	0.89

Every model is provided with the same pre-processed 1D image vector for fair evaluation, except 2D CNN is provided with the 2D images (1 band). XDeep is able to improve the classification accuracy by 10% as compared to SVM as shown in Table 4. It also performs well as compared to CNN models. LSTM can form the meaningful connections from the given 1D data as it forms a sequence. LSTM also contains the forget gate which only stores the relevant information in the next time step.

CONCLUSION

In this paper, we developed a framework XDeep which uses the LSTMs, deep learning recurrent networks for effectively classifying the covid positive patients based on the chest X-rays. The employed dataset is pre-processed and converted into 1D image vectors, due to which the LSTM is able to form sequential connections. When compared to existing state-of-the-art models, the proposed model is extremely precise and capable of achieving a maximum improvement in classification accuracy of 10% in comparison.

REFERENCES

Ahsan, M. M. E., Alam, T., Trafalis, T., & Huebner, P. (2020). Deep MLP-CNN model using mixed-data to distinguish between COVID-19 and non-COVID-19 patients. *Symmetry*, *12*(9), 1526. doi:10.3390ym12091526

Albawi, S., Mohammed, T. A., & Al-Zawi, S. (2017, August). Understanding of a convolutional neural network. In *2017 International Conference on Engineering and Technology (ICET)* (pp. 1-6). IEEE.

Apostolopoulos, I. D., & Mpesiana, T. A. (2020). Covid-19: Automatic detection from x-ray images utilizing transfer learning with convolutional neural networks. *Physical and Engineering Sciences in Medicine*, *43*(2), 635–640. doi:10.100713246-020-00865-4 PMID:32524445

Belchior, R., Vasconcelos, A., Correia, M., & Hardjono, T. (2021). *HERMES: Fault-Tolerant Middleware for Blockchain Interoperability*. Academic Press.

Chan, J. F. W., Yuan, S., Kok, K. H., To, K. K. W., Chu, H., Yang, J., & Yuen, K. Y. (2020). A familial cluster of pneumonia associated with the 2019 novel coronavirus indicating person-to-person transmission: A study of a family cluster. *Lancet*, *395*(10223), 514–523. doi:10.1016/S0140-6736(20)30154-9 PMID:31986261

Chen, L., Wang, S., Fan, W., Sun, J., & Naoi, S. (2015, November). Beyond human recognition: A CNN-based framework for handwritten character recognition. In *2015 3rd IAPR Asian Conference on Pattern Recognition (ACPR)* (pp. 695-699). IEEE.

Chen, Y., Jiang, H., Li, C., Jia, X., & Ghamisi, P. (2016). Deep feature extraction and classification of hyperspectral images based on convolutional neural networks. *IEEE Transactions on Geoscience and Remote Sensing, 54*(10), 6232–6251. doi:10.1109/TGRS.2016.2584107

Chung, J., Gulcehre, C., Cho, K., & Bengio, Y. (2014). *Empirical evaluation of gated recurrent neural networks on sequence modeling.* arXiv preprint arXiv:1412.3555.

COVID-19 coronavirus pandemic. (n.d.). Available: https://www.worldometers.info/coronavirus

Hemdan, E. E. D., Shouman, M. A., & Karar, M. E. (2020). *Covidx-net: A framework of deep learning classifiers to diagnose covid-19 in x-ray images.* arXiv preprint arXiv:2003.11055.

Hochreiter, S. (1998). The vanishing gradient problem during learning recurrent neural nets and problem solutions. *International Journal of Uncertainty, Fuzziness and Knowledge-based Systems, 6*(02), 107–116. doi:10.1142/S0218488598000094

Hochreiter, S., & Schmidhuber, J. (1997). Long short-term memory. *Neural Computation, 9*(8), 1735–1780. doi:10.1162/neco.1997.9.8.1735 PMID:9377276

Horry, M. J., Chakraborty, S., Paul, M., Ulhaq, A., Pradhan, B., Saha, M., & Shukla, N. (2020). *X-ray image based COVID-19 detection using pre-trained deep learning models.* Academic Press.

Huang, C., Wang, Y., Li, X., Ren, L., Zhao, J., Hu, Y., & Cao, B. (2020). Clinical features of patients infected with 2019 novel coronavirus in Wuhan, China. *Lancet, 395*(10223), 497–506. doi:10.1016/S0140-6736(20)30183-5 PMID:31986264

Kanne, J. P., Little, B. P., Chung, J. H., Elicker, B. M., & Ketai, L. H. (2020). *Essentials for radiologists on COVID-19: An update—radiology scientific expert panel.* Academic Press.

Li, Y., & Xia, L. (2020). Coronavirus disease 2019 (COVID-19): Role of chest CT in diagnosis and management. *AJR. American Journal of Roentgenology, 214*(6), 1280–1286. doi:10.2214/AJR.20.22954 PMID:32130038

Liu, C., Cao, Y., Alcantara, M., Liu, B., Brunette, M., Peinado, J., & Curioso, W. (2017, September). TX-CNN: Detecting tuberculosis in chest X-ray images using convolutional neural network. In *2017 IEEE international conference on image processing (ICIP)* (pp. 2314-2318). IEEE.

Liu, J., Li, W., Zhao, N., Cao, K., Yin, Y., Song, Q., & Gong, X. (2018, September). Integrate domain knowledge in training CNN for ultrasonography breast cancer diagnosis. In *International Conference on Medical Image Computing and Computer-Assisted Intervention* (pp. 868-875). Springer. 10.1007/978-3-030-00934-2_96

Liu, Q., Zhou, F., Hang, R., & Yuan, X. (2017). Bidirectional-convolutional LSTM based spectral-spatial feature learning for hyperspectral image classification. *Remote Sensing, 9*(12), 1330. doi:10.3390/rs9121330

MacLean, O. A., Orton, R. J., Singer, J. B., & Robertson, D. L. (2020). No evidence for distinct types in the evolution of SARS-CoV-2. *Virus Evolution, 6*(1).

Martins, A., & Astudillo, R. (2016, June). From softmax to sparsemax: A sparse model of attention and multi-label classification. In *International conference on machine learning* (pp. 1614-1623). PMLR.

Narin, A., Kaya, C., & Pamuk, Z. (2020). *Automatic Detection of Coronavirus Disease (COVID-19) Using X-ray Images and Deep Convolutional Neural Networks.* arXiv preprint arXiv:2003.10849.

Noble, W. S. (2006). What is a support vector machine? *Nature Biotechnology, 24*(12), 1565–1567. doi:10.1038/nbt1206-1565 PMID:17160063

Pan, F., Ye, T., Sun, P., Gui, S., Liang, B., Li, L., & Zheng, C. (2020). Time course of lung changes on chest CT during recovery from 2019 novel coronavirus (COVID-19) pneumonia. *Radiology.*

Rumelhart, D. E., Hinton, G. E., & Williams, R. J. (1986). Learning representations by back-propagating errors. *Nature, 323*(6088), 533-536.

Sethy, P. K., & Behera, S. K. (2020). *Detection of coronavirus disease (covid-19) based on deep features.* Academic Press.

Shi, H., Han, X., Jiang, N., Cao, Y., Alwalid, O., Gu, J., Fan, Y., & Zheng, C. (2020). Radiological findings from 81 patients with COVID-19 pneumonia in Wuhan, China: A descriptive study. *The Lancet. Infectious Diseases, 20*(4), 425–434. doi:10.1016/S1473-3099(20)30086-4 PMID:32105637

Singhal, T. (2020). A review of coronavirus disease-2019 (COVID-19). *Indian Journal of Pediatrics, 87*(4), 281–286. doi:10.100712098-020-03263-6 PMID:32166607

Wang, L., Lin, Z. Q., & Wong, A. (2020). Covid-net: A tailored deep convolutional neural network design for detection of covid-19 cases from chest x-ray images. *Scientific Reports, 10*(1), 1–12. doi:10.103841598-020-76550-z PMID:33177550

World Health Organization. (2020). *Pneumonia of unknown cause-China. Emergencies preparedness, response Web site*. WHO.

Wu, F., Zhao, S., Yu, B., Chen, Y. M., Wang, W., Song, Z. G., & Zhang, Y. Z. (2020). A new coronavirus associated with human respiratory disease in China. *Nature*, *579*(7798), 265–269. doi:10.103841586-020-2008-3 PMID:32015508

Xie, X., Zhong, Z., Zhao, W., Zheng, C., Wang, F., & Liu, J. (2020). Chest CT for typical 2019-nCoV pneumonia: Relationship to negative RT-PCR testing. *Radiology*. Advance online publication. doi:10.1148/radiol.2020200343

Zhang, Z., & Sabuncu, M. R. (2018, January). Generalized cross entropy loss for training deep neural networks with noisy labels. *32nd Conference on Neural Information Processing Systems (NeurIPS)*.

Zhao, W., Zhong, Z., Xie, X., Yu, Q., & Liu, J. (2020). Relation between chest CT findings and clinical conditions of coronavirus disease (COVID-19) pneumonia: A multicentre study. *AJR. American Journal of Roentgenology*, *214*(5), 1072–1077. doi:10.2214/AJR.20.22976 PMID:32125873

Zhao, X., Liu, L., Qi, S., Teng, Y., Li, J., & Qian, W. (2018). Agile convolutional neural network for pulmonary nodule classification using CT images. *International Journal of Computer Assisted Radiology and Surgery*, *13*(4), 585–595. doi:10.100711548-017-1696-0 PMID:29473129

Zou, L., Zheng, J., Miao, C., Mckeown, M. J., & Wang, Z. J. (2017). 3D CNN based automatic diagnosis of attention deficit hyperactivity disorder using functional and structural MRI. *IEEE Access: Practical Innovations, Open Solutions*, *5*, 23626–23636. doi:10.1109/ACCESS.2017.2762703

Chapter 3

Healthcare Management Intricacy, Governance, and Strategic Plan During the COVID–19 Pandemic (With Special Reference to India)

Astha Bhanot
Princess Nourah Bint Abdulrahman University, Saudi Arabia

Naila Iqbal Qureshi
ⓘD https://orcid.org/0000-0002-0352-5019
Princess Nourah Bint Abdulrahman University, Saudi Arabia

ABSTRACT

The COVID-19 pandemic has left the healthcare sector with a slew of problems, including a lack of capacity, supply restrictions, the need for service reform, and financial losses. According to complexity, healthcare delivery organizations are complex adaptive systems that function in extremely complicated and unpredictable situations. Many healthcare organizations suffered ambiguity and inconsistency that was not under control as per requirements. In this chapter, the authors look at an effective management system in the face of COVID-19. In order to tackle the pandemic, Word Health Organization (WHO) is bringing together scientists and health experts from all across the world to speed research and development. The governmental and private sectors in India are viewed as cooperating. Private Indian healthcare organizations stepped up and have been providing everything it requires, including testing, treatment isolation beds, medical professionals, and equipment to the government.

DOI: 10.4018/978-1-7998-9831-3.ch003

INTRODUCTION

Individual parts' discrete actions are typically less essential than the interactions within a complex adaptive system. COVID-19 has left the healthcare sector with a slew of problems, including a lack of capacity, supply restrictions, the need for service reform, and financial losses. Healthcare delivery organizations, according to complexity, are sophisticated adaptive systems that operate in exceedingly intricate and unexpected settings. Many healthcare organizations, according to this opinion, suffered ambiguity and inconsistency that was not under control as per requirements. This chapter refer to the context of the COVID-19 outbreak, we examine an efficient management method. Hospitals and health systems during the pandemic have emphasized effective communication, collaboration, and innovation techniques all carried out quickly and well informed by frontline workers. Word Health Organization (WHO) is bringing together scientists and health professionals from all around the world to accelerate research and development in order to combat the pandemic. The governmental and private sectors in India are viewed cooperating. Private Indian healthcare businesses have risen up to the mark, supplying the government with all it needs, including diagnostics, treatment isolation beds, medical specialists, and equipment at official COVID-19 sites and at home.

The highly infectious disease (coronavirus) pandemic has posed various issues for developed countries, which have been exacerbated in underdeveloped countries such as Asia and Africa. Due to a lack of knowledge and protective measures, the number of afflicted people was high. Various preventive techniques were established to aid in the fight against the pandemic crisis, and healthcare facilities around the world worked hard as frontline troops to safeguard patients, often with minimal hope of treatment. The pandemic wreaked havoc on countries with dense urban populations and extensive international travel ties. In countries previously assumed to be most at risk from COVID-19, mortality rates and degrees of restrictions – such as lockdowns and travel bans – were found to be lowest. To accelerate research and development, World Health Organization is bringing together scientists and global health professionals from around the world. It aided in the development of new norms and regulations to regulate the blowout of the coronavirus pandemic, as well as health-care resources for people impacted.

Italy was the first European country to acquire COVID-19 case. COVID-19, which is not the same as seasonal influenza, spread quickly, demonstrating its danger, which was previously underestimated (Indolfi, et al. 2020) COVID-19 is projected to have a burden of 121.449 disability-adjusted life years (DALYs) in Italy, showing enormity in terms of mortality and morbidity (Nurchis, et al. 2020). The role of healthcare workers has been critical in this scenario. In fact, they were both a high-risk group and a probable source of the outbreak (Nioi, el al. 2021 & D'Aloja, E, et al. 2020). During the last 40 years, previous epidemics have taught us a lot: To begin, strong public health infrastructure and protocols are needed at the national, intermediate, and local levels to prevent highly infectious disease (Coronovirus-19) from spreading (Smith, et al. 2014, Chiquoine, R. 2016). Second, community surveillance, early detection capabilities, and accurate information transmission to the entire population are essential. Finally, prepared healthcare services are required to respond appropriately and to restrict the spread of diseases and the number of persons sick (Belfroid, E et al. 2017).

The fundamental goal of the public health system was to reduce death and morbidity from different contagious and non-contagious illnesses by providing basic healthcare through community-based health initiatives. Basic health services are supplied by all healthcare organizations through sub-centres and primary health facilities, while secondary and tertiary care is offered in more advanced facilities. Many nations have achieved considerable breakthroughs in the delivery of healthcare globally during the previous few decades.

As the pandemic expanded across the country, all of the national and local governments issued statements aimed at halting the spread of the disease and coordinating patient care. These actions included social distance, lockdown, quarantine, epidemiological and microbiological surveillance, as well as national health service strengthening, health staff recruitment, equipment and consumables supplementation, and territory healthcare restructuring.

LITERATURE REVIEW

More than 800,000 instances of COVID-19 have been documented worldwide as of March 31, 2020, with 50, 000 patients and 3500 deaths confirmed in France. The pandemic is unlike any other disease because fast spread, lack of scientific proof, and importance of media attention (Shimizu, 2019). The pandemic required the institutions in charge of the cases to deal with a plethora of new problems (Hevmann & Shindo, 2020). The health system's resilience in the face of COVID-19 is a source of worry even in high-income countries (Legido, Q.H et al. 2020). The ability of healthcare staff, institutions, and individuals to prepare for and respond to catastrophes successfully, to keep key operations running during a crisis, and to restructure if required, based on what we've acquired from the catastrophe (Lruk. M.E et al. 2020).

Preparedness for emergencies and disasters was a major concern and a global issue. Due to the disaster-related resource scarcity, most hospitals were unable to continue their normal operations for a week (Vick, D. J et al. 2018). A prior evaluation emphasized the difficulty of acquiring standardized PPE supplies in an emergency (Patel, A et al. 2017). The hospital put in more effort to set up an emergency management system based on the risk of a danger. (W. N. Nasher and colleagues, 2018). Interim Personal protective equipment (PPE) readiness was impracticable owing to the epidemic's unpredictability, exclusively for less regularly used PPE, shielding equipment, and N95 respirators in routine employment. A flexible hospital contingency plan may be more realistic than maintaining a large stockpile of personal protective equipment.

The optimal architecture and high level isolation division facilities are created (Bannister, B et al. 2009), however the issue arises when one is not accessible. Following the COVID-19 catastrophe, management made changes to ensure that the finest facility possible could be built with the resources available. Despite the existence of standards for creating an infectious disease unit (Agarwal, A et al. 2019), implementation is a difficult process that need practical solutions. Space, inventory (supply), employees, and maintaining standards are the four main components in establishing a new facility (Goh, K J et al. 2015). We describe how, following the COVID-19 pandemic, we converted a normal healthcare facility into a specialized infectious disease center in this work. A quick overview of India's health-care system and reaction to the current pandemic follows.

The Obstacles to Achieving Equal, Accessible, and High-Quality Healthcare

The private sector is centered mostly in a few geographic regions. When injustices and difficulties related to equitable, reachable, and high-quality healthcare are investigated spatially, disparities and challenges emerge. National Health Policies have contributed in the development of a more inclusive healthcare system in the country throughout the years, with the objective of gradually achieving Universal Health Coverage (UHC).

Even the most modern healthcare systems improved their organizational working style in order to manage infected cases in a judicious way to testing the COVID-19 infection in patients. The shortage of resources necessitated a tremendous lot of patience on the part of health-care personnel to deal with the issue. Both the private and public sectors contributed to the overall response to the outbreak. Private Indian healthcare businesses have risen up to the mark, supplying the government with all it needs, including diagnostics, treatment isolation beds, medical specialists, and equipment at official COVID-19 sites and at home.

Healthcare organizations are complex systems with concerns like as intricacy, governance, and strategic planning. During the highly infectious illness COVID-19 Pandemic, the responsibility of healthcare organizations increased several fold, and there is a need to investigate some very excellent methods in private and public institutions, which is the focus of this research piece.

Scenario of Hospitals in India during COVID-19

Healthcare system are distinctive and intricate. Especially when we talk about Indian system its very unique and have both public and private sector working. The unexpected spread of pandemic lead to chaos and confusion. The overall objective is to understand the environment of hospitals and challenges faced by them due to sudden pandemic spread.

Hospital Management has been criticized by general public in developing facilitates, material and treating patients, which are key traits for the success of hospital in today's environment. This is because primarily traditional methods of hospitals were providing services to limited number of patients. The entire focus conventionally was to rely on doctors, being at the center, imparting the services with limited or no role of nurses. There is no relevance to the subject or skills required for understanding the topic. For years, this approach in the hospital environment has argued the significance of treating skills, and development of these skills through same issues solving learning method. Patients, today require knowledge and skills to synergize together the variety of ideas, to analyze and evaluate quickly their action in order to succeed in making well-informed decisions in their practical life. As the research focuses on Covid -19 era, it will further understand the foundation of hospital and the need to develop critical skills through problem-based method.

As we have limited hospitals and resources like facilities, Doctors, nurses etc. This is creating the stress on the healthcare center. As the disease is transferable, it became more difficult is management of limited resources. Another big challenge is to predict the number of patients affected by Covid-19. As times it increase by multiple fold and at times, it is very low. Biggest challenge again is lack of availability of proper treatments. Initially when Covid-19 began according to WHO, it took 67days to spread to 1 lakhs patients and the another 1 lakh got affected in just 12 days. Therefore, the patient's size and symptoms both were highly unpredictable.

As an experience, two hospitals in India performed a surgery on patients who infected by Covid-19. Tis lead too many healthcare professional getting further infected and spreading. The actually source of the disease spread was unidentified. However, this led to lockdowns and closure of hospital.

In India, it is predicted that the way the pandemic spread in month of July – August it was difficult to accommodate patients and provide necessary resources. If we pay attention to geographical demographic of India, we will find that 60-65% people are from rural area. This acted as a curse because of lack of awareness, ignorance, and lack of facilities. However, as rural is widely spread across the infection spread was low and slow. The suburbs in modern cities of India like Mumbai had very high spread as the space is less and people stay in closed dooms under one roof.

To enhance the overall healthcare management system experience and deliver better services to their consumers the government and private hospitals launched various models in Indian market. But due to poor network, inability of awareness and various global challenges could not build strong c base and failed at times to cater the wide variety of patients with different symptoms.

This chapter marks an attempt to empirically address the scenario and status of healthcare management system. From the study so far, we can see that healthcare faced too many challenges in times of pandemic. This is also evident by data analysis.

Effect of COVID-19 on Healthcare

Assessment of Current Healthcare Measurements

We may simply state that the healthcare necessities produced during the coronavirus pandemic will surpass our ability, based on a worldwide pattern. In the realm of contemporary medicine, India has 1154686 registered physicians. 10926 persons are now served by a single government allopathic doctor. India's rural population comprises 60 percent of the country's overall population. To deliver healthcare to people in rural India, the government has developed 25743 Primary Health Centers, 158417 Sub Centers, and 5624 Community Health Centers. There have been 713986 beds available in India's government hospitals, or 0.55 beds per 1000 people. Jharkhand, Assam, Haryana, Bihar, Gujarat, Odisha, Madhya Pradesh, Maharashtra, and Manipur, which account for more than 70% of India's population, have a lower population to bed ratio than the national average, whereas Kerala, Sikkim, and Tamil Nadu have a higher population to bed ratio than the national average.

Preparing for Increase in Covid-19 Cases

The circumstances of the nation was variance in the demand and availability of hospital equipment's and medical support like hospital beds, Intensive Care Unit (ICU) beds, qualified practitioners, etc. If just 0.1 percent of the population becomes ill in the next two months, and only 5% of those infected require ICU care, we will need 65000 ICU beds. When a patient is on a ventilator for 15 days, a demand for 975000 ventilator days is generated. If we use a 1% rate, we may imagine the demand produced by this pandemic.

Obtaining resources

In order to offer proper treatment and prevent infection transmission, each hospital must quickly train physicians, nurses, technicians, support staff, and sanitation employees. By bringing together skilled employees from frontline departments, a virtual disaster prevention and management department should be developed. Domestic production capacity ranged between 6000 and 7,000 PPE per day in April, but it has almost increased to more than 30 percent PPE per day. India is working hard to increase the number of ventilators available on the market. To save healthcare resources and minimize physician burnout from non-essential treatments, all normal surgeries and outpatient procedures have been suspended across the country.

RESEARCH DESIGN AND METHODOLOGY

Research and Aim of the Study

This study focuses on analysis and working strategies of healthcare organizational management intricacy, governance and strategic plans followed during COVID-19 Pandemic around the world with special reference to India.

Scope of the Study

The scope of the study includes 6 continents with 237 countries. Correlation was taken into consideration for analysis. As the research is, action oriented the researchers provided effective strategic plans that could enhance the working of the health organizations.

Selection of Problem

The research is based on inductive approach as the study begins with the selection of the problem followed by the data collection leading to final interpretation. The research evolves from general to specific country for the research study. The research was conducted for 6 continents including 237 countries. This research is based on the data collected from worldwide data source. Under the quantitative approach, this research study will use action-oriented research. Action oriented research is used because this research deals with the real-life problems and involves a lot of investigation, data collection, continuous monitoring and reflection of the collected data.

Identification of Problems Faced during Pandemic COVID-19

- Lack of separate arrangement for the Infectious Disease Hospital (COVID hospital)
- Lack of support for shifting of equipment from main hospital to COVID hospital
- Lack of organizing the movement of Patients and Healthcare Workers.

Data Collection Method

The quantitative approach for the research is used. The researchers focused on quantifying the collection from worldwide data source and done the analysis by finalising the variables for the study using Python Language. The data have been suitably prepared, in order, classified and tabulated according to the requirements of the study. The analysis is done on correlation basis. The data collected was based on Average of Daily report of the cases from August 2020 to August 2021. The sample area includes 6 continents consisting of 237 countries. It is represented by using statistical techniques such as bar chart, line chart and correlation.

The Variables under Study

- Cases with cumulative total, cumulative total per 100000 population, newly reported in last 7 days, newly reported in last 7 days per 100000 population, and newly reported in last 24 hours.
- Deaths with cumulative total, cumulative total per 100000 population, newly reported in last 7 days, newly reported in last 7 days per 100000 population, and newly reported in last 24 hours.

Study's Limitations are as Follows

- The scope of the study was vast; hence, it was difficult to take into consideration all the existing variables within the limited time.
- Due to dependency on secondary data numerous actual facts were overlooked.
- The research could be studied by extending the study by using regression analysis to understand the impact and role of each variable.

RESEARCH FINDINGS

Figure 1. Graph on regions under study

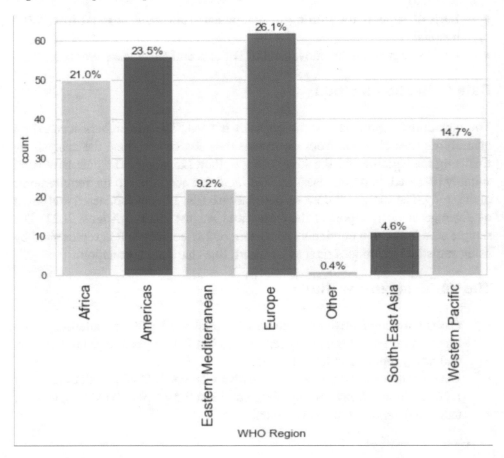

The figure 1 indicate that the study include the six major region for study and most of the country for the study belong to Europe region followed by America and Africa. The least count of countries belong to South East Asia.

Figure 2. Graphs shows the correlation between various variables

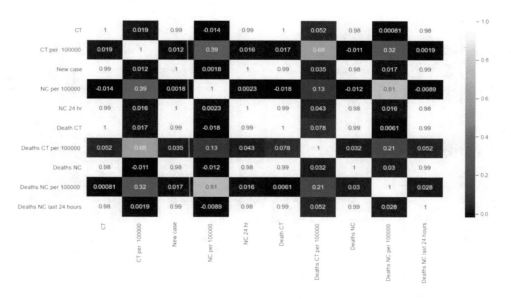

As shown in figure 2 the correlation Matrix we can conclude that there is high positive correlation between Cumulative cases and New cases, Cases reported in the previous 24 hours, Deaths recorded in the last 7 days, and Deaths reported in the last 24 hours Cases - newly reported in the last 7 days and Deaths - cumulative total, Deaths - newly reported in the last 7 days and Deaths - newly reported in the last 24 hours all had a strong positive association. Cases - newly reported in the last 24 hours and Deaths - cumulative total, Deaths - newly reported in the last 7 days and Deaths - newly reported in the last 24 hours all show a strong link. However, if Cases - cumulative total and Cases - cumulative total per 100000 population and Deaths - newly reported in the previous 7 days per 100000 population are identified, there is a very modest positive link. Finally, there is a negative association between Cases - cumulative total and Cases - newly reported in the previous 7 days per 100,000 people. We may deduce from the matrix that the deeper the color, the less the correlation between the variables, and the lighter the color, the stronger the connection.

Figure 3. Graph on relationship between new cases and deaths new cases

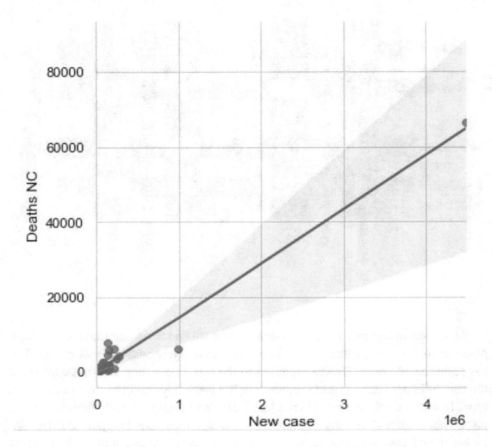

The figure 3 indicate that the new cases cumulative figures have positive upward relationship with the death new cases. It means as the new cases are rising it is also affecting the death cases. This is a cumulative figure representing the situation across the regions. As we can conclude that the overall the rise in cases are positively increasing the deaths.

SOLUTIONS OF THE PROBLEMS

The Infectious Disease Hospital does not have its own Layout (COVID Hospital)

The first challenge was finding a designated facility for COVID-19 patient. Choosing a hospital block that can be segregated from the key hospital is desirable (Bataille, J & Brouqui, P 2017). Lack of separate arrangement for the Infectious Disease Hospital (COVID hospital)

Otherwise, a physically separated area from regular services is preferable (Asperges, E wt al. 2020). Such temporary facilities, on the other hand, can only treat mild to moderate ailments, not those that require rapid medical treatment. Figure 4 depicts a hospital plan for COVID 19 patients so that they can be treated appropriately.

Managerial Control

- Workforce management, biological waste and laundry for impacted patients, food delivery to employees and patients, and communication and management with administrative agencies such as the Municipal Corporation, state and federal health authorities
- Single-point decision-making through the creation of a COVID-19 infection organization chart, including a timetable and staffing management for emergency departments, first detection clinics, and intensive care units. Along with keeping an eye on various departments engaged in policy implementation, troubleshooting, and swift corrective steps in the shortest period feasible.
- Healthcare worker surveillance, including a dedicated staff clinic and self-reporting of fever and respiratory symptoms.
- In hospitals, routine non-urgent work such as OPDs and consultations is being phased out. Telephonic/video consultations/WhatsApp, etc. were used to put up systems and processes.
- Using social media for internal communication, such as forming a hospital-wide WhatsApp group and forming the COVID-19 task force.
- The COVID-19 Team must be established, as well as its tasks, rotation policy, leave policy, and personnel backup buffer, as well as knowledge and resource improvements.

Figure 4. Hospital layout with COVID area in a normal hospital

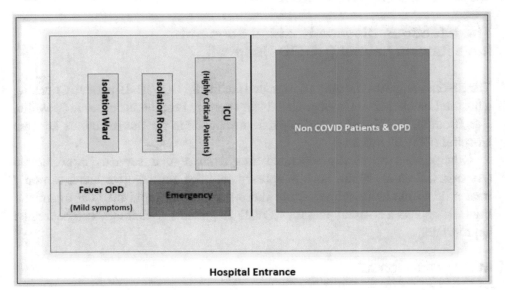

Lack of Support for Shifting of Equipment from Main Hospital to COVID Hospital

As a result of the lockdown, equipment procurement were delayed, and the newly built hospital lacked critical-care capabilities. An ICU checklist was developed in collaboration with the departments of anesthesiology and pulmonary medicine. Use existing inventories from several departments to store supplies and drugs for the future ICU. As a result, supplies were immediately transported from their original locations to the COVID region. ICU ventilators, defibrillators, monitors, crash carts, and other consumables were among them. In the patient care areas, use basic infection control procedures such as utilizing a separate stethoscope, thermometer, and other medical equipment's and instruments. There should be a separate authority to monitor and hand to mobilize the equipment as needed.

Extraordinary care was devoted to maintaining enough supply by keeping the track of daily stock list requirement.

- Medical equipment such as ventilators, defibrillators, backup power supply, oxygen supplies, and key medicine supplies were all updated on a regular basis to assure enough availability.

- Specific needs for alcohol-based disinfectants, personal protective equipment (PPE), N95 filtering face piece respirator (FFR), and other items, which were met by local manufacture.

Lack of Organizing the Movement of Patients and Healthcare Workers

The suspected patients should be examined and confirmed with COVID-19 at the hospitals. This will aid in limiting the virus's exposure to numerous physicians and effectively channeling pandemic care. This will help prevent unneeded pandemonium and patient admissions owing to fear in other specialties' doctors and surgeons. Cross contamination and illness among healthcare professionals will be avoided as a result of this.

- Planning hospital space with a focus on COVID 19 patients. Set up a clinic for patients with fever, emergency department, zone for suspicious patients, ICU, separate disease wards, and isolation rooms for the highly contagious sickness.
- To cope with serious situations, an emergency department should have all of the required amenities, as well as healthcare workers available 24 hours a day, seven days a week.
- Non-serious patients with fever, upper respiratory infection symptoms such as sore throat, cough, cold, etc., as well as travel history, may be seen in a fever OPD.
- A COVID ICU should have a separate air exchange unit with specific equipment for critically ill patients, such as ventilators, ultrasonography machines, and dialysis machines.
- A week-long rotation of dedicated teams allocated to emergency department, fever OPD, and COVID ICU care, followed by a one-week cooling period. The personnel should be divided into numerous groups and tasks should be distributed centrally.
- COVID ICU Management, which includes intensivist motivation and team development.
- Regular knowledge and training programs to upgrade the healthcare personnel on a variety of associated infections.
- A watchful Hospital Emergency Committee keeps a close eye on current infection control procedures and is ready to respond in an emergency.

CONCLUSION

COVID-19 sickness remained affirmed "pandemic" by the World Health Organization (WHO) in early March 2020. To counteract the outbreak's fast spread over the world, extraordinary measures were taken globally. Pandemics, like as COVID-19, put the healthcare system under strain. Healthcare organizations must have preparations in place to cope with big groups of patients affected with an infectious disease. Every big hospital in the world, should have a capacity to deal with the highly infectious disease with an isolation unit. An isolation division guarantees that medical personnel and the hospital are prepared to handle highly infectious disease outbreaks. Most hospitals, however, lack such facilities, especially in resource-constrained settings. In this circumstance, hospitals must convert their normal structure into special hospitals to handle the highly infectious disease. The writers hope to demonstrate their study expertise in converting a traditional clinic into a infectious disease unit by presenting successful solutions.

Hospitals should be advised not to use two products at the same time, and the recommendations should contain a clear declaration in contradiction of the usage of fabric or cloth masks. Despite the fact that four standards support reusing PPE or wearing it for longer periods of time, there are currently no rules to address hand hygiene and throw on/removing protocols should be followed for PPE and mask kit. The ECDC advises wearing PPE for up to 4–6 hours, whilst the UK standard suggests wearing PPE for 2–6 hours. Observation studies should be done if nations utilize these strategies, so that the results may be used to develop future standards for the benefit of the international community. Finally, the WHO guidelines provide no suggestion for fit testing. Finally, the WHO guidelines provide no suggestion for fit testing. Healthcare workers should be pushed to fit test working in the special units / wards because it is unrealistic to presume that they are fit.

This study demonstrates the critical necessity for all healthcare providers to undertake sporadic the knowledge and training programs on highly infectious diseases to prevent such pandemics in future. Conducting regular webinars for educating all healthcare workers, including non-clinical and managerial personnel. Training paramedical and nursing groups will be beneficial and safe was to increase awareness in future.

ASSISTIVE MEASURES

The greatest cause of death is infectious or contagious diseases. Pandemics pose a significant threat to public health and are a worldwide issue, and they are exceedingly difficult to contain. In these circumstances, the country's economic, social, and health factors are crucial; as a result, healthcare executives must effectively manage and support healthcare centers, as well as employ supportive procedures and methods for hospitals and healthcare workers, in order to offer the best available healthcare facilities. Providing a systematic foundation for health center management might be quite advantageous. The following management-supportive strategies are crucial during pandemics:

1. Involve leadership: Physician and nurse performance is influenced by leadership. Maintain good touch with employees by paying attention to and appropriately listening to them.
2. Select the appropriate motivations: Discuss the importance of employee work, express gratitude for their efforts, and support them.
3. Maintain a healthy work–life balance: Create a task that is appropriate and balanced for your personnel. Say that proper rest is the foundation for excellent performance to underline the requirement of re-energizing.
4. Inspire peer support: To protect your employees from extraneous pressures such as inappropriate or confusing demands from patients and others.
5. Offer mental health protection tools for employees: To prevent placing employees under even more stress, reduce hazardous working conditions and workplace stress.
6. Foster a pleasant community: To build a joyful workplace, foster great cooperation and strengthen working connections.
7. Give employees more control over their work: Establish clear expectations for your employees and create an environment in which they may complete vital tasks without being interrupted.
8. Regularly analysis your achievements: Talk to your co-workers about your development and accomplishments on a regular basis.
9. Withdraw meetings that aren't necessary: Try to minimize unnecessary gatherings at work. If you need to hold a meeting, use video conferencing.

ACKNOWLEDGMENT

The authors declare that there is no conflict of interests regarding the publication of this manuscript.

REFERENCES

Agarwal, A., Nagi, N., Chatterjee, P., Sarkar, S., Mourya, D., Sahay, R. R., & Bhatia, R. (2020). Guidance for building a dedicated health facility to contain the spread of the 2019 novel coronavirus outbreak. *The Indian Journal of Medical Research*, *151*(2), 177–183. doi:10.4103/ijmr.IJMR_518_20 PMID:32362643

AHA. (2020). *Leading during COVID-19: Lessons Learned from Clinical and Administrative Teams.* Available online at: https://www.aha.org/podcasts/2020-05-28-leading-during-covid-19-lessons-learned-clinical-and-administrative-teams

Ahmed, F., Ahmed, N., Pissarides, C., & Stiglitz, J. (2020). Why inequality could spread COVID-19. *The Lancet. Public Health*, *5*(5), e240. doi:10.1016/S2468-2667(20)30085-2 PMID:32247329

Allcorn, S. (1990). Using matrix organization to manage health care delivery organizations. *Hospital & Health Services Administration*, *35*, 575–590. PMID:10107388

Asperges, E., Novati, S., Muzzi, A., Biscarini, S., Sciarra, M., Lupi, M., Sambo, M., Gallazzi, I., Peverini, M., Lago, P., Mojoli, F., Perlini, S., & Bruno, R. (2020). Rapid response to COVID-19 outbreak in Northern Italy: How to convert a classic infectious disease ward into a COVID-19responsecentre. *The Journal of Hospital Infection*, *105*(3), 477–479. doi:10.1016/j.jhin.2020.03.020 PMID:32205162

Bannister, B., Puro, V., Fusco, F. M., Heptonstall, J., & Ippolito, G. (2009). Framework for the design and operation of high-level isolation units: Consensus of the European network of infectious diseases. *The Lancet. Infectious Diseases*, *9*(1), 45–56. doi:10.1016/S1473-3099(08)70304-9 PMID:19095195

Bataille, J., & Brouqui, P. (2017). Building an intelligent hospital to fight contagion. *Clinical Infectious Diseases*, *65*(suppl_1), S4–S11. doi:10.1093/cid/cix402 PMID:28859348

Bedford, J., Enria, D., Giesecke, J., Heymann, D. L., Ihekweazu, C., Kobinger, G., Lane, H. C., Memish, Z., Oh, M., Sall, A. A., Schuchat, A., Ungchusak, K., & Wieler, L. H. (2020). COVID-19: Towards controlling of a pandemic. *Lancet*, *395*(10229), 1015–1018. doi:10.1016/S0140-6736(20)30673-5 PMID:32197103

CBHI. (2019). *National Health Profile 2019.* Central Bureau of Health Intelligence. Directorate General of Health Services. Government of India. Available online at: http://www.cbhidghs.nic.in/showfile.php?lid= 1147

CDC. (2003). *CDC Guidelines for Environmental Infection Control in Health-Care Facilities*. Available online at: https://www.cdc.gov/infectioncontrol/ guidelines/ environmental/appendix/air.html

Cheney, C. (2020). *Coronavirus: 5 Lessons Learned from Temporary Hospitals in China*. Available online at: https://www.healthleadersmedia.com/clinical-care/ coronavirus-5-lessons-lear-temporary-hospitals-china

Chief Executives Board for Coordination (CEB) Human Resources Network Version 1.0. (2020). *Administrative Guidelines for Offices on the Novel Coronavirus (COVID-19) Outbreak*. Available online at: https://hr.un.org/sites/hr.un.org/ files/Administrative%20Guidelines%20-%20Novel%20Coronavirus %20Final_ Version%201.0_13%20February%202020_0.pdf

Chinese Center for Disease Control and Prevention. (2020). *Epidemic Update and Risk Assessment of 2019 Novel Coronavirus 2020*. Available online at: http://www. chinacdc.cn/yyrdgz/202001/P020200128523354919292. pdf

Chowell, G., & Mizumoto, K. (2020). The COVID-19 pandemic in the USA: What might we expect? *Lancet, 395*(10230), 1093–1094. doi:10.1016/S0140-6736(20)30743-1 PMID:32247381

Cucinotta, D., & Vanelli, M. (2020). WHO declares COVID-19a pandemic. *Acta Biomedica, 91*, 157–160. doi:10.23750/abm.v91i1.9397 PMID:32191675

Goh, K. J., Wong, J., Tien, J. C., Ng, S. Y., Duu Wen, S., Phua, G. C., & Leong, C. K.-L. (2020). Preparing your intensive care unit for the COVID-19 pandemic: Practical considerations and strategies. *Critical Care (London, England), 24*(1), 215. doi:10.118613054-020-02916-4 PMID:32393325

Gupta, A., Singla, R., Caminero, J. A., Singla, N., Mrigpuri, P., & Mohan, A. (2020). Impact of COVID-19 on tuberculosis services in India. *The International Journal of Tuberculosis and Lung Disease, 24*(6), 637–639. doi:10.5588/ijtld.20.0212 PMID:32553014

Heymann, D.L., & Shindom N. (2020). COVID-19: what is next for public health? *Lancet, 395*, 542-50. . doi:10.1016/S0140-6736(20)30374-3

Jog, S., Kelkar, D., Bhat, M., Patwardhan, S., Godavarthy, P., & Dhundi, U. (2020). Preparedness of Acute Care Facility and a Hospital for COVID-19 Pandemic: What We Did! *Indian Journal of Critical Care Medicine: Peer-Reviewed, Official Publication of Indian Society of Critical Care Medicine, 24*(6), 385–392. doi:10.5005/ jp-journals-10071-23416 PMID:32863628

Jones, L. (n.d.). *The Big Ones: How Natural Disasters Have Shaped Humanity.* New York, NY: Anchor Books Press.

Kruk, M.E., Myers, M., Varpilah, S.T., & Dahn, B.T. (2015). What is a resilient health system? Lessons from Ebola. *Lancet, 385,* 1910-2. . doi:10.1016/S0140-6736(15)60755-3

Lancet Infectious Diseases. (2020). Challenges of coronavirus disease 2019. *The Lancet. Infectious Diseases, 20*(3), 261. doi:10.1016/S1473-3099(20)30072-4 PMID:32078810

Legido-Quigley, H., Asgari, N., Teo, Y.Y., Leung, G.M., Oshitani, H., & Fukuda, K. (2020). Are high-performing health systems resilient against the COVID-19 epidemic? *Lancet, 395,* 848-50. . doi:10.1016/S0140-6736(20)30551-1

Listed, N. A. (2020). *Michigan National Guard Building Temporary Medical Station in Detroit to Support Coronavirus Patients.* Available online at: https://www.mlive.com/public-interest/2020/04/michigan-national-guard-building-temporary-medical-station-in-detroit-to-support-coronavirus-patients.html

MOHFW. (2020a). *Guidance Document on Appropriate Management of Suspect/ Confirmed Cases of COVID-19.* Available online at: https://www.mohfw.gov.in/pdf/FinalGuidanceonMangaementofCovidcases version2.pdf

MOHFW. (2020b). *Government of India. Ministry of Health and Family Welfare. Directorate General of Health Services (EMR Division). COVID-19: Guidelines on Dead Body Management.* Available online at: https://www.mohfw.gov.in/pdf/1584423700568_ COVID19GuidelinesonDeadbodymanagement.pdf

Muñana, C., Hamel, L., Kates, J., & Michaud, J. (2020). *The Public's Awareness of Concerns About Coronavirus. Global Health Policy.* Henry J. Kaiser Family Foundation, KFF Health Tracking Poll. Available online at: https://www.kff.org/global-health-policy/issue-brief/the-publicsawareness-of-and-concerns-about-coronavirus/

Naser, W. N., Ingrassia, P. L., Aladhrae, S., & Abdulraheem, W. A. (2018l). A study of hospital disaster preparedness in South Yemen. *Prehospital and Disaster Medicine, 33*(2), 133–138. doi:10.1017/S1049023X18000158 PMID:29455694

National Institute of Health. (2020). *News Release: NIH Clinical Trial Shows Remdesivir Accelerates Recovery From Advanced COVID-19.* Available online at: https://www.nih.gov/news-events/news-releases/nih-clinical-trialshows-remdesivir-accelerates-recovery-advanced-covid-19

Patel, A., D'Alessandro, M. M., Ireland, K. J., Burel, W. G., Wencil, E. B., & Rasmussen, S. A. (2017). Personal protective equipment supply chain: Lessons learned from recent public health emergency responses. *Health Security*, *15*(3), 244–252. doi:10.1089/hs.2016.0129 PMID:28636443

Pharmaceuticals, R. (2020). *News Release: Regeneron and Sanofi Provide Update on US Phase 2/3 Adaptive-Designed Trial of Kevzara R (Sarilumab) in Hospitalized COVID-19 Patients*. Available online at: https://investor. regeneron.com/news-releases/news-release-details/regeneron-and-sanofiprovide-update-us-phase-23-adaptive

Sengupta, M., Roy, A., Ganguly, A., Baishya, K., Chakrabarti, S., & Mukhopadhyay, I. (2021, June 1). Challenges Encountered by Healthcare Providers in COVID-19 Times: An Exploratory Study. *Journal of Health Management*, *23*(2), 339–356. doi:10.1177/09720634211011695

Seshadri, M. S., Seshadri, M. S., & John, T. J. (2020, April 4). Hospital Readiness for COVID-19: The Scenario from India with Suggestions for the world. *Christian Journal for Global Health*, *7*(1), 33–36. doi:10.15566/cjgh.v7i1.375

Shimizu, K. (2020). 2019-nCoV, fake news, and racism. *Lancet*, *395*(10225), 685–686. doi:10.1016/S0140-6736(20)30357-3 PMID:32059801

Taccone, S. F., Gorham, J., & Vincent, J. L. (2020). Hydroxy chloroquine in the management of critically ill patients with COVID-19: The need for an evidence base. *The Lancet. Respiratory Medicine*, *8*(6), 539–541. doi:10.1016/S2213-2600(20)30172-7 PMID:32304640

Unnithan, P. S. G. (2020). Kerala Reports First Confirmed Coronavirus Case in India. *India Today*. Available online at: https://www.indiatoday.in/india/ story/kerala-reports-first-confirmed-novel-coronavirus-case-in-india1641593-2020-01-30

USFDA Press Announcement. (2020). *Coronavirus (COVID-19) Update: FDA Issues Emergency Use Authorization for Potential COVID-19 Treatment*. Available online at: https://www.fda.gov/news-events/press-announcements/coronavirus-covid-19-update-fda-issues-emergency-use-authorizationpotential-covid-19-treatment

Vick, D. J., Wilsom, A. B., & Fisher, M. (2018). Assessment of community hospital disaster preparedness in New York State. *Journal of Emergency Management (Weston, Mass.)*, *16*, 213–227. doi:10.5055/jem.2018.0371 PMID:30234908

Vincent, J. L., & Taccone, F. S. (2020). Understanding pathways to death in patients with COVID-19. *The Lancet. Respiratory Medicine*, *8*(5), 430–432. doi:10.1016/S2213-2600(20)30165-X PMID:32272081

WHO. (2020a). *WHO Disease Outbreak News. Pneumonia of unknown cause – China.* Available online at: https://www.who.int/csr/don/05-january-2020pneumonia-of-unkown-cause-china/en/

WHO. (2020b). *WHO Director-General's Opening Remarks at the Media Briefing on COVID-19 - 11 March 2020.* Available online at: https://www.who.int/ dg/ speeches/detail/who-director-general-s-opening-remarks-at-the-mediabriefing-on-covid-19--11-march-2020

Wikipedia. (2020). *2020 Coronavirus Lockdown in India.* Available online at: https:// en.wikipedia.org/wiki/2020_coronavirus_lockdown_in_India

World Health Organization. (2020c). *WHO Director-General's Opening Remarks at the Media Briefing on COVID-19.* Available online at: https://www.who. int/dg/ speeches/detail/who-director-general-s-opening-remarks-at-themedia-briefing-on-covid-19---11-march-2020

World Health Organization. (2020d). *Coronavirus Disease 2019 (COVID-19) Situation Report-51.* Available online at: https://www.who.int/docs/defaultsource/coronaviruse/ situation-reports/20200311-sitrep-51-covid-19.pdf? sfvrsn=1ba62e57_10

World Health Organization. (2020e). *Modes of Transmission of Virus Causing COVID19: Implications for IPC Precaution Recommendations: Scientific Brief.* World Health Organization. Available online at: WHO/2019-nCoV/ Sci_Brief/ Transmission_modes/2020.2

World Health Organization. (2020f). *Coronavirus Disease 2019 (COVID-19) Situation Report-43.* Available online at: https://www.who.int/docs/defaultsource/coronaviruse/ situation-reports/20200303-sitrep-43-covid-19.pdf? sfvrsn=76e425ed_2

World Health Organization. (2020g). *Coronavirus Disease 2019 (COVID-19) Situation Report-47.* Available online at: https://www.who.int/docs/defaultsource/coronaviruse/ situation-reports/20200307-sitrep-47-covid-19.pdf? sfvrsn=27c364a4_4

World Health Organization. (2020h). *Coronavirus Disease 2019 (COVID-19) Situation Report–53.* Available online at: https://www.who.int/docs/defaultsource/ coronaviruse/situation-reports/20200313-sitrep-53-covid-19.pdf? sfvrsn=adb3f72_2

World Health Organization. (2020i). *Coronavirus Disease (COVID-19) Advice for the Public.* Available online at: https://www.who.int/emergencies/diseases/ novel-coronavirus-2019/advice-for-public

World Health Organization. (2020j). *Q & A on Coronaviruses (COVID-19).* Available online at: https://www.who.int/news-room/q-a-detail/q-acoronaviruses

World Health organization. (2020k). *Coronavirus Disease 2019 (COVID-19) Situation Report-153.* Available online at: https://www.who.int/docs/ defaultsource/coronaviruse/situation-reports/20200621-covid-19-sitrep-153.pdf? sfvrsn=c896464d_2

Wu, H., Huangc, J., Casper, J. P. Z., Zonglin, H., & Ming, W. K. (2020). Facemask shortage and the novel coronavirus disease (COVID-19) outbreak: Reflections on public health measures. *EClinicalMedicine, 21,* 100329. doi:10.1016/j. eclinm.2020.100329 PMID:32292898

Zaki, A. M., van Boheemen, S., Bestebroer, T. M., Osterhaus, A. D., & Fouchier, R. A. (2012). Isolation of a novel coronavirus from a man with pneumonia in Saudi Arabia. *The New England Journal of Medicine, 367*(19), 1814–1820. doi:10.1056/ NEJMoa1211721 PMID:23075143

Zhong, B. L., Luo, W., Li, H. M., Zhang, Q. Q., Liu, X. G., Li, W. T., & Li, Y. (2020). Knowledge, attitudes, and practices towards COVID-19 among Chinese residents during the rapid rise period of the COVID-19 out break: A quick online cross-sectional survey. *International Journal of Biological Sciences, 16*(10), 1745–1752. doi:10.7150/ijbs.45221 PMID:32226294

Zhu, N., Zhang, D., Wang, W., Li, X., Yang, B., Song, J., Zhao, X., Huang, B., Shi, W., Lu, R., Niu, P., Zhan, F., Ma, X., Wang, D., Xu, W., Wu, G., Gao, G. F., & Tan, W. (2020). A novel coronavirus from patients with pneumonia in China, 2019. *The New England Journal of Medicine, 382*(8), 727–733. doi:10.1056/NEJMoa2001017 PMID:31978945

APPENDIX

Table 1.

Abbreviations	Title
ICU	Intensive Care Unit
PPE	Personal Protective Equipment
OPD	Out Patient Department
ECDC	European Centre for Disease Prevention and Control
WHO Region	World Health Organization Region
CT	Cases - cumulative total
CT per 100000	Cases - cumulative total per 100000 population
New case	Cases - newly reported in last 7 days
NC per 100000	Cases - newly reported in last 7 days per 100000 population
NC 24 hr	Cases - newly reported in last 24 hours
Death CT	Deaths - cumulative total
Deaths CT per 100000	Deaths - cumulative total per 100000 population
Deaths NC	Deaths - newly reported in last 7 days
Deaths NC per 100000	Deaths - newly reported in last 7 days per 100000 population
Deaths NC last 24 hours	Deaths - newly reported in last 24 hours

Chapter 4
A Smartphone–Based Dermatological Disease Identification System Using Probabilistic Neural Networks

Siji A. Thomas
Mount Zion College of Engineering, Kerala, India

Mathew K.
Mount Zion College of Engineering, Kerala, India

Jerin Geo Jacob
Mount Zion College of Engineering, Kerala, India

Thomas George
Mount Zion College of Engineering, Kerala, India

Sini K. Thomas
VISAT Engineering College, Kerala, India

Arun M. S.
Mount Zion College of Engineering, Kerala, India

ABSTRACT

In this chapter, the different dermatological diseases are differentiated using the concept of probabilistic neural networks (PNN). There are different colour transformations for various dermatological diseases. This chapter mainly focuses on the differentiation of psoriasis and dermatitis with the normal one. The colour, shape, and textural features of the patches are studied and analysed for recognising the various dermatological diseases. The colour, texture, mean, median, entropy, standard deviations are considered for feature analysis. The pre-screening system uses the PNN algorithm after the feature extraction. The experimental results define the accuracy and effectiveness of the proposed algorithm, and the system scores sensitivity of 0.91, specificity of 0.94, with an accuracy rate of 96.25%.

DOI: 10.4018/978-1-7998-9831-3.ch004

INTRODUCTION

Dermatological diseases have major impacts and concerns on people's lives and are one of the most prevalent diseases which people are taken into consideration. According to the survey mentioned in Karimkhani *et al.* (2017) and Hay *et al.* (2010), almost one-third of the worldwide population suffer from skin diseases. Sometimes, the early diagnosis of dermatological disease is difficult, and it may enhance the severity if it is left undetected. Skin disease can be caused due to various reasons which include heredity, exposure to chemicals, lack of cleanliness, usage of cigarettes, drugs, alcohol, etc., and even the climatic change is also one of the factors. Though it does not have much relation with mortality rates in connection with dermatological abnormalities, these diseases have greater impacts on the quality of life. The skin covers the entire body and it acts as a protective barrier layer against the damage to internal tissues. It is having a total of 20 square feet of area with a weight of around 8 pounds. The detailed illustration of the skin anatomy is depicted in figure 1.

Figure 1. Anatomy of skin

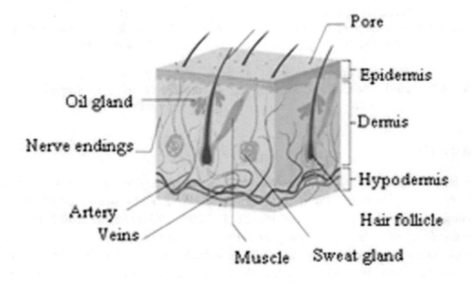

The skin has mainly three layers: Epidermis, Dermis and Hypodermis. The skin colouring pigment called melanocytes are located in the epidermis layer, the outermost part of our skin, and this layer creates the texture. Most of the symptoms are shown in this layer. The dermis layer contains tough connective tissues, hair follicles, sweat glands. Much deeper, there is another layer is called the Hypodermis layer which contains fat and other connective tissues.

People have a weak knowledge about the diseases, that they consult a dermatologist several weeks or months later after the skin irritation starts, causing the enhancement in the disease severity. In some cases, the doctors find it difficult to diagnose the disease symptoms at its early stage and it requires expensive tests in order to diagnose the disease and its severity level. Though lasers and photonics technology are available, the expensiveness of such laboratory tests is still a limitation. Here, the authors are proposing a neural network-based image processing algorithm, capable of correctly diagnosing the disease and its stage. This system can be effectively used by the dermatologists for their reference. Another peculiarity of the proposed system is that, it helps the patient to diagnose whether the abnormalities on the skin are the symptoms for normal flakes or rashes, by imputing the captured image taken from a smartphone into the Probabilistic Neural Network algorithm. Some of the skin infections include Rashes, Dermatitis, Psoriasis, Eczema, Acne, etc., even some of the abnormalities have the same visual characteristics.

Nowadays, the symptoms from the patient's skin are analysed manually by the Dermatologist based on his/ her experience, but it can also lead to misjudgements which in turn delay the proper treatments. Some people predict their dermatological infection, just by analysing its outer surface and considers to be a normal infection and finally leading the disease to reach at its intensive level. Biopsy procedures are also done clinically to identify the diseases, which in turn requires local anaesthesia to mitigate the stinging effects, and there are many risk factors too when it is to be examined on children under ten years. This chapter mainly focuses on the early detection of psoriasis and dermatitis to avoid the risk factors at its intense stage. Psoriasis is a chronic inflammatory skin condition that causes erythematous plaques with scaling and skin inflammation; which may be due to the enhancement in the growth of dermatological cells or even the abnormalities in the blood vessels. Dermatitis is a general term defined for skin irritation or sometimes; skin inflammation. Dermatitis is of different types namely; atopic dermatitis, contact dermatitis, dyshidrotic dermatitis, Seborrheic dermatitis etc. In some cases, there may be no indications of a skin disease and this may result in the ineffectiveness of the treatment as the disease escalates to its intense stage undetected. The mild stage of psoriasis is sometimes misinterpreted as dermatitis since the early mild indications shown by both diseases are almost the same. Rough scaly skin on the surfaces, including the scalp, are the main symptoms of both of these diseases. Dermatitis is not a serious condition and mainly occurs on the scalp portions but it may affect anywhere in the body. It is not a contagious condition but makes the skin uncomfortable. In most cases, people misunderstand psoriasis as dermatitis and they do not take much care of it. The other common symptoms include itching, reddened skin and the appearance of flakes. Figure 2 shows images of normal skin, dermatitis and psoriasis affected skin.

Figure 2. a) Normal skin b) Dermatitis affected skin c) Psoriasis affected skin

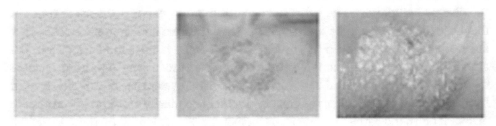

Early detection plays an important role in psoriasis treatment because it can be made into curative completely in most of the cases, if it is diagnosed earlier; the latter stage increases the risk of death. Thus, effective image processing algorithm helps the specialists to prescribe timely treatments. The term Dermoscopy is also known as epiluminescence microscopy which is a non-surgical skin examination technique that magnifies the lesion area making the abnormal surface more clearly visible. It is commonly used by dermatologists to examine suspicious abnormal lesions or any other expensive visual aid systems. But this equipment sometimes makes the medical experts difficult to use due to the lack of adequate training.

The algorithm described in this chapter only requires Smartphone and a Computer, the proposed system does not rely on dermatoscopy, which in turn, makes the algorithm very simple, robust and effective. It can also be used in the rural areas during campaigns for medical practitioners and in the hospitals or clinics where there is less access to the dermatology department.

LITERATURE REVIEW

Early diagnosis of dermatological diseases helps patients to take appropriate treatments that prevent skin infections to reach its severe stage. Current diagnosis can be costlier, tedious and time-consuming; this can lead to the development of automatic analysis so that doctors can save their valuable time to attend more critical medical issues. Even though there are many literature backgrounds available that dictate about the diagnosis of dermatological diseases, only the recent and relevant models are discussed here.

Vezhnevets *et al* (2003) proposed a system for the identification of skin diseases using colour images minimizing the dermatologist's intercession. The system uses k-means clustering and colour gradient procedures to differentiate between the infected and the normal skin, the authors adopted Artificial Neural Networks for the classification of the skin disease type. The authors in Bulent *et al* (2005) focuses mainly on the lesion segmentation, the borders were identified using Gradient Vector Flow (GVF) snakes. The authors considered 70 benign and 30 melanoma skin lesion images for the analysis. The algorithm developed by Bulent et al consists of mainly two steps: 1) the pre-processing step: in order to employ the GVF snake algorithm; firstly initialization of snake point is done and then the pre-processing. Gaussian filtering is adopted in order to reduce the noise level during the deformation process. It allows the snake to simply ignore all the edges the algorithm found weak. 2) a multi-step deformation was used in the second step. The authors used only 20 iterations during the deformation process. Linear interpolation was also employed during the deformation process if necessary; that is when it found that the Euclidian distance is greater than one pixel.

Nidhal *et al.* (2010) proposed a Psoriasis detection system using feed-forward neural networks by extracting the Gray Level Co-occurrence Matrix (GLCM) features from the input images. The algorithm considered colour and texture features for the GLCM procedure. The authors used a tan sigmoid function as the activation function in both hidden as well as the output layer. The activation function is generally used since non-linearity is added into neural networks, which in turn allows the neural networks to train under powerful operations. The authors, Rahat *et al.* (2014) developed a method for diagnosing different types of skin diseases; the authors employed a feed-forward ANN for pre-training and testing the images. The authors adopted different algorithms for extracting the features; they focussed on nine dermatological diseases with an accuracy rate of 90%. Prathamesh *et al.* (2015) discuss a comparative study of different methods used for automatic detection of hair and restoration of the texture-part is presented. The authors mainly focus on three methods which include linear interpolation, Partial Differential Equation (PDE) and the fast marching scheme algorithm. The advantages of using the fast marching method is that, it uses non-iterative PDE's and it utilizes structure tensor to accurately define the coherence direction that switches between diffusion and directional transport. Nafiul *et al.* (2016) proposed a system for the automatic diagnosis of eczema by extracting colour; texture and border features from the segmented image, the authors used Support Vector Machine (SVM) for classification. By calculating the body region score, the algorithm easily identifies the disease stages such as mild or severe. The performance was analysed on 85 images and achieved good classification accuracy.

An automated system for diagnosing the skin malignancy by using plain photographs of affected regions by employing the ABCDE rule has been put forward in the work done by Mustafat *et al.* (2018) for detecting melanoma. The main steps for detection are pre-processing, image segmentation, feature extraction and classification. Segmentation helps to separate the skin lesion and they employed a Grab cut segmentation method which is then post-processed by combining mean-shift filtering and median blurring. Finally, some morphological operations for the elimination of noise. The authors in Mohd Affandi *et al.* (2018), researches a ten-year review from the Malaysian Psoriasis Registry. About 2-6% of the people in Malaysia, affected by this, are registered in the Malaysian Dermatological Society. The authors mentioned the most common type of psoriasis is plaque psoriasis and it shows a percentage of 85.1%. But, there are many dermatological infections with the same symptoms or appearance that makes uncertainty in predictions.

Cruz *et al.* (2019) illustrates a dermatological diagnostic system to identify the skin diseases such as hives, eczema and psoriasis. The authors used a texture operator called Local Binary Pattern (LBP), RGH-HSV Colour Space, Colour Histogram and Support Vector Machine (SVM) to train the images. 30 images in the Dermnet database were taken into consideration for each of the diseases- eczema, hives and psoriasis. The system achieved 96.0560%, 95.8041%, and 98.5609% for the above mentioned three skin infections respectively. Manisha *et al.* (2019) developed an automatic method to enhance the accuracy of the disease detection using multiclass Probabilistic Neural Network (PNN). The authors in Manisha et al focussed mainly on two diseases as melanoma and vitiligo. As the first stage, removal of noises from the input image is done using median filter followed by the feature extraction. The features were extracted by considering the Gray Level Co-Occurrence Matrix (GLCM), Discrete Fourier Transformation (DFT) and intensity histogram. The GLCM features evaluate the textural features which include contrast, correlation, homogeneity and energy whereas the intensity histogram considers the features such as mean, variance, standard deviation, skewness, kurtosis; the extraction of feature vectors was done using the DFT technique. All the extracted features were used in the PNN classifier and finally the detection of the mentioned skin diseases. The performance of this algorithm was tested on 550 input images and achieved an accuracy rate of 86%.

Nawal *et al.* (2019) discuss an early diagnosis of skin disease detection system in which they pre-trained the images using Convolutional Neural Networks (CNN). After resizing the features were extracted using a deep CNN model called Alexnet, which consists of five convolutional layers. A ReLU layer is also used after each convolutional layer. Other than, max-pooling layers, the authors in Nawal et al used normalization layers, in order to enhance the training rate. Finally, the features were classified using Support Vector Machine (SVM). This algorithm mainly focussed on three different dermatological diseases such as eczema, melanoma and psoriasis, differentiating these from the healthy skin image. Bhavani *et al.* (2019) discuss another dermatological disease detection method where they used Inception_v3, MobileNet and Resnet algorithms for feature extraction and logical regression for training as well for testing. The authors designed a three model neural network in a single architecture. The images were collected from the Dermnet database and the method achieved a good classification rate. The authors suggest that adding more neural network models can improve the overall efficiency.

The authors in Velasco *et al.* (2019) established a model with the use of transfer learning to diagnose various skin diseases. The authors adopted oversampling and data augmentation techniques to improve the accuracy resulted in 94.4% output. The work done by Zhao *et al.* (2020) discusses the identification of Psoriasis with clinical images and developed a two-stage Convolutional Neural Network Model for the diagnosis. The first stage used a multi-label classifier and in the next stage, the authors utilized the output from its previous stage to differentiate between Psoriasis from other dermatological diseases. The authors in Rosniza *et al.* (2020) states that more than 125 million people across the globe affects by various dermatological abnormities. The authors evaluated the psoriasis diseases such as Plaque and Guttate using CNN. Exactly 187 images were taken into consideration for training as well as for testing purposes. After resizing the raw images, the features required are extracted using CNN procedures, where the image passes through three main layers namely the convolutional layer, pooling and the fully connected layer. The algorithm achieved good parameter rates for both Plaque and Guttate dermatological disease, 82.9% and 72.4% respectively. A survey was conducted by Saja *et al.* (2020) for the classification of skin diseases by different machine learning techniques, the authors found that most of the researches are using Convolutional Neural Networks for the classification of lesions, but one of the limitations highlighted is that the training and the processing time; also the system shows high accuracy only if the data set is strong. Briefly, the techniques which come under Artificial Neural Networks (ANN) requires large data set for the accurate and précised classification resulting in high true positive rates, but if the datasets are small, it results in low false positive and false negative rates. This turns out to be even more problematic because the accuracy and precision rate is lower in such cases. The authors point out another classification algorithm called Naïve Bayes, which results in good range of results, it does not affect even if the datasets are small.

Adegun *et al.* (2021) highlighted the usage of a Probabilistic model with fully connected Convolutional Neural Networks to analyse the skin lesion images for improving efficiency. The authors aimed to overcome the limitations that occur due to the interference of unwanted features in skin images. Srinivasu *et al.* (2021) developed a deep learning-based classification system using MobileNet V2 and

Long Short Term Memory (LSTM) and its performance was compared with other models. For analysing the intensive stage of the disease, the authors used a grey-level co-occurrence matrix and the algorithm achieved more than 85% accuracy.

Elngar *et al.* (2021) achieved a good range of detection rate for Eczema, Melanoma, Psoriasis, Onychosis, Acne and Corn respectively wherein the authors used a CNN pre-trained model and a statistical analysis algorithm, called SVM. As a pre-processing step, the authors used smoothening and filtering technique, since these steps plays a crucial role while classifying an image. The authors extracted mainly two features for the classification purpose especially the colour and the texture of the infected area. There are various methods such as, Sobel, Canny and Prewitt, for the detection of edges. The Sobel edge detection is a widely used edge detection method though it has two shortcomings. Firstly it is sensitive to noise. Secondly, the Sobel threshold has to be determined by the user. The Sobel algorithm takes advantage of the horizontal and vertical directional gradient differences of the adjacent pixel. The Sobel edge detection determines whether the point is a border point or not by comparing gradient and threshold differences. If the result is higher than the threshold, the point is an edge. If the result is below the threshold, the point is not an edge. The authors in this chapter thus uses, Sobel operator as one of the pre-processing steps to detect the edge perfectly. The various filtering techniques for the removal of skin hairs are described in Amarathunga *et al.* (2015), Zaqout *et al.* (2019) and Jana *et al.* (2017) which includes Gaussian filter, various morphological operations (erosion and dilation, thresholding techniques) and median filtering.

From the above mentioned backgrounds, the following inferences were considered for reference.

- For dermatological disease identification, neural networks play a pivotal role; as the number of works prove that, the false rate while extracting the features can be reduced by using the same.
- For the result analysis, most of the researchers used the parameters like accuracy, sensitivity and specificity.
- The experimental results depend upon the clarity of the dermatological images used.
- The accuracy of prediction level depends upon the pre-processing steps done before the feature extraction.
- Most of the traditional classification techniques are time-consuming.

The purpose of this work is to automatically identify whether the captured image is Normal, Dermatitis or Psoriasis infected ones. In this work, PNN is used for classification purposes and is a widely used classifier for getting the promising results in biomedical applications. The images used for the analysis of the algorithm were collected from hospitals as well as from publically available databases since the outcome is heavily dependent on the data. The proposed algorithm also, works well with Smartphone-based test images also. And, as far the authors know, no previous research papers have investigated much on PNN for the classification of dermatological diseases.

ARCHITECTURE AND METHODOLOGY

In this section, the methodology of the proposed system is discussed. After the image acquisition, the whole architecture can then be subdivided into three main sections comprising Pre-processing, Feature Extraction and Classification. The dermatological library is comprised of 100 skin images of size 256 x 256 pixels, out of which 50 samples are normal, 24 are Psoriasis affected ones and remaining dermatitis affected. The algorithm is also tested for the images captured using Smartphones. The block diagram of the proposed methodology is shown below in figure 3.

Figure 3. Block diagram of the proposed procedure

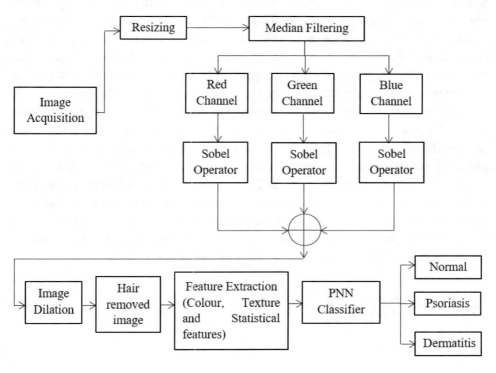

The below section describes the experimental approach and its interpretations for the identification of skin diseases using image processing and the classification of different categories using neural networks.

Pre- Processing

The steps used for pre-processing stage plays a crucial role before extracting the features for image classification because the skin lesion analysis is sometimes complex and becomes tedious. In this methodology, the bicubic interpolation method is used for resizing the image and it does not affect the quality of the input, thereby resulting in uniformly sized data; image filtering is done for removing the unwanted noises and also to get the sharper details of the affected area. Then, median filtering is performed where a 3x3 neighbourhood was chosen for performing the filtering operation.

For getting better classification accuracy, the edges of the infected area need to be identified. The work described by Sangeetha *et al.* (2016) explains that the detection of edges as a pre-processing step plays an important role in computer vision, machine learning and many imaging applications. Edge defines the object limits within the image and occurs when discontinuities in the intensity of pixels are present. Thus, a Sobel operator is applied to the RGB channel since the combination of the red, green and blue channels always scores better efficiency. The edge detected image can be defined as 'optimal' if the distance between the actual edges of the dermatological image and the edges detected by the proposed algorithm is minimum. The dilation process is performed on the edge detected image to create a mask. The dilated mask images of three channels are combined to get the hair removed image. The segmentation procedures are done by using K- means clustering where the algorithm clusters data by iteratively computing a mean intensity for each class and segmenting the image by in which each pixel in the class is classified with the nearest mean. The segmentation procedure plays a significant role in dermatological disease identification because more than the majority of features that dealt with the identification depends upon the shape than other features. The new cluster is obtained by using the equation 4.1 given below where C_j denotes the sample set 'x' whose cluster centre is Z_j (k) and N_j is the number of samples in C_j (k).

$$Z_j \left(k + 1 \right) = \frac{1}{N_j} \sum_{x \in C_j(k)} x \text{ where; j=1, 2, 3 .... k.} \tag{4.1}$$

Feature Extraction

The main parameters considered for feature analysis in the proposed algorithm are colour, texture, mean, median, entropy and standard deviations since the content-based image retrieval is an important tool in the classification of images. Among these, the colour and texture features are the important features that perform well in classification. This process reduces the number of variables and it contains the most discriminatory information. The colour histogram is one of the significant colour features used for extracting the features of an image. The Gray-Level Co-occurrence Matrix (GLCM) is mainly adopted for calculating the texture features wherein the texture analysis is done by computing the statistics of neighbouring pixels with the co-occurrence matrix. Thus, a GLCM matrix is created and the statistical relationship is extracted from this matrix. The statistical features computed from the images are mean, median, standard deviation, entropy and skewness. The mean value is the average value of the colour values and it gives the contribution of the individual pixel intensity. Median aids the separation of high-intensity values from the lower intensity pixel values whereas standard deviation indicates the measure of data variability. Skewness is related to the measure of surface symmetry, its values can be positive or negative; even they can be zero or undefined.

Classification

For disease identification, the features taken from the dermatological images are fed to the PNN Classifier which classifies any given image into Normal, Psoriasis or Dermatitis. PNN comes under the class of Artificial Neural Networks (ANN) and is derived from the probabilistic graphical model called Bayesian network. It is a non-linear feed-forward neural network used for classification purposes. The authors used PNN for classification since it can be easily trained. Also, it greatly reduces the misclassifications since the basic principle employed in this model is the theory of probability. It can be defined as a flexible substitute for a back-propagation neural network algorithm. Mainly, PNN has four layers such as input layer, summation layer, pattern layer and output layer. The PNN framework is shown below in figure 4.4.

Figure 4. PNN framework

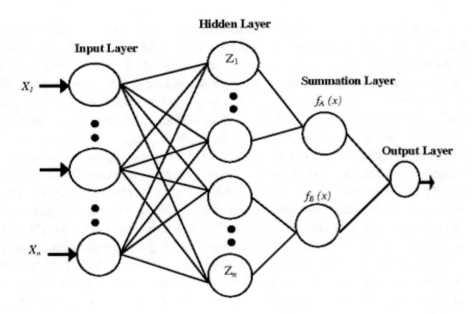

Description of PNN Layers

Input Layer: Each feature is represented as a node by the input layer. This layer calculates the distance between the input and the data which are trained, which in turn indicates the closeness between the two.

Hidden Layer: The core objective of the pattern layer is the identification of a class, based on its pattern, also known as the hidden layer. This layer contains the Gaussian function and it receives all feature vectors from the first layer and produces a net value of the probability vectors.

Summation Layer: The summation layer employs a sum operation from the hidden layer of each class. This layer performs the average output values from the previous layer for each class.

Output Layer: This is the final layer of neurons that does the actual classification. This layer does not have much learning process as well. It simply evaluates the output of the previous layer, i.e., the summation layer and computes the output. This final layer called the output layer which performs the actual identification of dermatological disease i.e., this layer differentiates the input image as Normal, Psoriasis or Dermatitis affected one by selecting the highest summation value from the previous layer, reducing the probability of misclassification between normal and abnormal lesions.

Highlights of Probabilistic Neural Networks

1) The main advantage of selecting PNN as the classification algorithm is its simplicity and intuitiveness.
2) It is comparatively high-speed and more accurate than multilayer perceptron networks.

RESULTS AND INTERPRETATIONS

This work scores well efficiency level since the PNN is much faster when compared to other multi-layered perceptron, and its approach is based on Bayes classification.

Figure 5. a) Original Image b) Sobel Operation c) Hair Removed Image

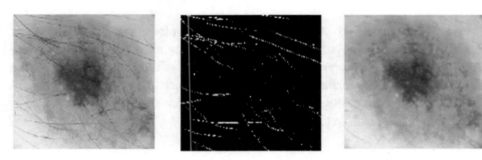

For implementation purposes and performance analysis, 127 images were taken into consideration from different publically available database such as dermnet, dermatological clinics as well real times samples captured using smartphones. The performance of the proposed procedure is validated based on the analysis of accuracy, sensitivity and specificity. The authors conducted three experiments which include: Normal- Psoriasis, Normal- Dermatitis and Normal- Psoriasis- Dermatitis. For the 3 classes, the same network classifier was used. The model has been trained on a non-dedicated Intel Core 5 PC with 4GB memory, the model also works well in the system with lower specifications. Figure 5 depicts the original image, the resultant image of the Sobel Operation and followed by the hair removed image after the dilation process. The database description and the validation sets are detailed in Table 1.

Table 1. Dataset details

	Dermnet	Images collected from hospital	Images captured using Smartphone	Total
Training Set				
Normal	41	7	2	50
Psoriasis	24	0	0	24
Dermatitis	24	2	0	26
Total	89	9	2	100
Validation Set				
Normal	6	5	2	13
Psoriasis	8	0	0	8
Dermatitis	4	2	0	6
Total	18	7	2	27

The performance and validity of the proposed algorithm was analysed by considering the following parameters mainly; sensitivity, specificity and accuracy to quantify how valid the proposed model is. Sensitivity is the measure of true positive rate whereas specificity for the true negative rate to predict different classes. Accuracy is defined as the ratio of the number of skin images that are perfectly diagnosed to the total number of skin images.

$$Sensitivity = \frac{TP}{TP + FN}$$

$$Specificity = \frac{TN}{FP + TN}$$

$$Accuracy = \frac{TP + TN}{TP + FP + FN + TN}$$

where TN, TP, FN and FP represents True Negative, True Positive, False Negative and False Positive respectively. The description of TP and FN are as following.

True Positive (TP): If the proposed algorithm predicts the dermatological image as 'Positive' for a person actually with Psoriasis or Dermatitis skin disease is termed as True Positive.

The TP accuracy rate can be calculated by the following equation:

$$TP= \frac{A}{B} \times 100$$

Where A defines the total number of dermatological images with Psoriasis or Dermatitis disease, which are truly diagnosed as actual images with Psoriasis or Dermatitis skin disease. B represents the total number of Psoriasis and Dermatitis affected images.

False Negative (FN): If the proposed algorithm predicts the dermatological image as 'Negative' for a person actually with Psoriasis or Dermatitis skin disease is termed as False Negative.

The FN accuracy rate can be calculated by the following equation:

$$FN= \frac{A}{B} \times 100$$

Where A defines the total number of dermatological images with Psoriasis or Dermatitis disease which are not truly diagnosed as actual images of Psoriasis and Dermatitis skin disease. B represents the total number of Psoriasis and Dermatitis affected images.

Table 2. Performance analysis on various datasets

Database	PNN Classifier								
	Normal- Psoriasis			Normal- Dermatitis			Normal- Psoriasis-Dermatitis		
	Ac.	Se.	Sp.	Ac.	Se.	Sp.	Ac.	Se.	Sp.
Dermnet	88.88%	0.83	1	90%	1	0.83	92.5%	0.83	0.88
Hospital images	87.5%	1	1	87.5%	1	0.85	100%	1	1

Table 2 gives the performance analysis of the proposed methodology with three experimental models, achieved an average scores of specificity and sensitivity of 0.94, 0.91 with an accuracy rate of 96.25%. Cross-validation was also performed with a skin specialist for analysing the algorithm's capability to differentiate the diseases. 20 images were taken from the database and are given to the skin specialist for the classification.

Table 3. Classification of developed system with benchmarked scores of a dermatologist

Dataset	Image Count	Dermatologist Analysis		Proposed System	
		Normal	Abnormality	Normal	Abnormality
Dermnet	15	10	5	9	6
Hospital images	3	2	1	2	1
Smartphone	2	2	0	2	0

The score has been recorded in Table 3 and are compared with the values obtained with the developed PNN algorithm. Though there are a number of advantages, the limitations include the requirement of more memory space for storing the model and is slower on comparing with the multilayer perceptron.

CONCLUSION AND FUTURE SCOPES

In this chapter, a diagnostic model has been presented which could automatically recognize the skin diseases. The efficiency of the algorithm can be proven by analysing the algorithm using the input image captured using Smartphone. Current methods of detection or assessments are time-consuming and require trained dermatologists. Even the trained specialists may also find difficulty in its diagnosis at its initial stage. Early detection can potentially reduce the risk of irritations and other complications that might occur at its severe stage. The developed algorithm differentiates between the normal and pathological skin images using a simple automatic diagnosis procedure. The technique is fully automated and the obtained result provides useful information for the classification and detection of dermatological diseases. The trained model is capable of achieving the average scores namely accuracy (96.25%), sensitivity (0.91), specificity (0.94) respectively. The simplicity of the algorithm makes this method, efficient as well as a significant tool for the diagnosis of diseases. As a future scope, deep learning techniques can be incorporated instead of PNN to improve the classification efficiency, also more images with various dermatological abnormalities, any dysplastic conditions or any other pigmented skin lesions can be trained to make the algorithm more advanced. The methodology discussed in the chapter can also effectively rely on teledermatology smart care system using mobile applications for a second opinion; rather than consulting a skin specialist through a normal referral pathway. The developed system would be advantageous to the medical practitioners and dermatologists, which helps them to assist their prediction, it also reduces the requirement of a big inter-professional team-based works especially during rural campaigns.

However, there are a few concerns that need to be monitored.

1. It is a prerequisite that the camera of the capturing medium must be of good resolution for the diagnosis to be done perfectly.
2. Adding a new skin abnormality to the proposed algorithm will result in computational demands, as the database needs to be retrained.

As a part of future work:

1. The authors are experimenting with the research on extracting more features from the raw image of the skin lesion, to identify and predict various dermatological infections using the same algorithm without affecting the accuracy and the precision rate.
2. The adaptive Wiener filter can be incorporated in future works in order to avoid the blurring effects and also to get sharp edges.
3. More hybrid techniques can also be incorporated into the model to enhance computational performance.
4. The model can be modified and made so common to the people that it may help them to self-check and become cautious about the skin irritations or allergies due to the over usage of cosmetics and other chemicals these days.
5. Efficient image augmentation technique can be incorporated with a deep learning approach.
6. The Enhanced Probabilistic Neural Network (EPNN) can also be incorporated to outperform the algorithm.
7. Convolutional Neural Networks (CNN) can be used to enhance the disease identification accuracy further, where the raw pixels can be directly processed without any detailed pre-processing steps.
8. Standalone systems can be designed to improve the accuracy and precision of the proposed model to a higher rate.

REFERENCES

Karimkhani, C., Dellavalle, R. P., Coffeng, L. E., Flohr, C., Hay, R. J., Langan, S. M., Nsoesie, E. O., Ferrari, A. J., Erskine, H. E., Silverberg, J. I., Vos, T., & Naghavi, M. (2017). Global skin disease morbidity and mortality: An update from the Global Burden of Disease Study. *JAMA Dermatology*, *153*(5), 406–412. doi:10.1001/jamadermatol.2016.5538 PMID:28249066

Hay, R. J., Johns, N. E., & Williams, H. C. (2014). The global burden of skin disease in 2010: An analysis of the prevalence and impact of skin conditions. *The Journal of Investigative Dermatology*, *134*, 1527–1534. doi:10.1038/jid.2013.446 PMID:24166134

Vezhnevets, V., Sazonov, V., & Andreeva, A. (2003). A Survey on Pixel-based Skin Colour Detection Techniques. *Proceedings of International Conference Graphicon*, 85-92.

Erkol, B., Moss, R. H., Stanley, R. J., Stoecker, W. V., & Hvatum, E. (2005). Automatic Lesion Boundary Detection in Dermoscopy Images Using Gradient Vector Flow Snakes. *Skin Research and Technology*, *11*(1), 17–26. doi:10.1111/j.1600-0846.2005.00092.x PMID:15691255

Nidhal, K. (2010). Psoriasis Detection Using Skin Colour and Texture Features. *Journal of Computational Science*, *6*(6), 648–652. doi:10.3844/jcssp.2010.648.652

Rahat Yasir, R., Rahman, M. A., & Ahmed, N. (2014). Dermatological Disease Detection Using Image Processing and Artificial Neural Network. *8th International Conference on Electrical and Computer Engineering*, 687-690. 10.1109/ICECE.2014.7026918

Prathamesh, Somnathe, & Gumaste. (2015). A Review of Existing Hair Removal Methods in Dermoscopic Images. *IOSR Journal of Electronics and Communication Engineering*, 73- 76.

Alam, M. Tavakolian, MacKinnon, & Fazel-Rezai. (2016). Automatic Detection and Severity Measurement of Eczema Using Image Processing. *38th IEEE Engineering in Medicine and Biology Society Conference,* 1365-1368.

Mustafat, S., & Kimura, A. (2018). A SVM-Based Diagnosis of Melanoma Using Only Useful Image Features. *International Workshop on Advanced Image Technology (IWAIT)*, 1-4.

Mohd Affandi, A., Khan, I., & Ngah Saaya, N. (2018). Epidemiology and Clinical Features of Adult Patients with Psoriasis in Malaysia: 10-Year Review from the Malaysian Psoriasis Registry (2007-2016). *Dermatology Research and Practice*.

Cruz, Garcia, Dimaunahan, Labaclado, Reyes, Riomero, Salamatin & Patrisha. (2019). Eczema, Color histogram, Support vector machine, Psoriasis, RGH-HSV color space, Skin disease, Local binary pattern, Hives. *Proceedings of the 2019- 9th International Conference on Biomedical Engineering and Technology*, 160-165.

Barman, M., Chaudhury, J. P., & Biswas, S. (2019). Automated Skin Disease Detection Using Multiclass PNN. *International Journal of Innovations in Engineering and Technology*, *14*(4), 19–24.

Soliman, N. (2019). A Method of Skin Disease Detection Using Image Processing and Machine Learning. *Procedia Computer Science*, *163*, 85–92.

Bhavani, R., Prakash, V., Kumaresh, R. V., & Sundra Srinivasan, R. (2019). Vision-Based Skin Disease Identification Using Deep Learning. *International Journal of Engineering and Advanced Technology*, *8*(6), 3784–3788.

Velasco, Pascion, Alberio, Apuang, Cruz, & Gomez, Molina, Tuala, Thio-ac, & Jorda. (2019). A Smartphone-Based Skin Disease Classification Using MobileNet CNN. *International Journal of Advanced Trends in Computer Science and Engineering*, *8*(5), 2632–2637.

Zhao, S., Xie, B., Li, Y., Zhao, X., Kuang, Y., Su, J., He, X., Wu, X., Fan, W., Huang, K., Su, J., Peng, Y., Navarini, A., Huang, W., & Chen, X. (2020). Smart Identification of Psoriasis by Images Using Convolutional Neural Networks: A case Study in China. *Journal of the European Academy of Dermatology and Venereology*, *34*(3), 518–524.

Roslan, Razly, Sabri, & Ibrahim. (2020). Evaluation of Psoriasis Skin Disease Classification using Convolutional Neural Network. *IAES International Journal of Artificial Intelligence, 9*(2), 349-355.

Mohammed & Al-Tuwaijari. (2020). Skin Disease Classification System Based on Machine Learning Technique: A Survey. *IOP Conference Series: Materials Science and Engineering (ISCES), 1076*, 1-13.

Adegun, A. A., Viriri, S., & Yousaf, M. H. A. (2021). Probabilistic-Based Deep Learning Model for Skin Lesion Segmentation. *Applied Sciences (Basel, Switzerland)*, *11*(7), 3025–3038.

Srinivasu, SivaSai, Ijaz, Bhoi, Kim, & Kang. (2021). Classification of Skin Disease Using Deep Learning Neural Networks with MobileNet V2 and LSTM. *Sensors (Basel)*, *21*(8), 2852–2879.

Elngar, A. A., Kumar, R., Hayat, A., & Churi, P. (2020). Intelligent System for Skin Disease Prediction using Machine Learning. *6th International Conference on Advanced Computing and Communication Systems (ICACCS)*, 599-605.

Amarathunga, A. A., Ellawala, E. P., Abeysekar, G. N., & Amalraj, C. R. (2015). Expert System for Diagnosis of Skin Diseases. *International Journal of Scientific and Technology Research*, *4*(1), 174–178.

Zaqout, I. (2019). *Diagnosis of skin lesions based on Dermoscopic Images Using Image Processing Techniques*. In *Pattern Recognition Selected Methods and Applications*. Intech Open.

Jana, E., Subban, R., & Saraswathi, S. (2017). Research on Skin Cancer Cell Detection using Image Processing. *IEEE International Conference on Computational Intelligence and Computing Research (ICCIC)*, 1-8.

Sangeetha, D., & Deepa, P. (2016). An Efficient Hardware Implementation of Canny Edge Detection Algorithm. *29th International Conference on VLSI Design and 2016 15th International Conference on Embedded Systems (VLSID)*, 457-462.

Chapter 5
Machine Learning

Khalid Ahmed AlAfandy

(iD) https://orcid.org/0000-0003-1465-4446
ENSA, Abdelmalek Essaadi University, Morocco

Hicham Omara
Abdelmalek Essaadi University, Morocco

Mohamed Lazaar
ENSIAS, Mohammed V University in Rabat, Morocco

Mohammed Al Achhab
NTT, ENSATE, Abdelmalek Essaadi University, Tetouan, Morocco

ABSTRACT

This chapter provides a comprehensive explanation of machine learning including an introduction, history, theory and types, problems, and how these problems can be solved. Then it shows some of the most used machine learning algorithms that are used in image classification, ending with the evaluation matrices calculations that are used to assess the performance of the learning models. The open source libraries also mentioned in this chapter facilitate the used codes for building any learning model with the use of machine learning.

INTRODUCTION

Artificial intelligence is a broad discipline of computer science concerned with developing intelligent machines that can accomplish activities that would normally need human intelligence by mimicking human intelligence (Shinde & Shah, 2018). Artificial intelligence is a multidisciplinary subject with many techniques, but

DOI: 10.4018/978-1-7998-9831-3.ch005

advances in machine learning and deep learning are causing a paradigm shift in almost every field (Shinde & Shah, 2018; Bowling et al., 2006). The relationship between artificial intelligence, machine learning, and deep learning is depicted in figure 1. Machine learning is an artificial intelligence portion that relies on the utilization of real data to train computers, which qualifies computers to reach strong predictions for a particular data type as a human expert and without modular programming. That means it is a process of importing dataset features and exporting output classes or results depending on the used machine learning algorithm type. These data features can be linear data, images, videos, audios, or any other used data type in our human life. So, machine learning is an attempt to make computers learn as humans using commonly used data in our human life (Alpaydin, 2020). Machine learning can be divided into two types; supervised and unsupervised machine learning. The supervised machine learning is based on training computers using given data that have known correct outputs where the unsupervised machine learning is based on given data without outputs or cleared results to build the learning models. The supervised machine learning can be categorized into two branches; classification and regression. The regression problem is based on the predictions within continuous outputs where there is a relation between inputs and outputs within continuous function. The classification problem is based on the predictions in discrete outputs where the outputs are limited to two or more known categories or classes (Alloghani et al., 2020). The learning model must count on a mathematical model where it can be different according to the learning type which is called the hypothesis function. In supervised machine learning, the cost function or loss function must be used through a training process which is built according to the used mathematical model; it must be minimized to achieve a high accuracy prediction model. The lowest cost value can be achieved by updating the model parameters. Thus, the main goal to build a high performance learning model is selecting model parameters values that result in the lowest cost function. There are two main problems that can occur in learning models; the over-fitting problem and the under-fitting problem, and then there are more ways to solve these problems (Alpaydin, 2020; Alloghani et al., 2020).

This chapter outlines the machine learning history, types, problems, and how learning problems can be solved, then shows some of the most used machine learning algorithms, the open sources library which is ease the used codes for building any learning model with the use of machine learning, ending with the evaluation matrices calculations that are used in the learning models performance assessment.

Figure 1. The relation between the artificial intelligence, machine learning, and deep learning
(Shinde & Shah, 2018; Bowling et al., 2006)

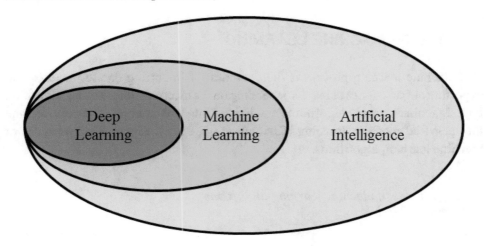

HISTORY OF MACHINE LEARNING

Machine learning started in 1943 with building the first mathematical model of the neural networks which was presented in (Mcculloch & Pitts, 1990). In 1950, Arthur Samual developed a computer program for playing checkers, he initiated the alph-beta pruning that measures the chance of winning to overcome the low available memory in this time, and then he designed the scoring function called minimax algorithm which is used in game programming till now (ElNaqa & Murphy, 2015). Arthur Samuel defined machine learning in 1959. His definition is "The machine learning is the field of study that gives computers the ability to learn without being explicitly programmed" (ElNaqa & Murphy, 2015). In 1965, Aleksei Ivakhnenko and Valentin Lapa created a hierarchical representation of polynomial activation function neural networks that were trained with the GMDH. It is widely regarded as the first multi-layer perceptron, and Ivakhnenko is frequently referred to as the "Father of Deep Learning." (Ivakhnenko & Lapa, 1966). In 1979, Kunihiko Fukushima created a hierarchical multilayered network for pattern recognition and inspiration for convolutional neural networks (Fukushima et al., 1983). In 1998, the problem of learning was also defined by Tom Mitchell as "a computer program is said to learn from experience E with respect to some task T and some performance measure P" (Mitchell, 2006). ImageNet, a vast visual database of labeled images founded by Fei-Fei Li in 2009, is a massive visual database of tagged images. She believed that in order to be genuinely practical and effective, machine learning needed appropriate training data that reflected the actual world (J. Deng et al., 2009).

THEORY OF MACHINE LEARNING

The machine learning process is the operation of importing dataset features and exporting output classes or results depending on the used machine learning algorithm type. Machine learning algorithms are divided into two categories: supervised and unsupervised machine learning (Khanum et al., 2015). Figure 2 shows types of machine learning algorithms.

Figure 2. Types of machine learning algorithms
(Khanum et al., 2015)

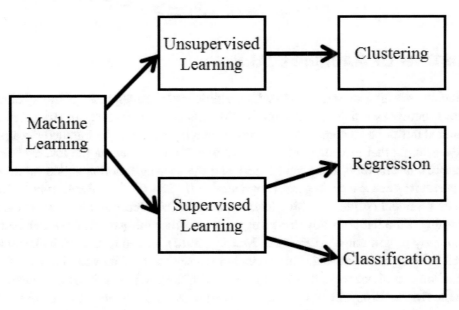

The supervised learning relies on a given data set with the known correct outputs, where there is relevance among the input and the output. Supervised learning models are assorted to regression and classification models. In a regression model, the results are tried to predict within a continuous output, which means that the input variables are tried to map to some continuous function. In a classification model, the results are tried to predict in a discrete output, which means that the input variables are tried to map into discrete categories or classes (Sen et al., 2020).

The unsupervised learning is based on approaching results with little or no idea about the results. The data structure can be deduced without necessarily knowing the effect of the variables. So, the data structure can be deduced by clustering the data based on relationships between the variables in the data. In unsupervised learning, there is no feedback based on the prediction results (Khanum et al., 2015).

UNSUPERVISED MACHINE LEARNING

The unsupervised machine learning counts on given data that doesn't have any labels. So, the learning algorithm attempts to find some structure in the given data. After the learning algorithm succeeds in structuring this given unlabeled data, the algorithm grouped these data into separate clusters. Then the main unsupervised machine learning algorithm is called the clustering algorithm (Smola & Vishwanathan, 2008). The k-means algorithm is the commonly used clustering algorithm. It based on the division of *m* objects into *k* clusters where each object is affiliated to the nearest mean cluster. This approach results perfectly *k* various clusters with greatest possible variation. Till now, it is not known the best number of clusters *k* that leads to the greatest variation as a priority, thus it must be reckoned from the data. The input features of dataset are given $X=\{x_1,\ldots,x_m\}$. The goal of k-means algorithm is to structure the given dataset into *k* clusters where every point in a cluster looks like the points from its own cluster than with the points from other clusters. To achieve this goal, realize the prototype vectors $\mu 1 \ldots,\mu k$ and an indicator vector r_{ij} which is 1, if and only if, is assigned to cluster j. To cluster our dataset we will minimize the following objective function $J(r,\mu)$, which minimizes the distance of each point from the prototype vector (Smola & Vishwanathan, 2008).

$$J\left(r,\mu\right) = \frac{1}{2}\sum_{i=1}^{m}\sum_{j=1}^{k} r_{ij}\left\|x_i - \mu_j\right\|^2 \tag{1}$$

where $r=\{r_{ij}\}$, $\mu=\{\mu j\}$ and $\|.\|^2$ denotes the usual Euclidean square norm.

To achieve the high performance learning model, it must be minimize the value of objective function $J(r,\mu)$ in (1), on the other hand to build this model it must to find r and μ values. So, practically it is very difficult to minimize objective function $J(r,\mu)$ with respect to both r and μ values, then two stages strategy must be adapted; the first stage is to determine r with fixing μ. The xi can be found by setting rj=1 i_j:

$$J\left(r,\mu\right) = \operatorname*{argmin}_{j}\left\|x_i - \mu_j\right\|^2 \qquad (2)$$

and 0 otherwise (Smola & Vishwanathan, 2008).

The second stage is to determine μ with fixing r. So, J *is* a quadratic function of μ, and it can be minimized by setting the derivative to be 0 with respect to μj fo$_r$ all j (Smola & Vishwanathan, 2008):

$$\sum_{i=1}^{m} r_{ij}\left(x_i - \mu_j\right) = 0 \qquad (3)$$

By rearranging, it is obtained (Smola & Vishwanathan, 2008):

$$\mu_j = \frac{\sum_i r_{ij} x_i}{\sum_i r_{ij}} \qquad (4)$$

Where $\sum_i r_{ij}$ counts the numbers of points that assigned to cluster j and μj is basically set to be the sample mean of points that assigned to cluster j. Figure 3 shows the unsupervised learning (Smola & Vishwanathan, 2008).

Figure 3. The unsupervised learning
(Smola & Vishwanathan, 2008)

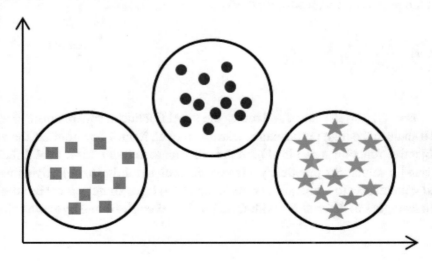

SUPERVISED MACHINE LEARNING

The supervised machine learning is based on given data with known correct results or outputs. The supervised machine learning can be categorized into two types; regression and classification. In the regression learning models, the given dataset inputs and its outputs must have a mathematical relation where the outputs are predicted within continuous function. In the classification learning models, the given dataset inputs and outputs also must have a mathematical relation but the outputs are predicted within discrete function. In these two types, the mathematical model is necessary but it can be different according to the learning model type (regression or classification), the used dataset, and the learning algorithm, this mathematical model is called hypothesis function $h_{\theta(}x)$. The model parameters $\{\theta0,...,\theta n\}_m$ ust be well selected and updated according to the dataset input features $\{x1,... xn\}$,o achieve the lowest cost or loss value that calculated using the cost function J (Verdhan, 2020). The main difference between the regression and classification algorithm is the hypothesis function where the cost function and updating model parameters are almost the same. Figure 4 shows the supervised learning (regression and classification).

Figure 4. The supervised Learning
(Verdhan, 2020)

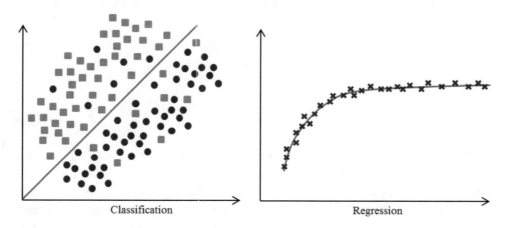

| Classification | Regression |

In regression, the hypothesis function can be calculated for each input in the dataset inputs by using the model parameters and the input features. This hypothesis function can be a linear function or any other mathematical function according to the nature of the used dataset (Gutenbrunner et al., 1993; Shanthamallu et al., 2017). It can be calculated by (Gutenbrunner et al., 1993; Shanthamallu et al., 2017):

$$h_\theta\left(x\right)=\theta_0 +\theta_1 x_1 +\theta_2 x_2 +\ldots +\theta_n x_n \tag{5}$$

where $h_\theta(x)$ is the hypothesis function, $\{\theta 0, \ldots ,\theta n\}$ is the model parameters, and $\{x1,\ldots xn\}$ is the nth input features for the dataset input .

It can be reformulated as matrix multiplication form by (Gutenbrunner et al., 1993; Shanthamallu et al., 2017):

$$h_\theta\left(x\right)=\begin{bmatrix}\theta_0 & \theta_1 & \theta_2 & \ldots & \theta_n\end{bmatrix}\begin{vmatrix}1\\x_1\\x_2\\\vdots\\x_n\end{vmatrix}=\theta^T x \tag{6}$$

In classification, the hypothesis function can be calculated for each input in the dataset inputs by using the model parameters and the input features. The most used hypothesis function in classification is the sigmoid function (Shanthamallu et al., 2017). The hypothesis function can be calculated by (Shanthamallu et al., 2017):

$$h_e\left(x\right) = g(z) = \frac{1}{1+e^{-z}} \tag{7}$$

$$z = \theta T^x \tag{8}$$

The sigmoid function is $g(z)$ whose output is any real number in [0, 1] interval as shown in figure 5. If the output is less than 0.5 then the classification output is 0, and if the output is greater than or equal 0.5 then the classification output is 1. In case of more than two classes which $y=\{0,1,2,\ldots,n\}$, the problem is divided into $n+1$ binary classification problems; in classes predictions outputs, the highest probability for a class means that y belongs to this class (Shanthamallu et al., 2017; Zhao et al., 2010).

Figure 5. The sigmoid function graph
(Shanthamallu et al., 2017)

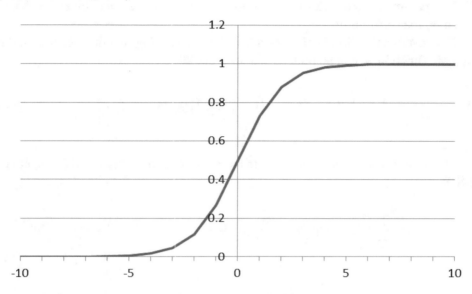

Through the training stage in supervised machine learning, two outputs can be utilized to build the learning model; the correct and predefined dataset outputs and the hypothesis outputs where the cost function is based on these two outputs. Thus, the cost function for regression learning can be built using the hypothesis function and the dataset known correct outputs by (F. Lubis et al., 2014):

$$J_{regression} = \frac{1}{2m} \sum_{i=1}^{m} \left(h_\theta \left(x^{(i)} \right) - y^{(i)} \right)^2 \qquad (9)$$

To enhance the learning model performance, a regularization term can be appended to the cost function. The regularization can be enforced to regression algorithms or classification algorithms. The cost function with regularization for regression algorithm can be represented by (Shi, 2013):

$$J_{regression} = \frac{1}{2m} \sum_{i=1}^{m} \left(h_\theta \left(x^{(i)} \right) - y^{(i)} \right)^2 + \frac{\lambda}{2m} \sum_{j=1}^{n} \theta_j^2 \qquad (10)$$

where λ or lambda is the regularization parameter. It determines how much the costs of theta parameters θ are elevated. It must be notice that the selection of λ value is based on the self-intuition.

The cost function for classification learning uses the log function because of the sigmoid function. It can be built by (Zhao et al., 2010):

$$J_{classification} = -\frac{1}{m}\sum_{i=1}^{m}\left[y^{(i)}\log\left(h_{\theta}\left(x^{(i)}\right)\right) - \left(1 - y^{(i)}\right)\log\left(1 - h_{\theta}\left(x\right)\right)\right] \tag{11}$$

The regularization term can be added as done in regression in (10) (Zhao et al., 2010).

$$J_{classification} = -\frac{1}{m}\sum_{i=1}^{m}\left[y^{(i)}\log\left(h_{\theta}\left(x^{(i)}\right)\right) - \left(1 - y^{(i)}\right)\log\left(1 - h_{\theta}\left(x\right)\right)\right] + \frac{\lambda}{2m}\sum_{j=1}^{n}\theta_{j}^{2} \tag{12}$$

To achieve the lowest cost value, it must estimate the model parameters that realize the minimum loss for this model, beginning with initializing these model parameters by random values which can't obtain the minimum loss for the learning model. So, it must update these parameters to achieve the targeted minimum loss value. This updating is done using the gradient descent which iterates this process until we reach the minimum loss (Ruder, 2016). The parameters can be updated by (Ruder, 2016):

$$\theta_{j} = \theta_{j} - \alpha\frac{\partial J}{\partial\theta_{j}} \tag{13}$$

where α is the learning rate, J is the cost function value, and $\theta j \in \{\theta 0, \dots \theta n\}$. It must be notice that the selection of α value is based on the self-intuition where it is preferred to select a small value that must be less than 1 (Ruder, 2016). By using (9) the updated parameters for regression learning can be calculated by (Ruder, 2016):

$$\theta_{j} = \theta_{j} - \alpha\frac{\partial\left(\frac{1}{2m}\sum_{i=1}^{m}\left(h_{\theta}\left(x^{(i)}\right) - y^{(i)}\right)^{2}\right)}{\partial\theta_{j}} \tag{14}$$

$$\theta_j = \theta_j - \alpha \left[2\frac{1}{2} \sum_{i=1}^{m} \left(h_\theta \left(x^{(i)} \right) - y^{(i)} \right) \right] \frac{\partial \left(\sum_{i=1}^{m} \left(h_\theta \left(x^{(i)} \right) - y^{(i)} \right) \right)}{\partial \theta_j} \tag{15}$$

$$\theta_j = \theta_j - \alpha \sum_{i=1}^{m} \left(\left(h_\theta \left(x^{(i)} \right) - y^{(i)} \right) x_j^{(i)} \right) \tag{16}$$

where $j = \{0, \ldots, n\}$ and $x_0 = 1$.

The parameters for classification learning can be updated by (F. Lubis et al., 2014; Ruder, 2016):

$$\theta_j = \theta_j - \frac{\alpha}{m} \frac{\partial \left(\sum_{i=1}^{m} \left[y^{(i)} \log \left(h_\theta \left(x^{(i)} \right) \right) - \left(1 - y^{(i)} \right) \log \left(1 - h_\theta \left(x \right) \right) \right] \right)}{\partial \theta_j} \tag{17}$$

$$\theta_j = \theta_j - \frac{\alpha}{m} \sum_{i=1}^{m} \left(\left(h_\theta \left(x^{(i)} \right) - y^{(i)} \right) x_j^{(i)} \right) \tag{18}$$

For training a supervised learning model even if this model is regression or classification, there are many steps to finalize the training process (Verdhan, 2020; Gutenbrunner et al., 1993; Shanthamallu et al., 2017; F. Lubis et al., 2014; Shi, 2013; Zhao et al., 2010; Ruder, 2016).

1. Divide the dataset into training dataset which is 80% from dataset records and the test dataset which is 20% from dataset records.
2. Initialize the model parameters to any random values.
3. Calculate the hypothesis function using the model parameters and the training dataset input features.
4. Calculate the cost function even if using regularization or not.
5. Update the model parameters values using the gradient descent.
6. Repeat steps from 3 to 5 to achieve the possible lowest cost value.
7. Calculate the hypothesis function using the final model parameters values and the test dataset input features.
8. Compare the hypothesis outputs with the test dataset known correct results to assess the learning model performance.

THE SUPERVISED MACHINE LEARNING PROBLEMS

Through running a learning algorithm, it is possible that it can't do as hoped almost all the time, it will be because it has either a high bias problem or a high variance problem, in other words, either an under-fitting problem or an over-fitting problem. These two problems are considered the main problems that can occur in supervised machine learning algorithms. To deal with these problems in the learning model, it is necessary to divide the used dataset into training dataset which is 60% from dataset records, validation dataset which is 20% from dataset records, and test dataset which is 20% from dataset records. After solving the problem, the training dataset and the validation dataset, which are 80% from the dataset records, are together the training dataset, and then retrain the model with the suggested problem solution (Hawkins, 2004; Jabbar & Khan, 2015).

The Over-Fitting Problem

The over-fitting problem is that the learning model can fit 100% of training data well through prediction after the training process but can't predict the test data well. In this problem, the training set cost function value will be low and the validation set cost function value will be much greater than the training set cost function value. There are two main solutions for these problems; the first solution is reducing the training features, thus it must fine select the features to be removed that can't affect the required data to train. This selection can be done manually or by model selection algorithm. The second solution is increasing the training set data. It can be done by getting more training data or using data augmentation. The data augmentation is selecting some data and adding these selected data as new data after doing mathematical or spatial modification on it, it will be explained in section 2. The third solution is the regularization where it must add the regularization term in the cost function calculations through the training process (Hawkins, 2004).

The Under-Fitting Problem

The under-fitting problem is that the learning model fails to predict the training data well after the training process. In this problem, the training set and the validation set cost function values will be high. There are two main solutions for these problems; the first solution is increasing the training features. It can be done by selecting some features and adding these features as new features after mathematical modification such as square or any other mathematical function. The second solution is increasing the training iterations to reduce under-fitting where stopping training too soon can also result in an under-fit learning model. The third solution is the decrease of the regularization parameter λ value if this value is high (Jabbar & Khan, 2015).

DATA AUGMENTATION

One way of preventing the over-fitting problems is increasing the training data, but sometimes there is no data available for use in training or providing additional data has high cost. Thus, the data augmentation is the solution in this situation. So, data augmentation, which is commonly used in computer vision, is a technique for increasing the amount of data by adding significantly changed copies of either existing data or new synthetic data derived from existing data (Shorten & Khoshgoftaar, 2019). The most well-known sort of data augmentation is image data augmentation, which entails transforming images in the training dataset into altered copies that belong to the same class as the original image. Shifts, flips, zooms, color modification, random cropping, rotation, noise injection, and many other operations from the field of image editing are all included in transforms. Typically, image data augmentation is only applied to the training dataset, not the validation or test datasets. This differs from data preparation tasks like image resizing and pixel scaling, which must be carried out uniformly across all datasets that interact with the model (Shorten & Khoshgoftaar, 2019).

THE MOST USED MACHINE LEARNING ALGORITHMS

In previous sections, the both of supervised machine learning and unsupervised machine learning techniques are explained with the most common used algorithm for each type of machine learning types; k-means or clustering algorithm for unsupervised machine learning, linear regression for supervised regression machine learning and logistic regression for classifying supervised machine learning. In this section some most common supervised machine learning algorithms are explained with its mathematical model; these algorithms are the Naïve Bayes, the K-nearest neighbors, the DT, the SVM, and the ANNs which is considered the base of the deep learning techniques.

The Naïve Bayes Algorithm

The Naïve Bayes algorithm is a machine learning algorithm which acts as a classifier. This classifier is based on the concept of the Bayes theorem where the Bayes theorem is one of the fundamental probability theorems. The Bayes theorem can be represented with a simple mathematical formula as (19) (Taheri & Mammadov, 2013).

$$P\left(A|B\right) = \frac{P\left(B|A\right)P\left(A\right)}{P\left(B\right)} \tag{19}$$

where *P(A|B)* is the probability of event A occurring given that B is true, *P(B|A)* is the probability of event B occurring given that A is true, and *P(A)* and *P(B)* are the probabilities of observing A and B respectively without any given condition.

So, if we have a given dataset to build a learning model using Naïve Bayes algorithm with input X with input features $(x_1, x_2, x_3, \ldots, x_n)$ where $X=(x_1,x_2,x_3,\ldots,x_n)$ and output y, the mathematical model of the Naïve Bayes learning algorithm can be represented as (Taheri & Mammadov, 2013):

$$P\left(y|X\right) = \frac{P\left(X|y\right)P\left(y\right)}{P\left(X\right)} \tag{20}$$

Using the input features the Naïve Bayes learning algorithm can be represented mathematically, for n features, as (Taheri & Mammadov, 2013):

$$P\left(y|x_1,x_2,x_3,\cdots,x_n\right) = \frac{P\left(x_1|y\right)P\left(x_2|y\right)P\left(x_3|y\right)\ldots P\left(x_n|y\right)P\left(y\right)}{P\left(x_1\right)P\left(x_2\right)P\left(x_3\right)\ldots P\left(x_n\right)} \tag{21}$$

By looking at the dataset and substituting the values into the equation, you can get the values for each. The denominator does not change for any of the entries in the dataset; it remains constant. As a result, the denominator can be eliminated and proportionality can be injected as (Taheri & Mammadov, 2013):

$$P\left(y|x_1,x_2,x_3,\cdots,x_n\right) \propto P\left(y\right)\prod_{i=1}^{n}P\left(x_i|y\right) \tag{22}$$

The output class (the value of y variable) can be given with maximum probability as (Taheri & Mammadov, 2013):

$$y = argmax_y\, P\left(y\right)\prod_{i=1}^{n}P\left(x_i|y\right) \tag{23}$$

There are three main types of Naïve Bayes classifier; the Multinomial Naïve Bayes, the Bernoulli Naïve Bayes, and the Gaussian Naïve Bayes (Singh et al., 2019; T. Wang & W. Li, 2010).

The Multinomial Naïve Bayes classifier is usually used for document classifications. It is used for discrete counts (Singh et al., 2019).

The Bernoulli Naïve Bayes classifier is useful in binary classification. One of most used applications is text classifications using a 'bag of words' paradigm, in which the 1s and 0s represent "word appears in the document" and "word does not appear in the document," respectively (Singh et al., 2019).

The Gaussian Naïve Bayes classifier works by using a Gaussian distribution to distribute the continuous values associated with each feature. So, the features likelihood is considered to be Gaussian, and then the conditional probability can be calculated by (T. Wang & W. Li, 2010):

$$P(X) = \frac{1}{\sqrt{2\pi\sigma^2}} e^{-\frac{(x-\mu)^2}{2\sigma^2}} \qquad (24)$$

where μ is the mean value and σ is the standard deviation value of X features; it can be given by (T. Wang & W. Li, 2010):

$$\mu = \frac{1}{n}\sum_{i=1}^{n} x_i \qquad (25)$$

$$\sigma = \left[\frac{1}{n-1}\sum_{i=1}^{n}(x_i - \mu)^2 \right]^{0.5} \qquad (26)$$

The KNN Algorithm

The KNN algorithm is a supervised machine learning algorithm. It is a simple algorithm and it can act as a regression or classification machine learning. This algorithm is facile to understand and facile to execute but has a major stumbling block, which is the significantly slowdown with the growth of used data size. This algorithm applies a rule that things that are comparable are close together (S. Zhang et al., 2017; A. Lubis & M. Lubis, 2020). Figure 6 shows the KNN algorithm which indicates that the nearest and closest points are classified as a corresponding class (S.

Zhang et al., 2017). The KNN algorithm is based on the calculation of the distances among a query and all the data examples, the specified number examples K selection which is closest to the query, then polls for the averages the labels (in the case of regression) or the most frequent label (in the case of classification) (S. Zhang et al., 2017; A. Lubis & M. Lubis, 2020). The K value is determined by iterations and test but it can be depended on the neighbors where the K can has high value in case of more neighbors and can has small value in case of fewer neighbors. Be careful that in the case of K = N, where N is the number of classes, over-fitting problem can be occurred (S. Zhang et al., 2017).

Figure 6. The KNN Machine Learning Algorithm
(S. Zhang et al., 2017)

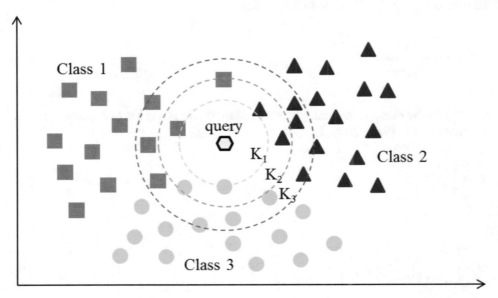

In mathematics, there are several distance calculation functions such as the Euclidean distance, the Manhattan distance, the Minkowski distance, the Jaccard distance, the Hamming distance… etc. The suitable function is elected according to the types of the used data. In this section, three of these functions are mentioned; the Euclidean distance, the Manhattan distance, and the Hamming distance. The most used function in the KNN machine learning algorithm is the Euclidean distance (A. Lubis & M. Lubis, 2020; Wu et al., 2002).

The Euclidean distance $D_e(x,y)$ is the calculation of the square root of the sum of the square differences between the coordinates (x,y) of n points as (A. Lubis & M. Lubis, 2020; Wu et al., 2002):

$$D_e\left(x,y\right)=\sqrt{\sum\nolimits_{i=1}^{n}\left(x_i-y_i\right)^2} \tag{27}$$

The Manhattan distance $D_m(x,y)$ is the calculation of the sum of the absolute values of the differences between the coordinates (x,y) of n points as (A. Lubis & M. Lubis, 2020):

$$D_m\left(x,y\right)=\sum\nolimits_{i=1}^{n}\left|x_i-y_i\right| \tag{28}$$

The Hamming distance $D_h(x,y)$ is the calculation of the distance between n given points is the maximum difference between their coordinates (x,y) on a dimension as (A. Lubis & M. Lubis, 2020; Wu et al., 2002):

$$D_h\left(x,y\right)=\sum\nolimits_{i=1}^{n}\left|x_i-y_i\right| \tag{29}$$

$$\text{With } D_h\left(x,y\right)=\begin{cases}0, & x=y\\ 1, & x\neq y\end{cases} \tag{30}$$

The DT Algorithm

The DT classifier is a supervised machine learning approach which can be utilized as a classifier. The DT is relied on building a tree structure with a root node and leaf nodes. The leaf nodes contain attribute test conditions to separate sample classes, and all of these nodes are assigned a class label yes or no. The data can be classified when the decision tree is constructed. Apply the test condition to the given data starting from the root node and follow the convenient flow based on the test results. Applying a new test condition can lead to another internal node or to a leaf node (Farid et al., 2014). The given data associated with the leaf node is assigned to the certain class when reaching the leaf node as shown in figure 7. This algorithm does not need training, and its computational efficiency is good but requires complex calculations. Accuracy depends on the tree design and the features selection (Farid et al., 2014).

Figure 7. The DT classifier
(Farid et al., 2014)

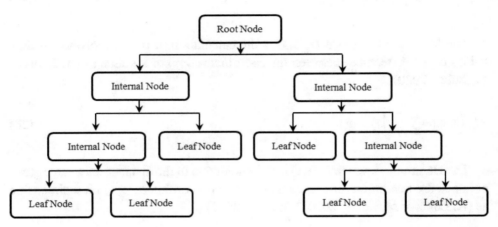

The SVM Algorithm

The SVM is a machine learning method that can be utilized in classification or regression prediction. When used as a supervised classifier, it provides an excellent separation of classes. The SVM classifier is based on small sample statistical theory that differentiates optimal hyper-planes from the training data. Decision planes determine decision boundaries, and these hyper-planes are formed by that decision planes (Guo & W. Wang, 2019; Chauhan et al., 2019; AlAfandy et al., 2020a). Those hyper-plans distinguish the various classes by constructing margins among classes. Maximizing those margins among classes, especially the closest classes, on both aspects of hyper-planes is the goal for reaching the most efficient SVM classifier. The SVM structure is difficult to understand. In the other words the SVM computational complexity is reduced. Figure 8 shows the SVM classifier (Chauhan et al., 2019). The SVM classifier cost function mathematical model can be achieved by deriving the classification cost function with regularization, which is represented in (12). The only way to do that by gets rid of these $\frac{1}{m}$ terms, it should give the same optimal value because $\frac{1}{m}$ is just a constant it gives (Chauhan et al., 2019; Vapnik, 2000; Koda et al., 2018):

$$J_{SVM} = -\sum_{i=1}^{m}\left[y^{(i)}\log\left(h_{\theta}\left(x^{(i)}\right)\right) - \left(1 - y^{(i)}\right)\log\left(1 - h_{\theta}\left(x\right)\right)\right] + \frac{\lambda}{2}\sum_{j=1}^{n}\theta_{j}^{2} \tag{31}$$

By multiplying the two terms (cost and regularization) of (22) by C where $C = \frac{1}{\lambda}$ and called the penalty parameter of the SVM classifier model, it gives (Chauhan et al., 2019; Vapnik, 2000; Koda et al., 2018):

$$J_{SVM} = -C\sum_{i=1}^{m}\left[y^{(i)}\log\left(h_{\theta}\left(x^{(i)}\right)\right) - \left(1 - y^{(i)}\right)\log\left(1 - h_{\theta}\left(x\right)\right)\right] + \frac{1}{2}\sum_{j=1}^{n}\theta_{j}^{2} \tag{32}$$

So the hypothesis function for the SVM classifier can be represented as (Chauhan et al., 2019; Vapnik, 2000; Koda et al., 2018):

$$h_{\theta}\left(x\right) = \begin{cases} 0, & \theta^{T}x \geq 0 \\ 1, & \theta^{T}x < 0 \end{cases} \tag{33}$$

Figure 8. The SVM classifier
(Chauhan et al., 2019)

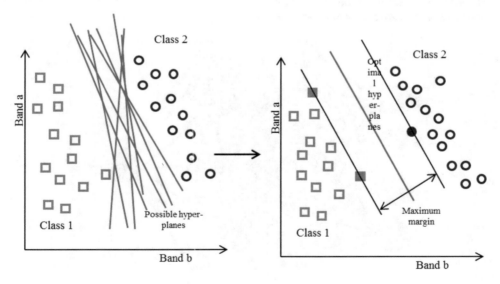

The ANNs

The ANNs algorithm is a machine learning approach which can act as a supervised or unsupervised machine learning algorithm; it can be utilized as a regression or classifier too. The use of the ANNs as a supervised classifier relies on the biological neural networks form. The definition of the ANNs approach is algorithms that attempt to imitate the human brain (Shanmuganathan, 2016; AlAfandy et al., 2019). The structure of the ANNs depends on the information that flows through this network. The ANNs are deemed as nonlinear applied mathematical information modeling tools whenever the complicated relationships between inputs and outputs are forged. The ANNs are formed of a sequence of layers; every layer contains a set of neurons. The input layer is the first layer wherever the output layer is the last layer; the internal layers are treated as the hidden layers. Neurons within the preceding and the succeeding layers are connected by weighted connections known as the weights (Srivastava et al., 2012). The accuracy and the performance of the ANNs are extremely looking at the network structure and the hyper-parameters values. The ANNs process rate is high however the network takes an enormous time for training and also needs a huge memory with advanced hardware; on the other hand there is some stiffness to set the network structure. Figure 9 shows the ANNs approach (Shanmuganathan, 2016; Srivastava et al., 2012).

Figure 9. The ANNs model classifier
(Shanmuganathan, 2016; Srivastava et al., 2012)

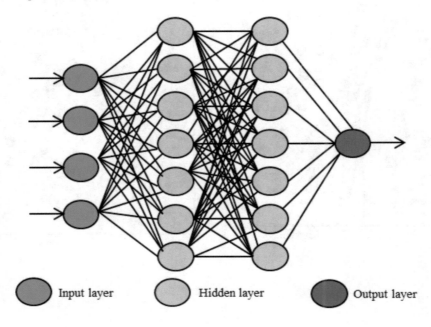

The ANNs structure with multilayers which each layer contains multiple nodes has input layer $X = A^{[0]}$, hidden layers from $A^{[1]}$ to $A^{[L-1]}$ to $\hat{y} = A^{[L]}$, and output layer $\hat{y} = A^{[L]}$ (Shanmuganathan, 2016; Srivastava et al., 2012; Bengio et al., 2017)

$$X = A^{[0]} = \begin{bmatrix} x_1 \\ x_2 \\ x_3 \\ \vdots \\ x_n \end{bmatrix} A^{[l]} = \begin{bmatrix} a_1^{[l]} \\ a_2^{[l]} \\ a_3^{[l]} \\ \vdots \\ a_{k^{[l]}}^{[l]} \end{bmatrix} and \ l = \left\{ 1,2,...,L \right\} \tag{34}$$

where L is the ANNs layers, n is the input features, and $k^{[l]}$ is the lth layer nodes.

Then, the lth layer output can be calculated as (Bengio et al., 2017):

$$A^{[l]} = \varnothing^{[l]} \left(Z^{[l]} \right) \tag{35}$$

$$Z^{[l]} = W^{[l]} A^{[l-1]} + b^{[l]} \tag{36}$$

$$b^{[l]} = \begin{bmatrix} b_1^{[l]} \\ b_2^{[l]} \\ b_3^{[l]} \\ \vdots \\ b_{k^{[l]}}^{[l]} \end{bmatrix}, \text{ and } W^{[l]} = \begin{bmatrix} w_{11}^{[l]} & \cdots & w_{1k^{[l-1]}}^{[l]} \\ \vdots & \ddots & \vdots \\ w_{k^{[l]}1}^{[l]} & \cdots & w_{k^{[l]}k^{[l-1]}}^{[l]} \end{bmatrix}, \text{ and } Z^{[l]} = \begin{bmatrix} z_1^{[l]} \\ z_2^{[l]} \\ z_3^{[l]} \\ \vdots \\ z_{k^{[l]}}^{[l]} \end{bmatrix}, \tag{37}$$

So, the right vectors dimensions are $W^{[l]} = \left(k^{[l]}, k^{[l-1]} \right)$, $b^{[l]} = (k^{[l]}, 1)$, $(k^{[l]}, 1)$, and $A^{[l]} = (k^{[l]}, 1)$. The $\varnothing^{[l]}$ is the activation function of the lth layer (Bengio et al., 2017). Then, the output of the ANN structure is calculated as (Bengio et al., 2017):

$$\hat{y} = A^{[L]} \tag{38}$$

THE OPEN SOURCE IMPLEMENTATIONS

Open source is an expression referred to open source software. Open source software is a code that is designed to be publicly accessible for free. So, anyone can see, modify, and distribute this code. In machine learning, a lot of researchers routinely open source their work on the Internet, such as on GitHub. On the other hand there are open source libraries for machine learning such as TF and Scikit-learn. These libraries are available and easy to deal with the widely used programming languages such as MATLAB and Python.

TF is an end-to-end open-source platform for creating machine learning and deep learning applications which is created by the Google Brain team. It's a symbolic math package that performs numerous tasks involving DNNs training and inference using dataflow and differentiable programming (Gad, 2018).

Scikit-learn was created as a Google summer of code project in 2007 by David Cournapeau. It's a Python-based machine learning package that includes supervised and unsupervised machine learning approaches. It is distributed under several Linux distributions and is licensed under a liberal simplified BSD license, allowing for academic and commercial use (Pedregosa et al., 2011).

THE PERFORMANCE ASSESSMENTS

There are several evaluation metrics for assessing the performance of the classification algorithms; some of them assess the performance of each class prediction and the others assess the predictive performance for the whole classifier.

This section illustrates the confusion matrix, precision, recall, and F1-score which are used to assess the performance of each class prediction, the OA and the kappa coefficient which are used to assess the predictive performance for the whole classifier (X. Deng et al., 2016; AlBeladi & Muqaibel, 2018; Banko, 1998; W. Li et al., 2017; C. Liu et al., 2007; Cohen, 1960).

The Confusion Matrix

The confusion matrix is a performance assessment for binary or multi-classes classifiers that rely on machine learning or deep learning (X. Deng et al., 2016). The confusion matrix is appeared as a table, each cell represents the number of times the model can correctly or wrongly predict the class. The TP, TN, FP, and FN may all be calculated using the confusion matrix (X. Deng et al., 2016). The TP denotes the number of predictions where the model correctly predicted a positive predetermined class, the TN denotes the number of predictions where the model correctly predicted a negative predetermined class, the FP denotes the number of predictions where the model incorrectly predicted a positive predetermined class, and the FN denotes the number of predictions where the model incorrectly predicted a negative predetermined class (X. Deng et al., 2016). Figure 10 shows the confusion matrix for binary classifiers which represent the TP, the TN, the FP, and the FN calculations (X. Deng et al., 2016).

Figure 10. The confusion matrix for binary classifiers
(X. Deng et al., 2016)

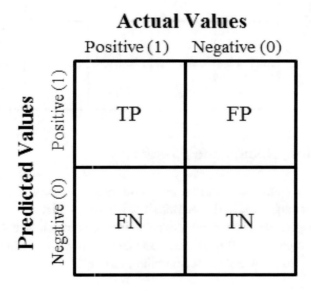

Figure 11 shows the confusion matrix for multi-classes classifiers.

Figure 11. The confusion matrix for multi-classes classifiers
(X. Deng et al., 2016)

		Predicted Values			
		C_1	C_2	...	C_n
Actual Values	C_1	N_{11}	N_{12}	...	N_{1n}
	C_2	N_{21}	N_{22}	...	N_{2n}
	⋮	⋮	⋮	⋮	⋮
	C_n	N_{n1}	N_{n2}	...	N_{nn}

The Precision, Recall, and F1-score

As a result of this confusion matrix, precision, recall, F1-score and the OA can be calculated (X. Deng et al., 2016; AlBeladi & Muqaibel, 2018).

Precision depicts the proportion of expected samples in a class that actually belong to that class compared to all predicted samples in that class; it can be expressed as (X. Deng et al., 2016; AlBeladi & Muqaibel, 2018):

$$Precision = \frac{TP}{TP + FP} \qquad (39)$$

Recall depicts the proportion of anticipated samples in a class that actually belong to that class to all actual samples in that class; it can be expressed as (X. Deng et al., 2016; AlBeladi & Muqaibel, 2018):

$$Recall = \frac{TP}{TP + FN} \qquad (40)$$

The F1-score is a single assessment that combines precision and recall; it is represented as (X. Deng et al., 2016; AlBeladi & Muqaibel, 2018):

$$F1-score = 2 \times \frac{Precision \times Recall}{Precision + Recall} = \frac{2 \times TP}{\left(2 \times TP\right) + FP + FN} \tag{41}$$

The OA

The OA basically informs us what percentage of the reference sites were correctly mapped out of all of them. The OA is usually reported as a percentage, with 100% accuracy indicating that all reference sites were properly categorized. OA is the simplest to compute and comprehend, but it only provides basic accuracy information to map users and producers. The OA is the major classification accuracy appreciation. The OA is calculated as (Banko, 1998; W. Li et al., 2017; AlAfandy et al., 2020b):

$$OA = \frac{\text{Number of correctly classified data}}{\text{Total number of checked data}} \tag{42}$$

The Kappa Coefficient

A statistical test is used to calculate the kappa coefficient, which is used to assess the correctness of a categorization. Kappa is a metric that measures how well a categorization worked as compared to assigning values at random. The Kappa Coefficient might be anything between -1 and 1. A classification with a value of 0 is no better than a random categorization. The categorization is much poorer than random if the number is negative. A value near to 1 suggests that the classification is superior to chance. The kappa coefficient (κ) is calculated as (C. Liu et al., 2007; Cohen, 1960):

$$\kappa = \frac{p_o - p_e}{1 - p_e} \tag{43}$$

where p_o is the relative observed agreement between raters (identical to accuracy), and p_e is the hypothetical probability of chance agreement. The calculations of p_o and p_e are based on predictions, p_o and p_e are calculated by (W. Liu et al., 2007; Cohen, 1960):

$$p_o = \frac{TP + TN}{TP + FP + FN + TN} \tag{44}$$

$$\mathrm{p_e} = \mathrm{p_{yes}} + \mathrm{p_{no}} \tag{45}$$

$$p_{yes} = \frac{TP + FP}{TP + FP + FN + TN} \times \frac{TP + FN}{TP + FP + FN + TN} \tag{46}$$

$$p_{no} = \frac{FN + TN}{TP + FP + FN + TN} \times \frac{FP + TN}{TP + FP + FN + TN} \tag{47}$$

REFERENCES

AlAfandy, K. A., Omara, H., Lazaar, M., & Al Achhab, M. (Eds.). (2019). Artificial Neural Networks Optimization and Convolution Neural Networks to Classifying Images in Remote Sensing: A Review. *Proceeding of The 4th International Conference on Big Data and Internet of Things (BDIoT'19)*. 10.1145/3372938.3372945

AlAfandy, K. A., Omara, H., Lazaar, M., & Al Achhab, M. (2020a). Investment of Classic Deep CNNs and SVM for Classifying Remote Sensing Images. *Advances in Science Technology and Engineering Systems Journal*, *5*(5), 652–659. doi:10.25046/aj050580

AlAfandy, K. A., Omara, H., Lazaar, M., & Al Achhab, M. (2020b). Using Classic Networks for Classifying Remote Sensing Images: Comparative Study. *Advances in Science Technology and Engineering Systems Journal*, *5*(5), 770–780. doi:10.25046/aj050594

AlBeladi, A. A., & Muqaibel, A. H. (2018). Evaluating Compressive Sensing Algorithms in Through-the-wall Radar via F1-score. *International Journal of Signal and Imaging Systems Engineering*, *11*(3), 164–171. doi:10.1504/IJSISE.2018.093268

Alloghani, M., Al-Jumeily, D., Mustafina, J., Hussain, A., & Aljaaf, A. J. (2020). A Systematic Review on Supervised and Unsupervised Machine Learning Algorithms for Data Science. In M. Berry, A. Mohamed, & B. Yap (Eds.), *Supervised and Unsupervised Learning for Data Science. Unsupervised and Semi-Supervised Learning*. Springer. doi:10.1007/978-3-030-22475-2_1

Alpaydin, E. (2020). *Introduction to Machine Learning*. MIT Press.

Banko, G. (1998). *A Review of Assessing the Accuracy of Classifications of Remotely Sensed Data and of Methods Including Remote Sensing Data in Forest Inventory. International Institution for Applied Systems Analysis (IIASA)*.

Bengio, Y., Goodfellow, I., & Courville, A. (2017). *Deep Learning*. MIT press.

Bowling, M., Furnkranz, J., Graepel, T., & Musick, R. (2006). Machine Learning and Games. *Machine Learning, Springer, 63*(3), 211–215. doi:10.100710994-006-8919-x

Chauhan, V. K., Dahiya, K., & Sharma, A. (2019). Problem Formulations and Solvers in Linear SVM: A Review. *Artificial Intelligence Review, Springer, 52*(2), 803–855. doi:10.100710462-018-9614-6

Cohen, J. (1960). A Coefficient of Agreement for Normal Scales. *Educational and Psychological Measurement, 20*(1), 37–46. doi:10.1177/001316446002000104

J. Deng, W. Dong, R. Socher, L. Li, K. Li, & L. Fei-Fei (Eds.). (2009). ImageNet: A Large-Scale Hierarchical Image Database. In *Proceeding of the 2009 IEEE Conference on Computer Vision and Pattern Recognition*. IEEE. 10.1109/CVPR.2009.5206848

Deng, X., Liu, Q., Deng, Y., & Mahadevan, S. (2016). An Improved Method to Construct Basic Probability Assignment Based on the Confusion Matrix for Classification Problem. *Information Sciences, Elsevier, 340-341*, 250–261. doi:10.1016/j.ins.2016.01.033

ElNaqa, I., & Murphy, M. J. (2015). What is Machine Learning? In I. Issam ElNaqa & M. J. Murphy (Eds.), *Machine Learning in Radiation Oncology* (pp. 3–11). Springer. doi:10.1007/978-3-319-18305-3_1

Farid, D. M., Zhang, L., Rahman, C. M., Hossain, M. A., & Strachan, R. (2014). Hybrid Decision Tree and Naive Bayes Classifiers for Multi-class Classification Tasks. *Expert Systems with Applications, Elsevier, 41*(4), 1937–1946. doi:10.1016/j.eswa.2013.08.089

Fukushima, K., Miyake, S., & Ito, T. (1983). Neocognitron: A Neural Network Model for a Mechanism of Visual Pattern Recognition. *IEEE Transactions on Systems, Man, and Cybernetics, SMC-13*(5), 826–834. doi:10.1109/TSMC.1983.6313076

Gad, A. F. (2018). Practical Computer Vision Applications Using Deep Learning with CNNs. Apress. doi:10.1007/978-1-4842-4167-7

Guo, H., & Wang, W. (2019). Granular Support Vector Machine: A Review. *Artificial Intelligence Review, Springer*, *51*(1), 19–32. doi:10.100710462-017-9555-5

Gutenbrunner, C., Jureckova, J., Koenker, R., & Portnoy, S. (1993). Tests of Linear Hypotheses Based on Regression Rank Score. *Journal of Nonparametric Statistics*, *2*(4), 307–331. doi:10.1080/10485259308832561

Hawkins, D. M. (2004). The Problem of Overfitting. *Journal of Chemical Information and Computer Sciences, ACM*, *44*(1), 1–12. doi:10.1021/ci0342472 PMID:14741005

Ivakhnenko, A. G., & Lapa, V. G. (1966). Cybernetic Predicting Devices. Technical Report, DTIC Document, Purdue University.

Jabbar, H. K., & Khan, R. Z. (2015). Methods to Avoid Over-fitting and Under-fitting in Supervised Machine Learning (Comparative Study). *Computer Science, Communication and Instrumentation Devices*, *2015*, 163–172. doi:10.3850/978-981-09-5247-1_017

Khanum, M., Mahboob, T., Imtiaz, W., Abdul Ghafoor, H., & Sehar, R. (2015). A Survey on Unsupervised Machine Learning Algorithms for Automation, Classification and Maintenance. *International Journal of Computers and Applications*, *119*(13), 34–39. doi:10.5120/21131-4058

Koda, S., Zeggada, A., Melgani, F., & Nishii, R. (2018). Spatial and Structured SVM for Multilabel Image Classification. *IEEE Transactions on Geoscience and Remote Sensing*, *56*(10), 5948–5960. doi:10.1109/TGRS.2018.2828862

Li, W., Fu, H., Yu, L., & Cracknell, A. (2017). Deep Learning Based Oil Palm Tree Detection and Counting for High-Resolution Remote Sensing Images. *Remote Sensing*, *9*(1), 22–34. doi:10.3390/rs9010022

Liu, C., Frazier, P., & Kumar, L. (2007). Comparative Assessment of the Measures of Thematic Classification Accuracy. *Remote Sensing of Environment, Elsevier*, *107*(4), 606–616. doi:10.1016/j.rse.2006.10.010

Lubis, A. R., Lubis, M., & Khowarizmi, A. (2020). Optimization of Distance Formula in K-Nearest Neighbor Method. *Bulletin of Electrical Engineering and Informatics*, *9*(1), 326–338. doi:10.11591/eei.v9i1.1464

F. F. Lubis, Y. Rosmansyah, & S. H. Supangkat (Eds.). (2014). Gradient Descent and Normal Equations on Cost Function Minimization for Online Predictive Using Linear Regression with Multiple Variables. In *Proceeding of the 2014 International Conference on ICT For Smart Society (ICISS)*. IEEE. 10.1109/ICTSS.2014.7013173

Mcculloch, W. S., & Pitts, W. (1990). A Logical Calculus of the Ideas Immanent in Nervous Activity. *Bulletin of Mathematical Biology, Springer*, *52*(1-2), 99–115. doi:10.1016/S0092-8240(05)80006-0 PMID:2185863

Mitchell, T. M. (2006). *The Discipline of Machine Learning*. Carnegie Mellon University, School of Computer Science, Machine Learning Department.

Pedregosa, F., Varoquaux, G., Gramfort, A., Michel, V., Thirion, B., Grisel, O., Blondel, M., Prettenhofer, P., Weiss, R., Dubourg, V., Vanderplas, J., Passos, A., Cournapeau, D., Brucher, M., Perrot, M., & Duchesnay, É. (2011). Scikit-learn: Machine Learning in Python. *Journal of Machine Learning Research*, *12*, 2825–2830.

Ruder, S. (2016). *An Overview of Gradient Descent Optimization Algorithms*. arXiv preprint arXiv:1609.04747.

Sen, P. C., Hajra, M., & Ghosh, M. (2020). Supervised Classification Algorithms in Machine Learning: A Survey and Review. In J. Mandal & D. Bhattacharya (Eds.), *Emerging Technology in Modelling and Graphics. Advances in Intelligent Systems and Computing* (Vol. 937). Springer. doi:10.1007/978-981-13-7403-6_11

Shanmuganathan, S. (2016). Artificial Neural Network Modelling: An Introduction. In Series in Artificial Neural Network Modelling (pp. 1-14). Springer. doi:10.1007/978-3-319-28495-8_1

U. S. Shanthamallu, A. Spanias, C. Tepedelenlioglu, & M. Stanley (Eds.). (2017). A Brief Survey of Machine Learning Methods and Their Sensor and IoT Applications. In *Proceeding of the 8th International Conference on Information, Intelligence, Systems & Applications (IISA)*. IEEE. 10.1109/IISA.2017.8316459

Shi, L. (2013). Learning theory estimates for coefficient-based regularized regression. *Applied and Computational Harmonic Analysis, Elsevier*, *34*(2), 252–265. doi:10.1016/j.acha.2012.05.001

Shinde, P. P., & Shah, S., Dr. (Eds.) (2018). A Review of Machine Learning and Deep Learning Applications. In *Proceeding of the 2018 Fourth International Conference on Computing Communication Control and Automation (ICCUBEA)*. IEEE. 10.1109/ICCUBEA.2018.8697857

Shorten, C., & Khoshgoftaar, T. M. (2019). A Survey on Image Data Augmentation for Deep Learning. *Journal of Big Data*, 6(1), 1–48. doi:10.118640537-019-0197-0

G. Singh, B. Kumar, L. Gaur, & A. Tyagi (Eds.). (2019). Comparison between multinomial and Bernoulli naïve Bayes for text classification. In *Proceeding of the 2019 International Conference on Automation, Computational and Technology Management (ICACTM)*. IEEE. 10.1109/ICACTM.2019.8776800

Smola, A., & Vishwanathan, S. V. N. (2008). *Introduction to Machine Learning*. Cambridge University.

Srivastava, P. K., Han, D., Rico-Ramirez, M. A., Bray, M., & Islam, T. (2012). Selection of Classification Techniques for Land Use / Land Cover Change Investigation. *Advances in Space Research, 50*(9), 1250–1265. doi:10.1016/j.asr.2012.06.032

Taheri, S., & Mammadov, M. (2013). Learning the Naïve Bayes Classifier With Optimization Models. *International Journal of Applied Mathematics and Computer Science*, 23(4), 787–795. doi:10.2478/amcs-2013-0059

Vapnik, V. N. (2000). *The Nature of Statistical Learning Theory*. Springer Science. doi:10.1007/978-1-4757-3264-1

Verdhan, V. (2020). Supervised Learning with Python. Apress. doi:10.1007/978-1-4842-6156-9

T. Wang, & W. H. Li (Eds.). (2010). Naïve Bayes Software Defect Prediction Model. In *Proceeding of 2010 International Conference on Computational Intelligence and Software Engineering*. IEEE. 10.1109/CISE.2010.5677057

Wu, Y., Ianakiev, K., & Govindaraju, V. (2002). Improved K-Nearest Neighbor Classification. *Pattern Recognition, Elsevier*, 35(10), 2311–2318. doi:10.1016/S0031-3203(01)00132-7

Zhang, S., Li, X., Zong, M., Zhu, X., & Cheng, D. (2017). Learning K for KNN Classification. *ACM Transactions on Intelligent Systems and Technology*, 8(3), 1–19. doi:10.1145/2990508

L. Zhao, M. Mammadov, & J. Yearwood (Eds.). (2010). From Convex to Nonconvex: A Loss Function Analysis for Binary Classification. In *Proceeding of the 2010 IEEE International Conference on Data Mining Workshops*. IEEE. 10.1109/ICDMW.2010.57

APPENDIX

Table 1.

ANNs	Artificial Neural Networks
BSD	Berkeley Software Distribution
DNNs	Deep Neural Networks
DT	Decision Tree
FN	False Negative
FP	False Positive
GMDH	Group Method of Data Handling
KNN	k-nearest neighbors
NNs	Neural Networks
OA	Overall Accuracy
SVM	Support Vector Machine
TF	Tensorflow
TN	True Negative
TP	True Positive

Section 2

From Artificial Intelligence to Good Healthcare: Review, Methods, and Healthcare

Chapter 6
Integration of ML and IoT for Healthcare Systems

Shruti Sharma

iD https://orcid.org/0000-0003-0056-8811
Ajou University, Suwon, South Korea

Gulab Singh Verma
Pt. Ravishankar Shukla University, Raipur, India

Kavita Thakur
Pt. Ravishankar Shukla University, Raipur, India

ABSTRACT

The internet of things (IoT) and machine learning (ML) are massive technologies that provide enhancement and better resolutions in our daily life, such as in industry, healthcare, space sector, defense, buildings, agriculture, traffic, and so on. The area of IoT has shown a boost over the past decades with the continuous development of the ML tools. The combination of IoT with ML tools has a high impact on medical devices. The application of ML and IoT can provide significant improvements in all parts of healthcare domain from diagnostics to treatment. It is generally believed that ML tools will simplify and boost human work. In this chapter, the authors present the overview of current advance integration IoT and ML application on healthcare care management listed with all benefits and uses. This chapter also supports healthcare professionals to detect and treat disease more efficiently and researchers for their understanding of growth in ML and IoT-based technology.

DOI: 10.4018/978-1-7998-9831-3.ch006

INTRODUCTION

Machine learning (ML) methods in healthcare use the increasing volume of health data carried by the Internet of Things (IOTs) for the improvement of patient outcomes. These methods provide auspicious applications as well as major challenges. More recently, IOTs and ML have joined to make several of things. IoT was firstly recommended to use radio frequency identification (RFID) systems to incorporate known objects and their electronic images into web architectures (Birje & Hanji, 2020; Lashkari et al., 2018; Liu et al., 2018). Ultimately, the IoT came in the form of sensors, GPS application, and mobile for health care domain (Dehkordi et al.,

Figure 1. Application of ML in hospitals (Bote-Curiel et al., 2019)

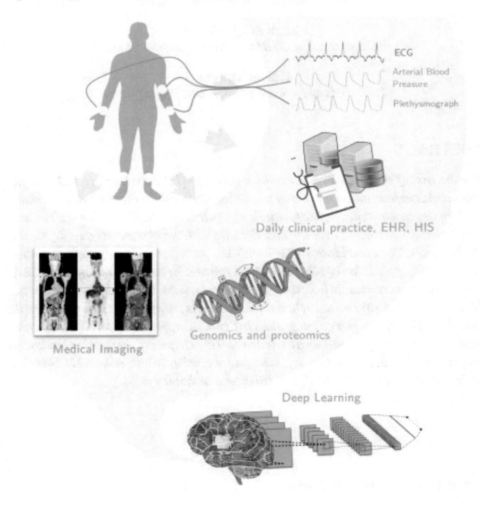

2020; Qi et al., 2017; Rodríguez-Mazahua et al., 2016). The endless integration in the global world and the supporting devices of these sensors has led to a number of discovery problems, from basic knowledge to processing and execution. In a transmission of wireless information, various appliances have been implemented. Regardless the ML-IoT in healthcare, there are challenge in about data security (Lee et al., 2018; Shahbazi & Byun, 2020). Accordingly, various studies have measured the integration of IoT -ML for checking patients with various medical disorders as a measure of data security. Today, IoT innovation has made rapid strides in multidisciplinary research (Kononenko, 2001; Yadav & Jadhav, 2019) in a myriad of scientific and mechanical controls, especially in medical services (Yadav & Jadhav, 2019). Multiobjective optimsation based research are an vital and effective methods for managing a health care problems. The article by (Fathollahi-Fard et al., 2021; Sharma & Yoon, 2018; Sharma & Yoon, 2019; Sharma & Yoon, 2021), in which used queuing theory based on multiobjective optimsation to examine waiting times and reservations in hospital outpatient departments.

Therefore, the combination of IoT technology and ML in healthcare development is now being shifted from the hospital to the home, as well as for routine medical testing for doctors and patients using medical devices. Thus by applying this technology we maintain the care for patients easier, especially in times of crisis. Furthermore, hospitals can ease the burden by moving some activities to the home environment (Otoom et al., 2015). Cost saving is one of the main benefits, patients can avoid hospital costs when they visit the doctor. Other limitations include the limitations of the existing network infrastructure incapable of handling sensitive applications in real time using IoT, so software-defined networks require a network infrastructure suitable for such applications (Aghdam et al., 2020; Evtodieva et al., 2020) Pharmacy containers can be used to increase the usability of the device through Android programs. IoT will improve people's lives. Aziz and Islam, 2020 Atiqur et al implemented an integrated device that will lead to many positive developments in administration services, arrangements and communications. There are areas that need to be addressed (Atiqur et al., 2020; Aziz & Islam, 2020; Ghose et al., 2014).

Different ways ML and IoT that change management in hospitals. Fig 1 show different application of ML in different field. Hospitals have vast amounts of data. Patient monitors record information such as heart beat rate, blood pressure, while doctors and specialists produce visual data in the form of MRI and CT scans report (Al-Fuqaha et al., 2015; Cook, 2006). All of this data can be hugely appreciated — but only if system of government access it at the exact time and have the tools to analyze it in a crisis.

Enhancement of Diagnostic Accuracy

Some common diseases, like breast and lung cancer, can be tough to analyze. Thus, doctors must identify tumors using images from a computed tomography scanner (CTS). Despite being the most effective means of diagnosis available, false positives and negatives are still common. Combination of ML and IoT can make this information convenient to doctors. As a result, they're transforming how hospitals run where adopted. Figure 2 shows architecture of ML and IOT where few different security threats are handled in daily operations in healthcare.

ML improves the quality of these scans as well as reads the scans themselves. In a few different studies, these ML algorithms have been more effective than radiologists at correctly identifying the signs of cancer in a CT scan.

Remote Patient Monitoring

Remote patient observing systems take to benefit of IoT sensors give update and provide information doctors and nurses on patient vitals. With the help of these sensors, it's conceivable to check a health of patient from anyplace aware staff and doctors to important health measures.

These IoT-ML healthcare diminish the worker to keep update of a patient's health while they're in the observation (Huang, 2011; Kan, 2019; Kohler et al., 2019; Lakshmi et al., 2016; Maskut et al., 2020). With an automated monitoring system, these vitals are automatically recorded and logged, freeing up staff for more critical work.

Reducing Need for Follow-Up Visits

Other applications of IoT and ML technology can monitor patients' health once they leave the hospital, reducing the need for follow-up visits. For example, healthcare providers use IoT devices to track the blood pressure of women with pregnancy-related hypertension. Generally, this would require follow-up visits, even though those with the issue notice it often goes away after birth.

Reducing Wait Times

ML and IoT technology also lessens wait times in hospitals. Automatic bed-tracking methods inform hospital workers when a bed is available, to admit emergency patients as rapidly as possible.

Figure 2. Smart security architecture of ML and IOT in healthcare (Michael et al., 2001)

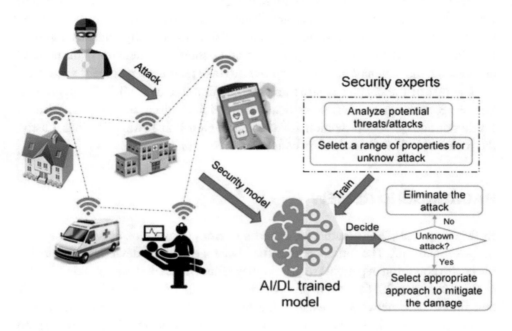

Isolating Critical Patients

When hospitals are stressed and reaching their capacity, identifying patients who need immediate attention becomes critical in providing the best possible care. This process isn't easy. Doctors and nurses must analyze vast amounts of patient information and make snap decisions, all while under significant pressure. Fortunately, AI and IoT systems provide a helping hand in situations like these. Hospitals are using new AI-powered virtual assistants to save their sickest patients (Boubiche et al., 2018; Ghate & Vijayakumar, 2018; Lee & Lee, 2015). These systems alert doctors when a patient's condition begins to deteriorate and provides them with an analysis of their vitals and conditions. In some cases, these AI hospital systems were able to catch problems that doctors missed.

Tracking Medical Tools

Lost medical equipment can be a significant expense for hospitals. Usually it's common for hospitals to lose 5-6 wound therapy pumps operated in negative pressure wound therapy every year. Cost of these pumps can be $20,000 to $30,000 each. With the accurate tracking systems and, organizations can greatly ease the risk of losing equipment, lowering costs and also confirming that pumps are available. Now mobile pump devices are invented with RFID and GPS so that people can track them while in the hospital and beyond if one is sent home with a patient (Cui et al., 2018; Ge et al., 2018). The RFID scanning system also automatically requests approval from insurance when a pump gets pulled off of the shelf for patient use. This process ensures that the patient will be pre-approved to take their device home if necessary.

The rest of the chapter is structured as: Section 2 shows ML-IoT integration. Section 3 presents the ML classification. Section 4 discusses the ML Disease Prediction and Detection. Section 5 discusses ML algorithm and applications. Lastly, the paper with further research is concludes in Section 6.

BACKGROUND REVIEW

In (Maskut et al., 2020) author designed a sensor comprise of different uses and purpose of utilities. The authors studied the advantages of these devices in monitoring the health condition of patients such as kidney failure, heart disease and skin disease. In (Fizi & Askar, 2016) authors proposed a sensor that relies on a wireless network and fuzzy logic network. Precisely, the researchers developed a microchip and integrated with wireless sensor to make a body sensor network that frequently checked the abnormal changes in body of patients. Particularly, the researchers studied by device like microcontroller, pulse, and temperature sensor to monitor a clinical data record (Keti & Askar, 2015; Miotto et al., 2018). Moreover, the proposed system was combined with various piece of equipment to detect the illness of patients as well as send the patient's data information to the doctor's via internet or phone. Notably, the organization can send messages to both the relative of the patient and hospital staff in emergency (Abdollahzadeh & Navimipour, 2016). Hence, the patients can obtain an instruction from medical staff via this scheme (Dang et al., 2019; Dhillon et al., 2019; Piccialli & Jung, 2017; Yuvaraj & SriPreethaa, 2017).

The predicted data is related to the quantity of massive data trained (Yuvaraj & SriPreethaa, 2017). Therefore, massive data improve the estimation techniques of ML utilized in healthcare domain. Fortunately, this method of prediction are based on ML algorithm for information sharing of patient among various hospitals. In a hospital and clinics, the historic information are taken and used to forecast and for research. ML methods with implanted IOT devices are used to detect specific health condition such as falls among old adult. The ML algorithms can successfully classify all activities among patients and warn to healthcare providers. In the same way, the daily patient daily activity is observed through device with IoT microchips. The data information is employed for noticing anomalies among the adults. They have examined their work based on different constraints and by their study compares existing literature, shortcomings, and highlights possible gaps to select procedures for enhancing model.

In 2020 authors (Shahbazi & Byun, 2021), proposed a algorithm based on a Long Short-Term Memory (LTSM) to identify COVID-19 spontaneously from X-ray images. Hence CNN methods is used in this agenda and LSTM is used for finding the same. In (Zabirul Islam et al., 2020), authors suggested an effective CNN based on AlexNet model for classifying COVID 19. In this model X-Ray image and CT image are used to identify the COVID-19. Moreover, the images (X-ray and CT) are achieved by different sources. Their accuracy are equal to 97-98% via training network and 94.5% precision by updated other CNN.

OVERVIEW OF ML- IOT IN THE HEALTHCARE

Machine learning (ML) is likewise it is regarded as one of our modern generation of revolution. The use of algorithms that can examine from the fact is machine learning. Machine learning in simplified terms is generally derived from outcomes. Grasp gaining knowledge of pursuits to acknowledge styles from the information and to use found out styles for beneficial inferences. Machine learning can be a comprehensive approach to many areas focusing on mathematics, algebra, data collection, mathematical testing, etc. The ML is a strategically important tool for extracting information on record training. (Banerjee & Das, 2020; Halgurd et al., 2020; Komal Kumar, 2020; Oyewo, 2020).

These days, machine studying applications are broadly applied in healthcare provider programs. Such system mastering algorithms are also implemented in lots of medical choice aid structures to set up superior learning fashions to improve the human health. Support vector machines (SVM) are example of the mixing of ML-IOT in healthcare domain. Traditional centralized learning is shown in Fig 3.

Pharmaceutical machine learning may be achieved in a couple of approaches such as

- Disease figuring out and analyzing
- Customized alternate of remedy/behavior
- Drug discovery/manufacture
- Clinical test result
- Treatment with radiology machine and radiation
- Electronic reports of patient health
- Epidemic outbreak forecast.

Figure 3. Traditional ML in the centralized form, collecting data from various domains

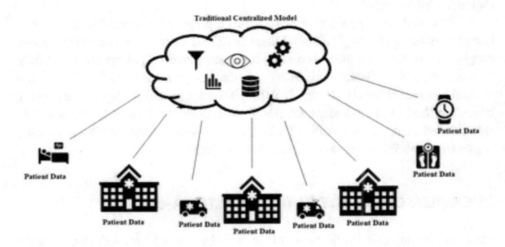

Data in ML

Figure 4 genuinely suggests that information have to be gathered from several sources for examine and using IOT-ML machinery. These data information represent a system unit. This system unit is being tested to create training data sets. Data point may show patient health information regarding a sample of cancerous tissue or something else. Details with the label are available an outstanding feature assigned to them, which can also be referenced such as output or response (Emu, 2020).

While most application can use both data, labeled and non-labeled, generally, labeled data are monitored in the supervised learning. On the contrary, no label data are observed under unsupervised learning, whereas both labeled data and no label data can be used in semi supervised learning.

Supervised Learning

The main ML method is a supervised learning. Used for real-world applications. The distinguishing characteristics of a supervised learning (SL) model is the individual's participation in it. Personal participation is important at first building a database, later works alone by adding and learning from the input examples. For the database construction, both inputs and optional outputs are given to machine learning model. This model then finds a way to work independently to produce results. The problem arises when a model has to predict the outcome of a new installation independently without human assistance. Therefore, make sure the accuracy of the suggested model is important.

122

Figure 4. Types of ML

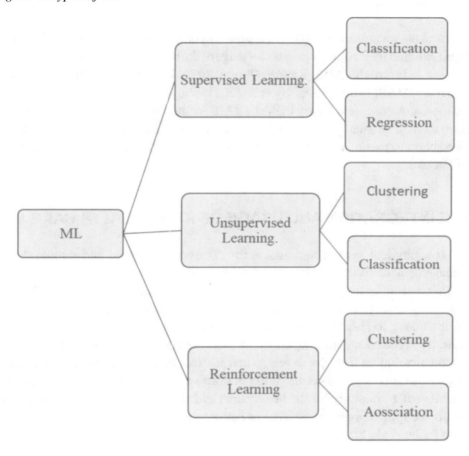

Unsupervised Learning

One of the purposes of ML is to identify unknown structures inside the unmarked data. Many successful programs have used these applications which are tough to study. owing to a lack of the use of unsupervised ML training knowledge (Dayanand & Neethi, 2020). Consequently, there is a lack of reward indicators for analyzing future solutions. Here, the reward value aids as a unique feature of the established and unattended. Unsupervised Learning includes database conversion and integration. In the process of change, data in the database is changed to present it in a different, new way so that it is easier to understand in humans and in machine algorithms. Collections of algorithms, on the other hand, divide data sets into important groups of related objects.

Reinforcement Learning

Researchers examines that RL is capable to computing ideal values by previous result, without requiring any prior knowledge of the biological systems (Basha, 2019; Cinaree & Emiroglu, 2019; Kaur & Oberoi, 2020; Moher et al., 2009; Olaković & Hadžialić, 2018; Paun, 1999; Roy et al., 2021; Vidya & Karki, 2020). RL methods are more progressive and easy than other ML method apply in health-care domains since it could be usually tough to build a correct application for the patient body and take action to treatments, owing to changing various interface between treatments and bodies.

THE INTEGRATION AND USAGE OF IOT IN HEALTH CARE

IoT is a physical system that allows for discovery, analysis, and remote device management. Computer design has been improved to connect to the edge computers so that portable sensors and smart devices can communicate well. Because processing data, Smart devices rely heavily on IoT's middleware layer. Any use of IoT includes good health, smart grid, smart cities, smart house, smart farming, wise movement, and so on. Three layers of IoT basic configurations include visualization, communication, and device layers. Then it expands to cover the most advanced construction and business crust. Without others portable and artificial devices that use ML-IoT technology for the healthcare field and personalization. Two types of healthcare application are shown below that demonstrate the essentials facts between them (Sahu et al., 2020).

Devices that we can Wear

Materials such as metal bracelets/smart watches, pendants, pins, shirts, smart bracelets, shoes, fitness material, and further health equipment i.e. moveable systems that may be installed the structure of the human body. A wearable device for direct communication can track illness, human health, and information found from a research institute. The machineries include wearable skills, such as sensors, computers, and screens. It is devices can produce natural information like, mobility, heart rate, blood stress, exercise time, etc. These machines have a significant impact and are very powerful that the physical health of the customer gets the best.

Devices can be Installed

Implant devices are implanted below the skin of the human and goal to repair the whole or part of the organic machine and its shape. Implants are certainly widely used for many programs, inclusive of neurons, radiology, coronary heart assault stent, microchips, etc., supporting a comfortable network for such services is critical. Any organic compounds, which include various metals like carbonates, silicon, titanium, etc. may be made from the inside of implantable devices. The content material can also be decided on in keeping with the human body section requirements and equipment for the implant tool. The various previous works done in the past is shown in Table 1.

Table 1. The previous work achieved by the researchers

Disease	Algorithm	Accuracy	Outcome	Ref./ year
Skin cancer	SVM and KNN	Precision SVM=97.8% and KNN= 86.25	SVM classifier betters with 97.7% correctness and 0.941 for textural features	52/2020
Thyroid disease	Naïve Bayes, KNN, and SVM algorithm	Accuracy:82% by SVM 83% by Naïve Bayes and 85% by KNN	The cure for thyroid patients is enhanced.	51/2020
Liver fibrosis	Random forests, MLP, logistic regression algorithm	Accuracy 97.228% by random forest, 98% by MLP, 97%by Logistic regression=	Good accuracy rate	50/2020
Cardio Vascular.	KNN, Logistic Regression, Decision Tree SVM	Precision Random forest=85.65%, decision tree =74.18%, Logistic Regression=74.2%, SVM=77.144 and KNN=68.58%	The random forest is beat by all the classifiers under the examination of classifying CVD patients.	19/2020
Lung cancer	SVM, Random Forest, ANN algorithms	Accuracy:70% by Random Forest 80.2% by SVM and ANN=96.1%.	Easy distinction between benign & malignant tumors with high accuracy.	18/2020
Brain Tumor	SVM, KNN, RF, algorithm	Accuracy KNN= 87%, SVM=90%, LDA=83% and RF=83%	Better and accurate to the other algorithm	53/2019
Prostate cancer	SVM, Decision Tree (DT), and MLP algorithm	Correctness of model 99.06%.	Effective in identifying both nonprostate and prostate cases	40/2020

Continued on following page

Table 1. Continued

Disease	Algorithm	Accuracy	Outcome	Ref./ year
Breast lesions	CNN algorithm	Accuracy CNN=90%	This motivates us to propose a novel hybrid approach by combining a convolution neural network (CNN) with connected component analysis (CCA) to segment malignant breast lesions without any pre-processing to avoid any distortion in image sharpness at the initial stages This motivates us to propose a novel hybrid approach by combining a convolution neural network (CNN) with connected component analysis (CCA) to segment malignant breast lesions without any pre-processing to avoid any distortion in image sharpness at the initial stages CNN component analysis show superior performance	60/2021
Lung nodules	Texture features ML	Accuracy = 89%, AUC-0.92	Progress in risk stratification by fusing shape & texture-based structures	60/2020
Breast Cancer	Back-propagation ANN	Accuracy of 98.56%	Highest precision is achieved when 18 relevant features were used	61/2021
Heart Syndrome	KNN, Naïve Bayes, DT, random forest, and SVM	Accuracy KNN, DT, Random forest, Naïve Bayes over 80%.	KNN algorithm has good Accuracy score compared to other algorithms	54/2019
Epilepsy detection	Support vector neural network (SVNN)	Accuracy =98.18% with 100% sensitivity	High accuracy with a fine Gaussian classifier over other algorithms	62/2021

MACHINE LEARNING IN DISEASE PREDICTION AND DETECTION

ML Algorithms and Classification

The study of ML classification in statistics is vast, and types of classification algorithms depend on the dataset. Below are the most common classification algorithms in machine learning as shown in Table 2.

Table 2. Classification of algorithms in ML

Name of ML algorithm	Use	Benefit	Drawback	Ref.
Supervised KNN	Classification used, Regression used	Nonparametric method. Easy and no training required, easily modified to changes in its set of labeled data	Long calculation. Low performance due to unnecessary datasets. The data might need to use same features.	30-31
Naïve Bayes	Probabilistic classification used	Data is scan individually.	Models that are trained and altered outperform.	65
DT	Prediction, Classification	Easy to handle and categorized attributes.	Long trees get hard to compute	67
Supervised Random Forest	Classification used, Regression	Low correlations value. Increased performance.	Need much time for training. Complexity	68
Supervised SVM	Binary, nonlinear classification	More active in large-dimensional space.	Hard to select a kernel function and does not work well under noise	69,71
Supervised Gradient Boosted DT	Used for Classification, Regression	Increases the estimation action iteratively.	Not work well in repeated construction of the tree	60

The aim of ML-IOT is to make technologies effective and reliable. In the healthcare domain, the machine's job is to help doctors and staff provides better service and care. Figure 5 shows application of ML. Hence, the usage of ML in healthcare domain is listed.

Personalization of Handling Disease

First step of ML in healthcare field is early treatment. The objective of analysis is to recover individual health services using personal data and examination techniques (Babar et al., 2018; Baker et al., 2017; Cortes & Vapnik, 1995; Latif et al., 2018; Pouryazdan et al., 2017). Furthermore, supervised learning algorithms permit the formation of modified treatment using the data of individual patients. Combination

Figure 5. Application of ML in healthcare

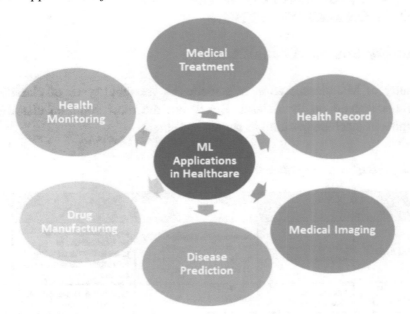

of various method like clinical, pharmaceutical, and socioeconomic data with ML-IOT, investigators can detect patterns in individual treatments and recognize genetic deviations that may be treated.

Virtual Aides to Patients

Virtual aides are gradually standard clarification in the healthcare sector many applications. In particular, the emergence of ML-IOT based application to support patients in all pathways of care. Hence, there are virtual nurses available used to answer patients' questions instantaneously, and providing advice (Dehkordi et al., 2020; Lashkari et al., 2018; Liu et al., 2018). These records are used at time of treatment and disease records so that physicians can use them in their treatment. Furthermore, the objective of these application is to save hospital visits or tension related to medical care.

The use of ML-IOT in initial stage of drug discovery has the possible for various services, from the first step of medicine to their success rate (Dehkordi et al., 2020; Lashkari et al., 2018). Additionally, it can help calculate safety of drugs and deliver information about new medicine.

DIAGNOSTICS

In the investigative stage, follow-up for patient is important. IOT-ML provide healthcare practitioner to save time and improve correct diagnoses (Rodríguez-Mazahua et al., 2016; Tsai et al., 2015). Furthermore, it offer novel perspectives method in the prediction of various syndromes. Scientists are studying ML algorithms to help identify heart disease.

Diabetes Diagnoses

Diabetes disease can harm many parts of the body like heart, kidneys, and nervous is tissue (Mohammadi et al., 2018). IOT-ML is thought to notice diabetes early to save patients' lives. Health care staff uses many ML algorithms to detect diabetes. Novel methods are also emerged for prolonged disease risk visualization.

Liver Disease Diagnoses

Concepts of data removal and ML have newly arisen to examine for a system to predict liver infection and disease. Examination of liver disease is a interesting one, because there are many diseases which affect the liver (Firouzi et al., 2018; Mahdavinejad et al., 2018). However, experts are performing well to solve these problems.

Optimizing Hospital Management

By initial prediction of each patient's diseases, demand for hospital assets like beds and operating rooms can be well predicted. Pattern detection methods are applied to notice regions of interest in digital pathology slides, and work surprisingly well to detect cancers.

Diagnosis of Breast Cancer

ML can identify different types of cancer. Since experts have enhanced the methods that can now detect and observe more diverse forms of cancer (Shirvanimoghaddam et al., 2017). These improvements now allow combination of IOT and ML to identify tumors with incredible precision.

FUTURE CHALLENGES AND ARGUMENTS

Adapting ML-IOT into all healthcare systems is inappropriately complicated. Many decision makers are senior person prefer simple systems like 'pen and paper' in which they have more comfortable and control. ML arrangements are complex and hence require simplest form. Additionally, many of the healthcares are not encouraged to spend their economical in financing in their staff and other ML models.

As with the growth of most IOT technologies and ML algorithm, ML gets hot discussion on ethics. When machines learn through our algorithms to 'think and work for themselves,' we have given up power and control and sometimes we don't know exactly what the machine learned, in that way pushing patients' lives in risk. Moreover, developments in ML-IOT can lead to problems about insurance coverage. Now days, insurance firms may start trying access to ML-IOT that is following a patient's records to check their health condition. Moreover, it is thinkable that when future investigation shows the achievement of ML, then hospitals might upsurge their fees.

CONCLUSION

Healthcare division is one of the growing field and it is becoming more expensive. Technologies such as artificial learning and ML provide better-quality treatment and lower the costs. The use of IoT technology provides medical practitioners and patients advance medical device environment. ML can also help healthcare system meet growing medical demands, improve operations and lower costs, healthcare specialists identify and treat disease more proficiently and with more accuracy. A many organization have already considered the first step in this ML field. Furthermore, the learning of the scheme influenced by huge data and algorithms available to classify data in certain category through combination of ML-IoT. Sometimes people have difficulties is taking decision and they rely on facts to take any action and IoT.

REFERENCES

Abdollahzadeh, S., & Navimipour, N. J. (2016). Deployment strategies in the wireless sensor network: A comprehensive review. *Computer Communications*, *91*, 1–16. doi:10.1016/j.comcom.2016.06.003

Aghdam, Z. N., Rahmani, A. M., Hosseinzadeh, M. J. C. M., & Biomedicine, P. I. (2020). *The Role of the Internet of Things in Healthcare: Future Trends and Challenges*. Academic Press.

Al-Fuqaha, A., Guizani, M., Mohammadi, M., Aledhari, M., & Ayyash, M. (2015). Internet of things: A survey on enabling technologies, protocols, and applications. *IEEE Communications Surveys and Tutorials, 17*(4), 2347–2376. doi:10.1109/COMST.2015.2444095

Athey, S. (2018). The impact of machine learning on economics. In *The economics of artificial intelligence: An agenda* (pp. 507–547). University of Chicago Press.

Atiqur, R., Liton, A., & Wu, G. (2020). Content Caching Strategy at Small Base Station in 5G Networks with Mobile Edge Computing. *International Journal of Science and Business., 4*(4), 104–112.

Atrey, K., Singh, B. K., & Bodhey, N. K. (2021). Feature Selection for Classification of Breast Cancer in Histopathology Images: A Comparative Investigation Using Wavelet-Based Color Features. In A. A. Rizvanov, B. K. Singh, & P. Ganasala (Eds.), *Advances in Biomedical Engineering and Technology. Lecture Notes in Bioengineering*. Springer. doi:10.1007/978-981-15-6329-4_30

Aziz, M. N., & Islam, A. (2020). Reviewing Data Mining as an enabling technology for BI. *International Journal of Science and Business, 4*(7), 46–51.

Babar, M., Khan, F., Iqbal, W., Yahya, A., Arif, F., Tan, Z., & Chuma, J. M. (2018). A secured data management scheme for smart societies in industrial internet of things environment. *IEEE Access: Practical Innovations, Open Solutions, 6*, 43088–43099. doi:10.1109/ACCESS.2018.2861421

Baker, S. B., Xiang, W., & Atkinson, I. (2017). Internet of things for smart healthcare: Technologies, challenges, and opportunities. *IEEE Access: Practical Innovations, Open Solutions, 5*, 26521–26544. doi:10.1109/ACCESS.2017.2775180

Banerjee, N., & Das, S. (2020). Prediction Lung Cancer. In *Machine Learning Perspective*. IEEE.

Basha, N. (2019). Early Detection of Heart Syndrome Using Machine Learning Technique. *4th International Conference on Electrical, Electronics, Communication, Computer Technologies and Optimization Techniques (ICEECCOT)*.

Birje, M. N., & Hanji, S. S. (2020). Internet of things based distributed healthcare systems: A review. *J. Data Inf. Manag, 2*(3), 149–165. doi:10.100742488-020-00027-x

Bote-Curiel, L., Muñoz-Romero, S., Gerrero-Curieses, A., & Rojo-Álvarez. José, L. (2019). Deep Learning and Big Data in Healthcare: A Double Review for Critical Beginners. *Applied Sciences (Basel, Switzerland)*, *9*(11), 2331. doi:10.3390/app9112331

Boubiche, S., Boubiche, D. E., Bilami, A., & Toral-Cruz, H. (2018). Big data challenges and data aggregation strategies in wireless sensor networks. *IEEE Access: Practical Innovations, Open Solutions*, *6*, 20558–20571. doi:10.1109/ACCESS.2018.2821445

Cinaree, & Emiroglu. (2019). *Classification of Brain Tumors by Machine Learning Algorithms*. IEEE.

Cook, D. (2006). Health monitoring and assistance to support aging in place. *JUCS*, *12*(1), 15–29.

Cortes, C., & Vapnik, V. (1995). Support-vector networks. *Machine Learning*, *20*(3), 23–297. doi:10.1007/BF00994018

Cui, L., Yang, S., Chen, F., Ming, Z., Lu, N., & Qin, J. (2018). A survey on application of machine learning for internet of things. *International Journal of Machine Learning and Cybernetics*, *9*(8), 1399–1417. doi:10.100713042-018-0834-5

Dang, L. M., Piran, M. J., Han, D., Min, K., & Moon, H. (2019). A Survey on Internet of Things and Cloud Computing for Healthcare. *MPDI. Electronics (Basel)*, *8*(7), 768. doi:10.3390/electronics8070768

Dayanand, J., & Neethi, P. (2020). Thyroid Disease Prediction Using Feature Selection And Machine Learning Classifiers. *The International Journal of Analytical and Experimental Modal Analysis*.

Dehkordi, S. A., Farajzadeh, K., Rezazadeh, J., Farahbakhsh, R., Sandrasegaran, K., & Dehkordi, M. A. (2020). A survey on data aggregation techniques in IoT sensor networks. *Wireless Networks*, *26*(2), 1243–1263. doi:10.100711276-019-02142-z

Dhillon, A., Singh, A. J., & World, T. (2019). *Machine learning in healthcare data analysis: a survey*. Academic Press.

Emu, M. (2020). *Assisting the Non-invasive Diagnosis of Liver Fibrosis Stages using Machine Learning Methods*. IEEE.

Evtodieva, T. E., Chernova, D. V., Ivanova, N. V., & Wirth, J. (2020). The internet of things: possibilities of application in intelligent supply chain management. In *Digital Transformation of the Economy: Challenges, Trends and New Opportunities* (pp. 395–403). Springer. doi:10.1007/978-3-030-11367-4_38

Fathollahi-Fard, A. M., Abbas, A., & Behrooz, K. (2021). Multi-Objective Optimization of Home Healthcare with Working-Time Balancing and Care Continuity. *Sustainability*, *13*(22), 12431. doi:10.3390u132212431

Firouzi, F., Rahmani, A. M., Mankodiya, K., Badaroglu, M., Merrett, G. V., Wong, P., & Farahani, B. (2018). Internet-of-Things and big data for smarter healthcare: From device to architecture, applications and analytics. *Future Generation Computer Systems*, *78*, 583–586. doi:10.1016/j.future.2017.09.016

Fizi, F., & Askar, S. (2016). A novel load balancing algorithm for software defined network based datacenters. *International Conference on Broadband Communications for Next Generation Networks and Multimedia Applications (CoBCom)*, 1-6. 10.1109/COBCOM.2016.7593506

Ge, M., Bangui, H., & Buhnova, B. (2018). Big data for internet of things: A survey. *Future Generation Computer Systems*, *87*, 601–614. doi:10.1016/j.future.2018.04.053

Ghate, V. V., & Vijayakumar, V. (2018). Machine learning for data aggregation in wsn: A survey. *International Journal of Pure and Applied Mathematics*, *118*(24), 1–12.

Ghose, A., Pal, A., Choudhury, A. D., Chattopadhyay, T., Bhowmick, P. K., & Chattopadhyay, D. (2014). *Internet of things application development*. U.S. Patent Application 14/286,068.

Halgurd, S., Maghdid, A. T., Asaad, K. Z., Ali Safaa, S., & Khurram Khan, M. (2020). *Diagnosing COVID-19 Pneumonia from X-Ray and CT Images using Deep Learning and Transfer Learning Algorithms*. arXiv preprint arXiv:2004.00038.

Huang, Y. H. (2011). DNA computing research progress and application. *The 6th International Conference on Computer Science & Education*, 232-235. 10.1109/ICCSE.2011.6028624

Hussain, W., Hussain, F. K., Hussain, O., Bagia, R., & Chang, E. (2018). Risk-based framework for SLA violation abatement from the cloud service provider's perspective. *The Computer Journal*, *61*(9), 1306–1322. doi:10.1093/comjnl/bxx118

Hussain, W., Hussain, F. K., Hussain, O. K., & Chang, E. (2016). Provider-Based Optimized Personalized Viable SLA (OPV-SLA) Framework to Prevent SLA Violation. *The Computer Journal*, *59*(12), 1760–1783. doi:10.1093/comjnl/bxw026

Kan, M. M. (2019). Digital technology and the future of health systems," Health Systems & Reform. *Reform*, *5*(2), 113–120.

Kaur, G., & Oberoi, A. (2020). Novel Approach for Brain Tumor Detection Based on Naïve Bayes Classification. In Data Management, Analytics and Innovation. Springer. doi:10.1007/978-981-32-9949-8_31

Keti, F., & Askar, S. (2015). Emulation of Software Defined Networks Using Mininet in Different Simulation Environments. *6th International Conference on Intelligent Systems, Modelling and Simulation*, 205-210. 10.1109/ISMS.2015.46

Kohler, J. E., Falcone, R. A. Jr, & Fallat, M. E. (2019). Rural health, telemedicine and access for pediatric surgery. *Current Opinion in Pediatrics*, *31*(3), 391–398. doi:10.1097/MOP.0000000000000763 PMID:31090582

Komal Kumar, N. (2020). Analysis and Prediction of Cardio Vascular Disease using Machine Learning Classifiers. *6th International Conference on Advanced Computing & Communication Systems*.

Kononenko, I. (2001). Machine Learning for Medical Diagnosis: History, State of the Art and Perspective. *Journal of Artificial Intelligence in Medicine*, *1*(1), 89–109. doi:10.1016/S0933-3657(01)00077-X PMID:11470218

Lakshmi, B., Indumathi, T., & Ravi, N. A. (2016). 5 decision tree classification algorithm for risk predictions during pregnancy. *Procedia Technol.*, *24*, 1542–1549. doi:10.1016/j.protcy.2016.05.128

Lashkari, B., Rezazadeh, J., Farahbakhsh, R., & Sandrasegaran, K. (2018). Crowdsourcing and sensing for indoor localization in IoT: A review. *IEEE Sensors Journal*, *19*(7), 2408–2434. doi:10.1109/JSEN.2018.2880180

Latif, S., Afzaal, H., & Zafar, N. A. (2018). Intelligent traffic monitoring and guidance system for smart city. In *International Conference on Computing, Mathematics and Engineering Technologies (iCoMET)*. IEEE. 10.1109/ICOMET.2018.8346327

Lee, I., & Lee, K. (2015). The internet of things (IoT): Applications, investments, and challenges for enterprises. *Business Horizons*, *58*(4), 431–440. doi:10.1016/j.bushor.2015.03.008

Lee, S. I., Celik, S., Logsdon, B. A., Lundberg, S. M., Martins, T. J., Oehler, V. G., Estey, E. H., Miller, C. P., Chien, S., Dai, J., Saxena, A., Blau, C. A., & Becker, P. S. (2018). A machine learning approach to integrate big data for precision medicine in acute myeloid leukemia. *Nature Communications*, *9*(1), 4. doi:10.103841467-017-02465-5 PMID:29298978

Liu, J., Shen, H., Narman, H.S., Chung, W., & Lin, Z. (2018). A survey of mobile crowd sensing techniques: A critical component for the internet of things. *ACM Transactions on Cyber-Physical Systems, 2*(3), 1–26.

Mahdavinejad, M. S., Rezvan, M., Barekatain, M., Adibi, P., Barnaghi, P., & Sheth, A. P. (2018). Machine learning for internet of things data analysis: A survey. *Digital Communications and Networks*, *4*(3), 161–175. doi:10.1016/j.dcan.2017.10.002

Mandal, S., Singh, B. K., & Thakur, K. (2021). Majority voting-based hybrid feature selection in machine learning paradigm for epilepsy detection using EEG. *International Journal of Computational Vision and Robotics*, *11*(4), 85–400. doi:10.1504/IJCVR.2021.116558

Maskut, S., Timur, S., Zhanar, B., Aigul, A., Marina, Z., & Nazym, A. (2020). *The Recent Progress and Applications of Digital Technologies in Healthcare: A Review. International Journal of Telemedicine and Applications*.

Michael, M., Sonoo, T. I., Andrew, A., Andrew, B., Paul, B., Wendy, C., & Seth, H. (2001). *Artificial Intelligence in Health Care:The Hope, the Hype*. National Academy of Medicine.

Miotto, R., Wang, F., Wang, S., Jiang, X., & Dudley, J. T. (2018). Deep learning for healthcare: Review, opportunities and challenges. *Briefings in Bioinformatics*, *19*(6), 1236–1246. doi:10.1093/bib/bbx044 PMID:28481991

Mohammadi, M., Al-Fuqaha, A., Sorour, S., & Guizani, M. (2018). Deep learning for iot big data and streaming analytics: A survey. *IEEE Communications Surveys and Tutorials*, *20*(4), 2923–2960. doi:10.1109/COMST.2018.2844341

Moher, D., Liberati, A., Tetzlaff, J., Altman, D., & The, P. (2009). Preferred Reporting Items for Systematic Reviews and Meta-Analyses: The PRISMA Statement. *PLoS Medicine, 6*(7), e1000097. doi:10.1371/journal.pmed.1000097 PMID:19621072

Olaković, A. Č., & Hadžialić, M. (2018). Internet of things (IoT): A review of enabling technologies, challenges, and open research issues. *Computer Networks*, *144*, 17–39. doi:10.1016/j.comnet.2018.07.017

Oshiro, T. M., Perez, P. S., & Baranauskas, J. A. (2012). How Many Trees in a Random Forest? In *International Workshop on Machine Learning and Data Mining in Pattern Recognition*. Springer. 10.1007/978-3-642-31537-4_13

Otoom, A. F., Abdallah, E. E., Kilani, Y., Kefaye, A., & Ashour, M. (2015). Effective Diagnosis and Monitoring of Heart Disease. *International Journal of Software Engineering and Its Applications*, *9*, 143–156.

Oyewo, O. (2020). Prediction of Prostate Cancer using Ensemble of Machine Learning Techniques. *International Journal of Advanced Computer Science and Applications*, *11*(3).

Paun, G. H. (1999). DNA Computing: New Computing Paradigms. Springer.

Piccialli, F., & Jung, J. E. (2017). Understanding customer experience diffusion on social networking services by big data analytics. *Mobile Networks and Applications*, *22*(4), 605–612. doi:10.100711036-016-0803-8

Pourghebleh, B., & Navimipour, N. J. (2017). Data aggregation mechanisms in the internet of things: A systematic review of the literature and recommendations for future research. *Journal of Network and Computer Applications*, *97*, 23–34. doi:10.1016/j.jnca.2017.08.006

Pouryazdan, M., Fiandrino, C., Kantarci, B., Soyata, T., Kliazovich, D., & Bouvry, P. (2017). Intelligent gaming for mobile crowd-sensing participants to acquire trustworthy big data in the internet of things. *IEEE Access: Practical Innovations, Open Solutions*, *5*, 22209–22223. doi:10.1109/ACCESS.2017.2762238

Qi, J., Yang, P., Min, G., Amft, O., Dong, F., & Xu, L. (2017). Advanced internet of things for personalised healthcare systems: A survey. *Pervasive and Mobile Computing*, *41*, 132–149. doi:10.1016/j.pmcj.2017.06.018

Rodríguez-Mazahua, L., Rodríguez-Enríquez, C.-A., Sánchez-Cervantes, J. L., Cervantes, J., García-Alcaraz, J. L., & Alor-Hernández, G. (2016). A general perspective of big data: Applications, tools, challenges and trends. *The Journal of Supercomputing*, *72*(8), 3073–3113. doi:10.100711227-015-1501-1

Roy, A., Singh, B. K., Banchhor, S.K., & Verma, K. (2021). *Segmentation of malignant tumours in mammogram images: A hybrid approach using convolutional neural networks and connected component analysis*. doi:10.1111/exsy.12826

Sahu, S. P., Londhe, N. D., Verma, S., Singh, B. K., & Banchhor, S. K. (2020). Improved pulmonary lung nodules risk stratification in computed tomography images by fusing shape and texture features in a machine-learning paradigm. *International Journal of Imaging Systems and Technology*, *31*(3), 1503–1518. doi:10.1002/ima.22539

Shahbazi, Z., & Byun, Y.-C. (2020). Towards a Secure Thermal-Energy Aware Routing Protocol in Wireless Body Area Network Based on Blockchain Technology. *Sensors (Basel)*, *20*(12), 3604. doi:10.339020123604 PMID:32604851

Shahbazi, Z., & Byun, Y.-C. (2021). Improving Transactional Data System Based on an Edge Computing–Blockchain–Machine Learning Integrated Framework. *Processes (Basel, Switzerland)*, *9*(1), 92. doi:10.3390/pr9010092

Sharma, S., & Yoon, W. (in press). *Multiobjective Reinforcement Learning Based Energy Consumption in C-RAN enabled Massive MIMO*. Academic Press.

Sharma, S., & Yoon, W. (2018). Multi-objective energy efficient resource allocation for WPCN. International Journal of Engineering Research and Technology, 11(12), pp. 2035-2043. ISSN 0974-3154.

Sharma, S., & Yoon, W. (2019). Multiobjective Optimization for Energy Efficiency in Cloud Radio Access Networks. International Journal of Engineering Research and Technology, 12 (5), pp. 607-610. ISSN 0974-3154.

Sharma, S., & Yoon, W. (2021). Multiobjective Optimization for Resource Allocation in Full-duplex Large Distributed MIMO Systems. *Advances in Electrical and Computer Engineering*, *21*(2), 67–74. doi:10.4316/AECE.2021.02008

Shirvanimoghaddam, M., Dohler, M., & Johnson, S. J. (2017). Massive non-orthogonal multiple access for cellular IoT: Potentials and limitations. *IEEE Communications Magazine*, *55*(9), 55–61. doi:10.1109/MCOM.2017.1600618

Singh, A., Thakur, N., & Sharma, A. (2016). A review of supervised machine learning algorithms. *Proceedings of the 2016 3rd International Conference on Computing for Sustainable Global Development*, 1310–1315.

Tsai, C.-W., Lai, C.-F., Chao, H.-C., & Vasilakos, A. (2015). Big data analytics: A survey. *Journal of Big Data*, *2*(1), 21. doi:10.118640537-015-0030-3 PMID:26191487

Vidya, M., & Karki, M. V. (2020). *Skin Cancer Detection using Machine Learning Techniques*. IEEE.

Yadav, S., & Jadhav, S. (2019). Machine Learning Algorithms for Disease Prediction Using IoT Environment. *International Journal of Engineering and Advanced Technology*, *8*(6), 8. doi:10.35940/ijeat.F8914.088619

Ye, J., Chow, J.-H., Chen, J., & Zheng, Z. (2009). Stochastic gradient boosted distributed decision trees. *Proceedings of the 18th ACM conference on Information and knowledge management—CIKM'09*. 10.1145/1645953.1646301

Yu, W., Liu, T., & Valdez, R. (2010). Application of support vector machine modeling for prediction of common diseases: the case of diabetes and pre-diabetes. *BMC Med Inform Decis Mak, 10*, 16. doi:10.1186/1472-6947-10-16

Yuvaraj, N., & SriPreethaa, K. R. (2017). Diabetes prediction in healthcare systems using machine learning algorithms on Hadoop cluster. *Cluster Computing*, *22*(S1), 1–9. doi:10.100710586-017-1532-x

Zabirul Islam, Md., Milon Islam, Md., & Amanullah, A. (2020). *A combined deep CNN-LSTM network for the detection of novel coronavirus (COVID-19) using X-ray images*. Elsevier.

Chapter 7
Heavy Metals in Ground Water Affect the Human Health Global Challenge

Pramisha Sharma
M. M. College of Technology, Raipur, India

Ashima Sharma
National Institute of Technology, Raipur, India

ABSTRACT

This chapter is based on a review of heavy metals, high atomic weight, and high-density naturally occurring elements transition elements. In the periodic table, about 80 elements of them are called metals. These metals can be further classified into two categories, those that are essential for survival such as magnesium, potassium, calcium, etc. and those that are nonessential such as lead, mercury, bismuth, and cadmium. These nonessential metals are known as toxic metals. Trace elements such as selenium, zinc, copper, etc. are necessary for maintaining the human body metabolism. These essential elements can be toxic if present at high concentrations. On the other hand, some elements like Hg, Cd, Pb, Bi, Cr, As, etc. are usually toxic to the living organisms when absorbed in small quantities. The source of heavy metals is natural as well as manmade. The toxicity of heavy metals causes carcinogenic effects in human beings related to organ, renal, hepatic, neural, skeletal, and glandular problems.

DOI: 10.4018/978-1-7998-9831-3.ch007

INTRODUCTION

The environmental abundance of heavy metals contributes the sustainability and equilibrium in the ecosystem. But the availability of heavy metals in groundwater easily enters the ecosystem and its excessive amount cause toxic effect. Heavy metals are non-biodegradable and disrupt the whole ecological functions (Hawkes 1997). Toxicity is the capacity of a substance to poison or it may be defined as the extent or degree to which a chemical substance, which is poisonous, to produce deleterious or adverse effect, interferes physiological functions, destroy living cells, has serious health threats, causes health risks on a living organism and can eventually cause death (Duffus 2002). The toxicity of heavy metals is not solely responsible but its doses, entry routs, exposure level, age, gender, nutrition way, interaction with chemical species and weather conditions also affects its toxicity. Toxic metals as zinc, arsenic, chromium, cadmium, mercury etc., beyond its tolerance limit immensely damage the health of human being. The bad effects of heavy metals appear in human body in the form of multiple organ malfunctions. Even its trace amount can also affect the human health (Ali and Khan 2018). Toxic metals can substitute also other substances in another tissue's structures. These tissues, like vessels, joints, skeletons and muscles are damaged through the substitution method. Toxic metals can be deposited in many areas, responsible for local allergy and other toxic impacts (Ali et al., 2013). They can also give support growth of micro-organisms infections those are complicated or not possible to eliminate until this reason is eliminated. Now it becomes a major issue under environmental science and related with hydrochemistry (Dai et al., 2018, Edelstein and Ben-Hur 2018). Various parameters present to water correlatedly affect toxic metals present in environment. Heavy metals contaminated the surface and groundwater is the global issue. Mainly heavy metals are of anthropogenic in origin. Mostly, released from the process of metal extraction, purification, mining, smelting and refining. Heavy metals become toxic when body could not metabolize and deposited in the soft tissues. These are mainly carcinogens (Bagul et al.,2015, Liu et al., 2008, Armah et al.,2014). So, poor management and over misuses of water, are responsible for the endangerment of fresh water bodies in all around the world. The ecological dreadful condition is responsible too. The fresh water pollution can be attributed as the main source as release of wastes, industrial discharge and agricultural runoff water. The rural area is decreasing and uses of pure and organic products are diminishing which cause very bad impacts on fresh water bodies. It can be factually agreed that the developed countries are suffering from the serious problem of waste water discharged from industries into water bodies specially it affects the groundwater in other hand developing countries facing the mixing of agricultural waste water into water bodies. Chemicals present in water resources cause health issues and cause water borne diseases in living being, should be avoided by taking actions.

Drinking water is the fundamental needs of the living beings on the precious Earth. Although 884 million population in the global lives with contaminated drinking water. The population of 2.5 billion still do not access to enhanced hygiene, including 1.2 billion can't avail a simple latrine (UNICEF, 2008). In World Health Organization (WHO) approximately 88% of diarrheal disease is due to by polluted water inadequate sanitation and poor hygiene. Consequently, more than 4,500 kids die daily due to diarrhea and other diseases. Many children die, including older children and adults, suffering from malnutrition and chance for work and education. The global water crisis claims more lives through disease than any war claims through guns (UNDP, 2006). In India a large part of population is dependent on groundwater that is the only source of drinking water supply. Groundwater believed to be comparatively much clean free from pollution then surface water. But prolonged discharge of industrial effluents, domestic sewage and solid waste dump causes the groundwater to become polluted and creates health problems (Patil et al., 2001). The rapid growth of urban areas affects groundwater quality due to over exploitation of resources and improper disposal of waste. The mixing of many contaminants and nutritive through city drains, factory effluents, agricultural drains etc. in to the water bodies changes in the physicochemical quality and its characteristics. Several investigations have been done on this aspect (Milway, 1969: Olimax and Sikorska, 1975: Piecznska et al., 1975 and Vollenweidre, 1986). Spoilage of quality of water is improving sequentially and becomes a global problem (Mahanand et al., 2005). Thus, it is required the regular enhancement of water quality. (Lokeshwari et al., 2006).

Groundwater

The water resources found under the Earth's surface is groundwater, aquifers in soil and rock fractures. About 20% of the entire world's fresh water obtained from groundwater (Central Groundwater Board). It supports drinking water supply, livestock requirement, agriculture, factory and so many business activities (Veslind, 1993). Groundwater is generally free from pollutants and pollution in comparison to surface water bodies (Zaman, 2002). Also, the natural impurities in rain water which fulfill groundwater systems removed while filtering through soil layers. In India, where groundwater is consumed fastly, for agricultural and industrial purposes, a lot of land and water dependent human functions are responsible for pollution of this expensive resource (Trivedi, 1990).

Surface Water

River, Wetland, Streams, Oceans, Lakes, Sea, etc. are known as the surface water. The non-saline surface water is an important source of water apart from the groundwater. Comparatively, the possibility of contamination of surface water is more than groundwater due to several activities as mining, extraction, agriculture etc. In the last two decades it was reported that the surface water has been contaminated due to the enhanced man activities (Masood et aL 2009 and Patrick et al., 2005). Thus, the contamination of water especially surface water is of several types, and can be divided as biologically, physical, radiological and chemical scums (Gay and Proop, 1993). Eutrophication from ·'sheet flow'· on an agricultural land or a forest are also cited as examples of furtilizer pollution. (S.S. Dara, 1997).

It has been reported that several diseases have been spread by the use of dirty water. It is observed as approximately 50,000 population got death daily global as a result or water borne diseases (Nevondo and Cloete, 1999). There are 50 countries still report Cholera which is a water borne disease (World Health Organization). Millions are borne to dangerous levels or naturally distributed arsenic and fluoride in drinking water give carcinogenic effect and tooth/skeletal weakness or breakage. An estimated 260 million people are infected with schistosomiasis (WHO, 2004). In polluted water viruses, bacteria, intestinal parasites and other harmful microorganisms, cause waterborne diseases such as diarrhea dysentery, and typhoid. More than 1.5 million deaths, due to contaminated water, mostly among children less than 5 years of age (WHO, 2005). Samples were collected from 16 sampling locations and tested for Calcium (Ca), Sodium (Na), Potassium (K), Magnesium (Mg), Manganese (Mn), Nitrate and Nitrite, Sulphate (So/·), Phosphate (PO/} Fluoride (F) Chloride (Cl), Total Dissolved Solids (TDS), EC, alkalinity, hardness and turbidity parameters. The concentrations of most of the investigated parameters in the sources of drinking water samples from Kohdasht region were within the permissible limits of the World Health Organization drinking water quality guidelines (Jafari et al., 2008). Contan1inated drinking water is also a major source of hepatitis, typhoid and opportunistic infections that attack the immuno-compromised, especially persons living with HIV/AIDS (UNICEF, 2011). There are 35 metals that concern occupational or residential exposure and of them, 23 are the heavy elements. '·Heavy metals'· (HMs) are chemical elements with a specific gravity that is at least 5 times higher than the specific gravity of water and is toxic or poisonous at low concentrations. HM is natural components of the Earth's crust and some well-known toxic metallic elements with a specific gravity higher than 5 of water are arsenic, 5.7: cadmium. 8.65; iron 7.9: lead, 11.34: and mercury, 13.54. They include antimony arsenic, 5.7: cadmium, 8.65: iron, 7.9: lead, 11.34: and mercury, 13.54 they include antimony, arsenic, bismuth, cadmium. Cerium, Chromium. Cobalt, copper, gallium, gold, iron, lead, and zinc (Lide, 1992 and HilL 1997). Most of HMs is of ma made origin. The most important cause is the process of extraction and purification, mining, smelting and refining. Metals are mixed to lubricants and so enter into the environment. Besides, these many metals occur naturally in the earth crust in highly concentrated from, constituting ore deposits, (Devi. et al., 2008). They are essential for healthy environment, but huge quantity of any of them may be responsible for chronic toxicity. HMs becomes toxic when they cannot be consumed by the body and collected in the soft tissues. (Smith et. al. 1998). Various heavy metals present in groundwater its origin, other sources, toxic effects on living organisms and its exposure in global context have been described in this chapter.

IMPORTANT TOXIC HEAVY METALS AND ITS ADVERSE EFFECTS

Arsenic

Arsenic (As) is naturally occurring pinctogen (p-block) group element and its trace concentration determined in the all-environmental samples (Agency for toxic 2000). As is always found either in the form of trivalent arsenite and pentavalent arsenate. Sometimes present in organic compounds such as trimethylarsine oxide, monomethylarsonic acid and dimethylarsinic acid. The huge use of arsenic is in pharma industries as anticancer agent in promeylocytic anemia. Also used in the treatment of wormiform diseases, syphilis and dysentery (Techounwon et al.,1999). The industrial use of arsenic is in manufacture of pesticides, herbicides, fungicides wood preservatives and in dye industry too. Arsenic is used as veterinary medicines for treating filariasis in dog and used as vermicides for cattle. The global use of As in African sleeping sickness (Centeno et al.,2005).

Arsenic is found in two oxidation states Arsenic (III) and Arsenic (V). In both of them Arsenic (III) is 10 times more toxic than Arsenic (V). Arsenic (III) replaces thiol group present in protein molecule and responsible for deactivation of more than 200 enzymes (Centeno et al.,2005). Arsenic (III) diminish the DNA repair mechanism and responsible for chromosomal damage, neural disorder, deafness, fibrosis, cancer of renal, respiratory system and digestive system, bladder, renal took place due to Arsenic (III) (Techounwon et al.,2004). A syndrome Guillain-Barre an anti-immune disease is caused by arsenic toxicity in which nervous system disorder takes place. It is carcinogenic and found in the form of oxides or sulphides. Arsenic is fetal to the people. Arsenic generally enters in the body through inhaling dusts solutions, suicides or in taking polluted food or water. Arsenic affects reproductive system too. Diminish the level of testosterone in the human beings.

Cadmium

Cadmium is 12 [th] group transition metal of periodic table. It is found as bivalent ion and used as heavy metal. It is abundantly found with 0. 1mg/kg concentration in earth's crust. The maximum concentration of cadmium is found in sedimentary rock and in the bottom of the sea in combined with phosphate (Gesamp1987). The huge consumption of cadmium has been seen in industries for the synthesis of alloys, batteries and pigments (Wilson 1988). Recently the growth of battery production has been enhanced with the use of cadmium. Apart from that cigarette smokes also consists of cadmium (International Agency for Research on Cancer (IARC,1993). Cadmium toxicity case kidney damage (Gobe and Crane, 2010), chronic renal damage (Bawaskar et al.,2010). It enters in body through digestive system and affect the infants through placenta in pregnant lady cause early delivery. Severely affects DNA and membrane (Von Ehrenstein et al.,2006). Half- life of cadmium is 25 years and it is accumulated in plants and animals through groundwater used for drinking purpose. According to epidemiological data the environmental exposure is related to pulmonary, pancreas, kidney and prostate gland cancer. Cadmium is responsible for osteoporosis. Liver and kidney are prone to cadmium's toxic effect. Some cadmium inducible proteins are highly active and cause cadmium toxicity. Cadmium is also responsible for pathogenic risks and formation of reactive oxygen species. Some plants like sunflower, Indian mustards are used to remove cadmium from soil and groundwater. The trace level of cadmium could be determined by various analytical methods using many organic and inorganic reagents.

Bismuth

Bismuth is found in +3 and +5 oxidation states. It is very important for analytical chemistry (Busev & Tiptsova 1981, Yamani et al.,2002). Bismuth is widely used in different industries such as cosmetic, pharmaceutical, pigment industries and used as semiconductors too. The tremendous use of bismuth in various fields, results in enhancement of bismuth concentration in the environment. Bismuth toxicity cause neurological disorder in human being as severe confusion, myoclonus, mental imbalance, loss of brain and body co-ordination etc. (Loiseau et al., 1976). Language problem and diarrhea, reduce the testosterone level and affect the reproductive system (Hutson 2005). As a secondary constituent, Bi occurs in some lead, copper and tin minerals and obtained as by product during the extraction of these metals. Bismuth minerals infrequently occur alone and are mostly found with other ores. Bismuth is used in the manufacture of pigments, cosmetics, semiconductors, metallurgical additives for casting and galvanizing (Pistofidis et al., 2007), bismuth alloys, solders, and in the processing and reuse of uranium nuclear fuels. Bismuth compounds are important in the context of medicine as it is used in desiccators, local astringents, antiseptics, antacids and as radio-opaque media for X-rays (http://www.eudra.org/vedocs). Bismuth enters in our environment through various process like weathering, combustion of fossil fuels, metallurgical process etc. Bismuth is an uncommon metal and might be poisonous when it is taken in excess. Several cases of neurotoxic, nephrotoxic and kidney damage symptoms were assigned from the utilization of bismuth bearing pharmaceutical formulations (Tomas 1991; Shemirani et al., 2005). The toxic effects of bismuth on human being are decrease appetite, weakness, rheumatic pain, diarrhea, dermatitis etc. (Frederick 1979). The trace level of bismuth could be determined by various analytical methods using many organic and inorganic reagents.

Lead

Lead is a p-block element naturally found in earth. Lead is bluish-grey in color and used in making of lead acid battery, some ammunitions, solders and pipes. About 1.52 million metric ton lead are used in industries. Lead is also used with fuels, glass, pigments and lead sheets (Gabby 2006, Gabby 2003). It is found in bivalent and tetravalent forms. Lead is the most important toxic heavy metal and globally abundant due to its dangerous physio-chemical properties (Mahaffey 1990). It is non-biodegradable in nature thus, its concentration is increasing continuously in the environment and became hazardous. Lead is highly poisonous metal and severely affects child growth and adults. It caused the damage of organ system. The lead toxicity has been affected even at low level to the children more than adults because the organ system in children is too delicate. Prolong exposure of lead cause behavioral problem as learning disability, low IQ level etc(Rubin & Strayer,2008). Lead is also responsible for kidney and brain damage, results in death also. Led also causes anemia, male and female infertility and blood disorder found (Sokol & Berman, 1991).

Lead is broadly dispersed toxic heavy metals found in many ores including anglesite, cerrosite and galena, (Ensafi et al., 2009). Lead is mainly used in batteries, cable sheath, lead plumbing, glazed pottery. It is also used in petrol as antiknock compound. Lead solder used in tin cans and lead based paints (Sharma and Agrawal, 2009). Lead is simply absorbed into the body through ingestion, inhalation and skin and cause many fatal diseases including dysfunction of renal, blood and neurological system (Saritha et al., 2014). Symptoms of severe lead poisoning in man are severe defects in the kidney, brain, liver, reproductive system, central nervous system and cause death [Steenland and Boffetta, 2000). The trace level of lead could be determined by various analytical methods using many organic and inorganic reagents.

Chromium

Chromium with atomic number 24 the most important toxic heavy metal of transition group element. Chromium is found in various valences ranges from +2 to +6. Chromium metal is abundantly distributed in earth crust. It's zero oxidation state is biologically inert and due to industrial activities chromium is converted in +3 and +6 oxidation state. In +2 oxidation state it is found in combined state with halides, oxides and sulphides which unstable and immediately converted into +3 oxidation state when reacts with air (Shekhawat et al.,2015).

Chromium with their different forms get absorbed in body through various ways, respiratory, dermal and oral pathways. Cr (IV) is more absorbed than Cr (III). The concentration of Cr (IV) found in excess in the liver, kidney and bones due to it's easily penetration property (Yamaguchi et al., 1983; Edel and Sabbioni, 1985; NTP, 2007). In human beings it causes oral cancer, ulcer, tissue damage, kidney failure and event it is lethal (Beaumont et al., 2008). In animals, various types of cancers such as skin, digestive system and reproductive organs cancers due to various forms of chromium have been seen (Costa and Klein, 2006). The trace level of chromium could be determined by various analytical methods using many organic and inorganic reagents.

Mercury

Mercury is well known disastrous and highly poisonous heavy metal. Mercury is obtains in different forms like inorganic and organic mercury. In the category of inorganic mercury, it is found in metallic as well as vapor form (Hg^0), mercurous (Hg^{2+}) and mercuric (Hg^+) salts. The organic mercury in which mercury is bonded with carbon atom of organic compounds. These all forms of mercury are very important. The vapor form of elemental mercury is breath in and absorbed via phelgm membranes and pulmonary organs and changes into other forms by oxidation process. Some amount of organic mercury is deposited in the brain.

Mercury salts are stable than organic mercury, insoluble and rarely absorbed. The different forms of mercury affect human body in various ways. Primarily it affects brain. +1 and +2 oxidation state of mercury salts severely affect the inner wall of gut and damage kidney (Berlin et al.,2007). The doses, exposure rate and timing decide the effect of mercury with various forms (Robin and Bernhoft 2012).

Mercury is one and only most harmful heavy metal in the earth, found in nature at low and ultra-trace amounts in the +1 and +2 oxidation states in environment. It is generally obtained in free in nature and mainly found as cinnabar ore. Anthropogenic activities are responsible for mercury, which is become extensive into the environment mainly (Martinis et al., 2009) in the form of metallic, inorganic and organic compounds through various industries like pulp, paper, cellulose and electrical, plastic industries, and pharma industries etc. Mercury is used in fungicides and pesticides which also mix mercury to the environment (Ahmad and Alam, 2003). Mercury is used in electrical gazettes, fluorescent light bulbs and mercury lamps. Its ease in amalgamating with gold is used in the recovery of gold from its ore. Mercury amalgam is used in dental fillings (Kaiser 2000; Holmes et al., 2009; Leermakers et al., 2005). Mercury is found as organic mercury compounds are more toxic than inorganic mercury. Indications of mercury (methyl mercury) poisoning cause's immediate neurological disorder particularly hearing loss, brain deterioration, language disorder, impaired sight, hearing dysfunction and autism (Gopal 2003). "Minimata disease" is one of the examples of acute poisoning of mercury which causes mental disturbance, loss of hearing, degeneration of brain etc. (Venugopal and Lucky, 1978). According to "World Health Organization" (WHO) the permissible bound for mercury in drinking water is restricted to 1 µg L^{-1} (Ebdon et al., 2002). The trace level of mercury could be determined by various analytical methods using many organic and inorganic reagents.

Figure 1. shows the adverse effects of toxic metals in human body.

Figure 1.

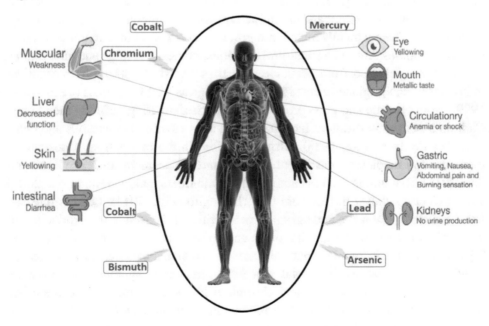

SOURCES OF HEAVY METALS AS POLLUTANTS FOR GROUNDWATER

The common categories of source of heavy metals are point and nonpoint sources. Point sources are identifiable but nonpoint sources cannot be identified easily. The main sources of origin of heavy metal which can contaminate groundwater through naturally as well as manmade, described as follows;

Natural Resources

Heavy metals are found in various form in the nature due to weathering of rocks, volcanic eruption, leaching to the groundwater and other water bodies (Bagul et al., 2015). Mining activities are responsible for reaching heavy metal waste into the natural water (Liu et al., 2008).

Manmade Sources

Human beings are the most responsible factor for spreading heavy metals as contaminant in the environment. Through mining activities low number of heavy metals released and huge amount is released by open fires. Due to enhancement of industries, metal extractions and mining activities are also increasing simultaneously. Consequently, heavy metals mixed into groundwater. Traces of heavy metals enter in to water bodies through agricultural activities, domestic sewage and auto drains.

Arsenic is released from pesticide industries (ATSDR 2000), pharmaceutical industries which produces drugs for human beings as well as animals (Techouwou 1999), from ceramic and glass producing industries, smelting, refining metal ores. Cadmium is used in different industries as in alloys synthesis, batteries and color pigments (Wilson et al., 1988). Bismuth is used in the production of cosmetics, pigments and medicines, casting of printing and replacement for lead (Kean and Sam 2011). Bismuth is used as catalyst for acrylic fibers making (Hammond 2004) and as electro catalyst in CO from CO_2 (Dimeglio et al., 2013). Lead is released from industrial, domestic and agricultural activities. It is used in the production of ammunitions, metallic things like pipes and solders, batteries production (Gabby 2006). Chromium is found via naturally as well as manmade processes. It is released heavily from industries like metal processing, tanneries, synthesis of chromate, welding of steel, ferrochrome and chromium pigment synthesis. The main use of mercury is in electrical industry for making switches, batteries, thermostats, in pharmaceutical industries for making dental amalgams. The mercury is also discharged from other industrial activities where it is used in preparation of caustic soda, in nuclear reactor, as solvent for precious metals, as antifungal as preservatives of medicinal products (Techounwou 2003).

Heavy Metal's Effect in Groundwater and its Toxicity as a Global Challenge

Arsenic was identified 768 hazardous waste sites out of 1300 sites and declared by U.S. EPA in the national priority list. In recent report Arsenic is found at high concentration level in Bangladesh, Thailand, Taiwan, China, Mexico, Argentina, Waste Bengal, Hungary etc. in drinking water through groundwater and many health-related disorders have been seen as diabetes, cancers, circulatory system damage, neurological and hematological disorders (ATSDR 2002, Techounwou 1999, Techounwou 2004). Cadmium is main content of cigarettes and enters in environment through smoking and many other ways even in batteries also it is obtained and recently the use of batteries has been increased but due to environmental concern its profitable usage was diminished in well-established countries. In U.S. the daily consumption of cadmium is 0.4µg/kg/day (EPA 2006). It is linked with limited entry of effluents from plating works and restricted in many countries. Cadmium burden is measured in blood and urine level, is found very high in cigarette smoking persons, medium in earlier smokers and minimum in nonsmokers, studied in U.S. population, proved dangerous for environmental health (Becker et al., 2002, Mannino et al., 2004). The safe level of Chromium 5µg/m^3 has been established by OSHA (Occupational Safety and Health Administration) for an 8 hr time bound average, this level has found as carcinogenic risk (OSHA 2006). Generally, atmospheric level should be 1-100ng/cm^3. But more than range Chromium cause disorder of organ systems. Cr toxicity, mainly inhaled through drinking water means groundwater pollution in river and lake (Jacobs and Testa 2005). Lead is used in many industries with estimated value 1.52 million metric tons in United States in year 2004. 83 percent lead is used in battery industry and 3.5% in ammunition industry, 2.6% in paint, pigments glass and chemicals. In a study NHANES (National Health and Nutrition Examination survey) found lead in blood in U.S. community and assessed by age, income, gender and industrialization (Pirkle et al., 1994). The results revealed that since 1970 the lead level in blood is increased more in children(>10µg/dL). Hence U.S is facing lead poisoning as pediatric health problem today (CDC 1991). In many countries bismuth is found as co product of metal ores processing as zinc, lead, copper etc. But in Bolivia and China bismuth is produced as major products via mining activities. An estimated value 320,000 tons of bismuth is reserved in all over the world. In year 2018, 16,000 tons of bismuth has been produced. China is the most leading producer of refined bismuth with 79.9% of the total population of the world. (Runming and Hongzhe 2019). In 18th and 19th century the emperor of unify China was died in

"Mad Hatter diseases which was by mercury poisoning (Waldron 1983). In 1950s Mercury poisoning was due to industrial spill in Minamata and Niigat Japan and popular as "Minamata Disease" (Hunter et al., 1940). The poisoning of mercury in rural area of Iraq in 1972 due to use of mercury-based fungicides (Engler 1985). In current study, it is revealed that mercury present 6.0% in skin lightening products (Hamann et al., 2014) and 47% of total products found in Somalia with mercury (Adawe and Oberg 2013). The long term effect of mercury has been seen in California Gold mine activities and eating habit of mercury laden fish increased the mercury in blood level of human beings (Nunes eta l., 2014, Rodriguez et al., 2014).

CONCLUSION

Proposed chapter based on the description of the main heavy metals, its exposure and effect of their toxicity in human as well as animals. The heavy metals severely affect the organ system damage in the form of cancers of different organs. The sources, from which these toxic heavy metals have been originated, naturally as well as due to human activities are explained. Various industries, mining activities and other ways are responsible for discharging of heavy metals to the atmosphere and contaminate because of severe toxicity. These heavy metals are responsible for adverse effects in animal as well as animal kingdom and arises many health issues due to more than tolerance limit values of heavy metals. Mainly carcinogenic effects of heavy metals found in different organs such as hepatic, renal, brain, heart etc. The global contact of toxic major heavy metals has been successfully described here. The world -wide reports of various organizations as WHO and UNICEF has been used for the showing the global data. Mainly, this review involves the update of heavy metals responsible for intercellular and microbial alterations. Many developed countries taking protective measures for avoiding huge consumption of heavy metals containing goods by a large population in the world. It is essential to taking actions by developing and ill developed countries.

ACKNOWLEDGMENT

Authors do not have any conflict of interest.

REFERENCES

Adawe, A., & Oberg, C. (2013). Skin-lightening practices and mercury exposure in the Somali community. *Minnesota Medicine*, *96*(7), 48–49. PMID:24133891

Ahmad, M. J., & Alam, M. S. (2003). A rapid spectrometric method for the determination of mercury in environmental biological, soil and plant samples using diphenylthiocarbazone. *Spectroscopy (Springfield, Or.)*, *17*, 45–52.

Ali, H., & Khan, E. (2018). Bioaccumulation of non-essential hazardous heavy metals and metalloids in freshwater fish. Risk to human health. *Environmental Chemistry Letters*, *16*(3), 903–917. doi:10.100710311-018-0734-7

Ali, H., Khan, E., & Sajad, M. A. (2013). Phytoremediation of heavy metals-concepts and applications. *Chemosphere*, *91*(7), 869–881. doi:10.1016/j.chemosphere.2013.01.075 PMID:23466085

Armah, F. A., Quansah, R., & Luginaah, I. (2014). Agency for Toxic Substances and Disease Registry (ATSDR). Toxicological Profile for Arsenic. *International Scholarly Research Notices*, 1–37. doi:10.1155/2014/252148

Centers for Disease Control. (1991). *Preventing Lead Poisoning in Young children*. Centers for Disease Control.

Bagul, V. R., Shinde, D. N., Chavan, R. P., Patil, C. L., & Pawar, R. K. (2015). New perspective on heavy metal pollution of water. *Journal of Chemical and Pharmaceutical Research*, *7*(12), 700–705.

Bawaskar, H. S., & Bawaskar, P. H. (2010). Chronic renal failure associated with heavy metal contamination of drinking water: A clinical report from a small village in Maharashtra. *Clinical Toxicology (Philadelphia, PA)*, *48*(7), 768–768. doi:10.31 09/15563650.2010.497763 PMID:20615151

Beaumont, J. J., Sedman, R. M., Reynolds, S. D., Sherman, C. D., Li, L. H., Howd, R. A., Sandy, M. S., Zeise, L., & Alexeeff, G. V. (2008). Cancer mortality in a Chinese population exposed to hexavalent chromium in drinking water. *Epidem*, *19*(1), 12–23. doi:10.1097/EDE.0b013e31815cea4c PMID:18091413

Becker, K., Kaus, S., Krause, C., Lepom, P., Schulz, C., Seiwert, M., & Seifert, B. (2002). German Environmental Survey (1998) (GerES III): Environmental pollutants in blood of the German population. *International Journal of Hygiene and Environmental Health*, *205*(4), 297–308. doi:10.1078/1438-4639-00155 PMID:12068749

Berlin, M., Zalups, R. K., & Fowler, B. A. (2007). Mercury. IN Handbook on the Toxicology of Metals. Elsevier. doi:10.1016/B978-012369413-3/50088-4

Busev, A. I., Tiptsova, V. G., & Ivanov, M. V. (1981). *Analytical Chemistry of Rare Elements*. Rusian Edn.

Centeno, J. A., Gray, M. A., Mullick, F. G., Tchounwou, P. B., & Tseng, C. (2005). Arsenic in drinking water andhealth issues. In T. A. Moore, A. Black, J. A. Centeno, J. S. Harding, & D. A. Trumm (Eds.), *Metal Contaminants in New Zealand* (pp. 195–219). Resolution Press.

Centeno, J. A., Tchounwou, P. B., Patlolla, A. K., Mullick, F. G., Murakat, L., Meza, E., Gibb, H., Longfellow, D., & Yedjou, C. G. (2005). Environmental pathology and health effects of arsenic poisoning: acritical review. In R. Naidu, E. Smith, J. Smith, & P. Bhattacharya (Eds.), *Managing Arsenic Inthe Environment: From Soil to Human Health* (pp. 311–327). CSIRO Publishing Corp.

Costa, M., & Klein, C. B. (2006). Toxicity and carcinogenicity of chromium compounds in humans. *Critical Reviews in Toxicology*, *36*(2), 155–163. doi:10.1080/10408440500534032 PMID:16736941

Dai, L., & Wang, L., Li. (2018). Multivariate geostatistical analysis and source identification of heavy metals in thesediment of Poyang Lake in China. *Science of EeTotalEnvironment*, *621*, 1433–1444. PMID:29056381

Dara, S. S. (1997). Environmental Chemistry and Pollution Control. S. Chand & Company Ltd.

Devi, R., Alemayehu, E., Singh, V., Kumar, A., & Mengistie, E. (2008). Removal of fluoride, arsenic and coli form bacteria by modified homemade filter media from drinking water. *Bioresource Technology*, *99*, 2269–2274.

DiMeglio, J. L., & Rosenthal, J. (2013). Selective conversion of CO2 to CO with high efficiency using an bismuth-based electrocatalyst. *Journal of the American Chemical Society*, *135*(24), 8798–8801.

Duffus, J. H. (2002). Heavy metals-a meaningless term? *Pure and Applied Chemistry*, *74*(5), 793–807. doi:10.1351/pac200274050793

Ebdon, L., Foulkes, M. E., Roux, S. L., & Munoz-Olivas, R. (2002). Cold vapour atomic fluorescence spectrometry and gas chromatography-pyrolysis-atomic fluorescence for routine determination of total and organometallic mercury in food samples. *Analyst (London)*, *127*(8), 1108–1114. doi:10.1039/B202927H PMID:12195954

Edel, J., & Sabbioni, E. (1985). Pathways of Cr (III) and Cr (VI) in the rat after intra tracheal administration. *Human Toxicology*, *4*(4), 409–416. doi:10.1177/096032718500400407 PMID:4018821

Edelstein, M., & Ben-Hur, M. (2018). Heavy metals and metalloids:sources, risks and strategies to reduce their accumulation inhorticultural crops. *Scientia Horticulturae*, *234*, 431–444. doi:10.1016/j.scienta.2017.12.039

Engler, R. (1985). Technology out of control. *Nation (New York, N.Y.)*, *240*(16), 488–500.

Ensafi Ali, A., Katiraei Far, A., & Meghdadi, S. (2009). Highly selective optical-sensing film for lead(II) determination in water samples. *Journal of Hazardous Materials*, *172*(2-3), 1069–1075. doi:10.1016/j.jhazmat.2009.07.112 PMID:19709813

Frederick, W. O. (1979). *Toxicity of heavy metals in the environment*. Part I & II Marcel Dekker, Inc.

Gabby, P. N. (2003). Lead. In *Environmental Defense "Alternatives to Lead-Acid Starter Batteries."* Pollution Prevention Fact Sheet. Available at http://www.cleancarcampaign.org/FactSheet_BatteryAlts.pdf

Gabby, P. N. (2006). Lead. In *Mineral Commodity Summaries* (pp. 92–93). U.S. Geological Survey. Available https://minerals.usgs.gov/minerals/pubs/commodity/lead/lead_mcs05.pdf

Gay & Proop. (1993). *Aspects of river pollution*. Butterworth's Scientific Publication.

Gobe, G., & Crane, D. (2010). Mitochondria, reactive oxygen species and cadmium toxicity in the kidney. *Toxicology Letters*, *198*(1), 49–55. doi:10.1016/j.toxlet.2010.04.013 PMID:20417263

Gopal, K. V. (2003). Neurotoxic effect of mercury on auditory cortex networks growing on microelectrode arrays: A preliminary analysis. *Neurotoxicology and Teratology*, *25*(1), 69–76. doi:10.1016/S0892-0362(02)00321-5 PMID:12633738

Hamann, C.R., Boonchai, W., Wen, L., Sakanashi, E.N., Chu, C.Y. & Hamann, K. (2014). *Spectrometric analysis of mercury content in 549 skin-lightening products: Is mercury toxicity a hidden global health hazard?* Academic Press.

Hawkes, S. J. (1997). What is a heavy metal? *Journal of Chemical Education*, *74*(11), 1374. doi:10.1021/ed074p1374

Hill, S. J. (1997). Speciation of trace metals in the environment. *Chemical Society Reviews*, *26*(4), 291–298. doi:10.1039/cs9972600291

Holmes, P., James, K A F., & Levy, L. S. (2009). Is low-level environmental mercury exposure of concern to human health? *The Science of the Total Environment*, *408*(2), 171–182. doi:10.1016/j.scitotenv.2009.09.043 PMID:19850321

Hunter, D., Bomford, R.R., & Russell, D.S. (1940). *Poisoning by methylmercury compounds*. Academic Press.

Hutson, J. C. (2005). Effects of Bismuth Citrate on the Viability and Function of Leydig Cells and Testicular Macrophages. *Journal of Applied Toxicology*, *25*(3), 234–238. doi:10.1002/jat.1060 PMID:15856528

International Agency for Research on Cancer (IARC). (2003). Monographs – Cadmium. Its toxicopathologic implications for public health. *Environmental Toxicology*, *18*, 149–175. PMID:12740802

Jafari, A., Mirhossaini, H., Kamareii, B., & Dehestani, S. (2008). Physicochemical Analysis of Drinking Water in Kohdasht City Lorestan, Iran. *Asian Journal of Applied Sciences*, *1*(1), 87–92. doi:10.3923/ajaps.2008.87.92

Kaiser, J. (2000). Toxicology-mercury report backs strict rules. *Science*, *289*(5478), 371–372. doi:10.1126cience.289.5478.371a PMID:10939938

Kean & Sam. (2011). *The Disappearing Spoon (and other true tales of madness, love, and the history of the world from the Periodic Table of Elements)*. Back Bay Books.

Shekhawat, K., Chatterjee, S., & Joshi, B. (2015). Chromium Toxicity and its Health Hazards. *International Journal of Advanced Research*, *3*(7), 167–172.

Leermakers, M., Baeyens, W., Quevauviller, P., & Horvat, M. (2005). Mercury in environmental samples: Speciation, artifacts and validation. *Trac-Trend. Analytical Chemistry*, *24*, 383–393.

Lide, D. (1992). *'CRC Handbook of Chemistry and Physics* (73rd ed.). CRC Press.

Liu, H., Li, L., Yin, C., & Shan, B. (2008). Fraction distribution and risk assessment of heavy metals in sediments of Moshui Lake. *Journal of Environmental Sciences (China)*, *20*(4), 390–397. doi:10.1016/S1001-0742(08)62069-0 PMID:18575121

Loiseau, P., Henry, P., Jallon, P., & Legroux, M. (1976). Iatro- genic Myoclonic Encephalopathies Caused by Bismuth Salts. *Journal of the Neurological Sciences*, *27*(2), 133–143. doi:10.1016/0022-510X(76)90056-3 PMID:1249582

Lokeshwari, H., & Chandrappa, G. T. (2006). Impact of heavy metal contamination of Bellandur Lake on soil and cultivated vegetation. *Current Science*, *91*(5), 584.

Mahaffey, K. R. (1990). Environmental lead toxicity: Nutrition as a componentof intervention. *Environmental Health Perspectives*, *89*, 75–78. doi:10.1289/ehp.908975 PMID:2088758

Mahananda, H. B., Mahanand, M. R., & Mohanty, B. P. (2005). Studies on the physicochemical and biological parameters of fresh water pond water ecosystem as an indicator of water pollution. *Ecol. Env. And Cons.*, *11*(3-4), 537–541.

Mannino, D.M., Holguin, F., Greves, H.M., Savage-Brown, A., Stock, A.L. & Jones, R.L. (2004). *Urinary cadmium levels predict lower lung function in current and former smokers: Data from the Third National Health and Nutrition Examination Survey*. Academic Press.

Martinis, E. M., Bertón, P., Olsina, R. A., Altamirano, J. C., & Wuilloud, R. G. (2009). Trace mercury determination in drinking and natural water samples by room temperature ionic liquid based-preconcentration and flow injection-cold vapor atomic absorption spectrometry. *Journal of Hazardous Materials*, *167*(1-3), 475–481. doi:10.1016/j.jhazmat.2009.01.007 PMID:19233554

Med, J. Am., Assoc. (1994). Blood lead levels in the United States. *The National Health and Nutrition Examination Surveys*, *272*, 284–291. PMID:8028141

Milway, C. P. (1969). Education in large lakes and impounds. *Proc. Upplasale Symp. DECO.*

Nevondo, T.S., & Cloete, T.E. (1999). *Bacterial and chemical quality of water in Dertig village settlement water SA*. Academic Press.

NTP. (2007). Technical Report on the Toxicity Study of Sodium Dichromate Dihydrate Administered in Drinking Water to Male and Female F344/N Rats and B6C3F1 Mice and Male BALB/c and am3 - C57BL/6 Mice. National Toxicology Program Toxicity Report Series.

Nunes, E., Cavaco, A., & Carvalho, C. (2014). Children's health risk and benefits of fish consumption: Risk indices based on a diet diary follow-up of two weeks. *Journal of Toxicology and Environmental Health. Part A.*, *77*(1-3), 103–114. doi: 10.1080/15287394.2014.866926 PMID:24555651

Ozimek, T. (1975). Field experiment on the effect of municipal sewage on macrophytes and epifauna in the lake littoral. *Bull. Acad. Pol. Sc. Clii*, *23*, 445–447.

Patil, P. R., Badgujar, S. R., & Wark, A. M. (2001). Evolution of groundwater quality in Ganesh Colony area of Jalgaon City, Maharashtra, India. *Oriental Journal of Chemistry*, *17*(2), 283.

Debels, P., Ricardofigueroaoberto, U. R. B., & Niel, X. (2005). Evaluation of Water Quality in the Chillán River (Central Chile) Using Physicochemical Parameters and a Modified Water Quality Index. *Environmental Monitoring and Assessment*, *110*(1-3), 301–322. doi:10.100710661-005-8064-1 PMID:16308794

Piecznska, E., Usikorna, & Olimak, T. (1975). The influence of domestic sewage on the littoral oflakes. *Polskie Archiwum Hydrobiologii*, *22*, 141–146.

Pistofidis, N., Vourlias, G., Konidaris, S., Pavlidou, E., Stergiou, A., & Stergioudis, G. (2007, February). The effect of bismuth on the structure of zinc hot-dip galvanized coating. *Materials Letters*, *61*(4-5), 994–997. doi:10.1016/j.matlet.2006.06.029

Rodríguez Martín-Doimeadios, R. C., Berzas Nevado, J. J., Guzmán Bernardo, F. J., Jiménez Moreno, M., Arrifano, G. P. F., Herculano, A. M., do Nascimento, J. L. M., & Crespo-López, M. E. (2014, March 5). Comparative study of mercury speciation in commercial fishes of the Brazilian Amazon. *Environmental Science and Pollution Research International*. Advance online publication. doi:10.100711356-014-2680-7 PMID:24590602

Rubin, R., & Strayer, D. S. (Eds.). (2008). *Environmental and Nutritional pathology. Rubins pathology; Clinico pathologic Foundations of Medicine* (5th ed.). LippincotWilliams & Wilkins.

Saritha, B., Giri, A., & Reddy, T. S. (2014). Direct spectrophotometric determination of Pb (II) in alloy, biological and water samples using 5-bromo-2-hydroxyl -3-methoxybenzaldehyde-4-hydroxy benzoichydrazone. *Journal of Chemical and Pharmaceutical Research*, *6*(7), 1571–1576.

Sharma, R. K., Agrawal, M., & Marshall, F. M. (2009). Heavy Metals in Vegetables Collected from Production and Market Sites of a Tropical Urban Area of India. *Food and Chemical Toxicology*, *47*(3), 583–591. doi:10.1016/j.fct.2008.12.016 PMID:19138719

Shemirani, F., Baghdadi, M., Ramezani, M., & Jamali, M. R. (2005). Determination of ultra trace amounts of bismuth in biological and water samples by electrothermal atomic absorption spectrometry (ET-AAS) after cloud point extraction. *Analytica Chimica Acta*, *534*(1), 163–169. doi:10.1016/j.aca.2004.06.036

Smith, A., Goycolea, M., Haque, R., & Bigs, M. L. (1998). Marked increase in bladder and lung cancer mortality in a region of northern Chile due to arsenic in drinking water. *American Journal of Epidemiology*, *147*(7), 660–669. doi:10.1093/oxfordjournals.aje.a009507 PMID:9554605

Sokol, R. Z., & Berman, N. (1991). The effect of age of exposure on lead-inducedtesticular toxicity. *Toxicology*, *69*(3), 269–278. doi:10.1016/0300-483X(91)90186-5 PMID:1949051

Steenland, K., & Boffetta, P. (2000). Lead and cancer in humans: Where are we now. *American Journal of Industrial Medicine*, *38*(3), 295–299. doi:10.1002/1097-0274(200009)38:3<295::AID-AJIM8>3.0.CO;2-L PMID:10940967

Tchounwou, P. B., Centeno, J. A., & Patlolla, A. K. (2004). Arsenic toxicity, mutagenesis and carcinogenesis – a health risk assessment and management approach. *Molecular and Cellular Biochemistry*, *255*(1/2), 47–55. doi:10.1023/B:MCBI.0000007260.32981.b9 PMID:14971645

Tchounwou, P. B., Wilson, B., & Ishaque, A. (1999). Important considerations in the development of public health advisories for arsenic and arsenic-containing compounds in drinking water. *Reviews on Environmental Health*, *14*(4), 211–229. doi:10.1515/REVEH.1999.14.4.211 PMID:10746734

Tchounwou, P. B., Wilson, B., & Ishaque, A. (2000). *Important considerations in the development of public TP-92/09. Georgia*. Center for Disease Control.

Trivedi, R. K. (1990). Physicochemical characteristic and Phytoplankton of the river Panchganga near Kolhapur, Maharashtra. In K. Trivedi (Ed.), *River pollution on India* (pp. 159–178). Ashish Publishing House.

UNDP (United Nations Development Programme). (2006). *Human Development Report 2006. Beyond scarcity Power, Povertyh and the global water crises*. Available at http//hdr.undp.org/hdr2006/

UNICEF. (2008). *UNICEF Hnad book on Water Quality*. Available at: www.uniceforg/wes/files/WQ_Handbook_final_signed_16_April_2008.

UNICEF. (2011). *Official Homepage of UNICEF Promotion of household water treatment and safe storage m UNICEF wash programmes 2011*. http.www.unicef.org

Venugopal, B., & Lucky, T. D. (1978). *Metal Toxicity in Mammals*. Plenum Press.

Veslind, P. J. (1993). '·National Geographic Senior Writer. *National Geographic*, *5*, 183.

Vollenweidre, R. A. (1986). *Scientific fundamental of the eutrophication of lakes and flowing waters v-rith special reference to nitrogen and phosphorus as factoring eutrophication*. OECD.

Von Ehrenstein, O. S., GuhaMazumder, D. N., Hira-Smith, M., Ghosh, N., Yuan, Y., Windham, G., Ghosh, A., Haque, R., Lahiri, S., Kalman, D., Das, S., & Smith, A. H. (2006). Pregnancy outcomes, infant mortality, and arsenic in drinking water in west Bengal, India. *American Journal of Epidemiology, 163*(7), 662–669. doi:10.1093/aje/kwj089 PMID:16524957

Waldron, H. A. (1983). Did the Mad Hatter have mercury poisoning? *British Medical Journal (Clinical Research Ed.), 287*(6409), 1961. doi:10.1136/bmj.287.6409.1961 PMID:6418283

WHO. (2004). *Guidelines for Drinking-Water Quality, Recommendations.* WHO.

Wilson, D. N. (1988). Cadmium - market trends and influences. *Proceedings of the 6th International Cadmium Conference*, 9-16.

Yamaguchi, S., Sano, K., & Shimojo, N. (1983). On the biological half-time of hexavalent chromium in rats. *Industrial Health, 21*(1), 25–34. doi:10.2486/indhealth.21.25 PMID:6841147

Zaman, C.L. (2002). A Nested Case control study of Methanoglobinemia risk factor in children of Transilvania Romania. *Env. Health Perspt., 110*(B).

Chapter 8
Study of Behavioral Changes and Heart Rate Variability Through Speech Signal Analysis in COVID–19 Patients

Anjali Deshpande
M. M. College of Technology, Raipur, India

Kavita Thakur
RSU, India

Prafulla Vyas
Disha College, India

G. R. Sinha
Ⓘ https://orcid.org/0000-0003-2384-4591
Myanmar Institute of Information Technology, Mandalay, Myanmar

ABSTRACT

This work shows the behavioral and heart condition monitoring of the patients during the COVID-19 infection. As the COVID-19 infection spreads very easily through contact, this work introduces a noninvasive technique to monitor such patients. The heart condition monitoring can be done through the analysis of acoustical cardiogram (ACG) as well as the behavioral changes observed through the Formant analysis. The speech of the patient is recorded, digitized, and its analysis is done using the PRAAT software. The required information from the speech samples is extracted and subjected to the analysis. The spectrogram of each utterance is plotted, and its first and second formants are analysed to form the vowel triangle. These vowel triangle provides behavioral monitoring. The monitoring of heart condition can be done using ACG. The Formant analysis of utterance of 12 Hindi consonants provides the assessment technique of the patient heart condition.

DOI: 10.4018/978-1-7998-9831-3.ch008

INTRODUCTION

Since speech reflects essential information regarding human emotion, it can be extracted in the form of speech features from the recorded speech samples by applying various speech processing techniques. Multiple analysis approaches are applied to these retrieved speech features. Acoustic vowel triangle analysis can be used to detect and predict a patient's emotions and behavior. Recently, special attention has been brought to speech as a modality to automatically deduct information on human emotions and behavioral prediction (A. Deshpande et.al.,2014; G.Fant, 1960; J.Benesty,2008). Emotion detection and classification play an essential role in user-friendly human-machine interaction. Human speech is influenced by a variety of factors, including posture. As a result, a human can be said to communicate using his breathing system, bodily muscles, and head. Speech is produced as a result of physical and vocal efforts. Speech processing techniques are being developed to provide a non-invasive, less expensive, and speedier method for assessing and diagnosing physiological conditions and behavioral abnormalities during COVID-19 infection.

The required information from the speech samples is extracted and subjected to the analysis. The spectrogram of each utterance is plotted and its first and second formants are analyzed to form the vowel triangle (Berstein A. et.al.,1985; E. Dmitrity et.al., 2009, L.Rabiner et.al., 1978; R.F. Orlikoff et.al., 1989). Various parameters like Euclidean distance, area of the vowel triangle, length of the base of the triangle, size of the vowel triangle, inclination of the triangle is used to predict emotional state of the persons. The stress, fear, anger, happiness, irritation is some of the common emotions which vary day by day in the COVID patients. Speech samples of some COVID patients has been recorded regularly for fourteen days daily and subjected to speech signal analysis. From these recorded speech samples, the F1 and F2 formants of the three particular Hindi vowels "aa", "ee" and "oo" have been determined to plot their vowel triangles (L.Rabiner et.al., 1978; R.F. Orlikoff et.al., 1989). These vowel triangles provide the behavioral information of patients.

Medical experts usually use an electrocardiogram (ECG) to monitor the heart condition. This ECG has various important parameters like heart rate, RR-duration or RR-cycle, PQ, QR, PQR, QRS duration, which are used to predict various heart diseases (K. Charles Friedberg,1966). The pattern of the various peaks is also used to diagnose many heart diseases. The patient's heart condition can be monitored using an acoustical cardiogram (ACG). Acoustical cardiogram (ACG) is a tool that can be an alternative to an electrocardiogram (ECG) for some cases. The speech signal processing techniques are used to extract the required information from the recorded speech sample of the COVID patients. The Formant analysis of utterance of twelve Hindi consonants' ka', 'kha', 'ga', 'gha', 'anga', 'cha', 'chha', 'ja', 'jha', 'yan', 'ta', 'tha' is used to determine the acoustical-cardiogram. Almost all heart parameters can be obtained using an acoustical cardiogram (ACG), in addition to those calculated using a regular electrocardiogram (ECG). This acoustical cardiogram (ACG) is used to determine the patient's cardiac status (A. Deshpande et.al.,2014; Nader Salari,2020). ACG can be used to forecast a variety of cardiac problems.

The autonomic nervous system regulates heart rate variability (HRV), a physiological trait or statistic (ANS). It is used to assess overall human well-being in various therapeutic contexts. Because the ANS reacts swiftly to changes in physiological conditions, it may provide signals, such as HRV, that warn of an imminent cytokine storm before another pathological testing can. Early detection of clinical deterioration and earlier therapeutic interventions are likely to improve the chances of favorable results (Bernard T. et.al., 1967; D.Kaliyaperumal et.al., 2021; Robert Drury et.al.,2021; V. Gemignani et.al., 2008)Further, this method can be developed and implemented in rural areas and in isolation wards where laboratory setups are unavailable. The monitoring of the physiological condition of the human heart can be possible using speech signal processing techniques. Speech samples of some COVID 19 patients has been regularly recorded for their infection period. Each sample contains utterances of 52 Hindi vowels and consonants. After noise removal from each sample, its Formant analysis has been carried out to determine its first and second formant. These formants are then used to plot vowel triangle and Acoustical- Cardiogram (ACG). This Acoustical - cardiogram analysis is used to determine the Heart Rate Variability of the patient (A.Deshpande et.al.,2014).

RELATED WORK

At the moment, the most effective strategies for avoiding or minimizing COVID-19 transmission in the community are prevention, precaution, and vaccination. However, monitoring such individuals' health becomes highly perilous even for medical specialists and experts. The majority of current procedures for monitoring the health of COVID-19 patients are intrusive, harmful, expensive, time-consuming, and require a quality laboratory setup. In this experiment, changes in speech formants were associated with the various stages of COVID-19 infection. Speech processing techniques are being developed to provide a non-invasive, low-cost, and straightforward tool for screening and diagnosing physiological problems in patients with COVID-19 infection, as well as monitoring behavioral changes (Bernard T. et.al., 1967).

COVID 19 can spread via personal contact, droplet, blood, mother-to-child, and animal-to-human transmission. COVID-19 infection can cause mild to severe respiratory problems and even death. Some infected people have no symptoms or no fever. Most infected patients have mild to severe illnesses and recover without hospitalization. COVID-19 includes fever, dry cough, fatigue, and loss of taste and smell. Other symptoms include aches and pains, sore throat, diarrhea, conjunctivitis, headache, and loss of taste or smell. Symptoms include difficulty breathing, chest pain, headache, and lack of speech or movement. Patients with moderate or no symptoms, on the other hand, can be healed with correct medicine and home isolation. For asymptomatic patients, recovery from the illness takes 5–6 days, although it might take up to 14 days in some situations. Patients who exhibit the following symptoms should get medical help right away, or they risk developing significant respiratory problems:

- rapid or shallow breathing
- chest pain or discomfort
- blue or discolored lips, nails, or skin
- a high fever
- low blood pressure
- a weak pulse

COVID-19 was once thought to be a respiratory illness, but it has since been found to damage the heart, kidneys, ANS, and other body parts. Experts say a severe COVID-19 infection can induce myocarditis or heart muscle inflammation. It's vital since severe myocarditis can be fatal. COVID-19 is a mild sickness treated at home or in a hospital. Around 20% of infected patients have severe symptoms and consequences, increasing their risk of hospitalization and, in extreme cases, death. Conditions include heart blockage, coronary artery disease (CAD), cardiomyopathy, obesity, and others that might make COVID 19 symptoms worse. COVID-19 is also more likely to impact people with high blood pressure (hypertension: a common illness affecting the blood vessels and heart). An infected patient with a weak heart or circulatory system may develop the following symptoms -

- Low blood pressure
- Low blood oxygen levels
- Fever-induced heart rate alterations
- Excessive inflammation
- Blood clot risk
- Foam

Overcoming COVID-19 generated cardiac difficulties is difficult for anyone with a healthy heart. However, COVID-19 infection causes more severe issues and can cause mortality in people with heart disease. Second, heart disease is commonly linked to other health conditions like diabetes and obesity. Obesity, for example, increases inflammation, and diabetes increases blood clot risk even without an infection. These pre-existing issues may worsen the effects of COVID-19 on an already strained heart. COVID-19 may cause direct or indirect damage to several organs, including the heart. The immune system can overreact to an infection, causing a "cytokine storm" that floods the body, causing inflammation in the heart. Indirect injury is more common than direct harm. Myocarditis is an inflammation of the heart muscle caused by a coronavirus infection. Right-sided heart failure is caused by fluid accumulating in the liver and kidneys. Swelling and fluid build-up in the legs and abdomen are also side effects. Also, COVID-19 can irritate blood vessel linings, transporting blood and nutrients. That can increase the formation of blood clots, which can attach to blood vessel walls, increasing the risk of heart attack or stroke and reducing blood oxygenation. The cardiac muscle cannot operate due to a lack of oxygen in the circulation.**2.**1 COVID-19 and Respiratory & Heart Diseases.

Many people experience a quick heartbeat or palpitations as a result of the COVID -19 effect. A brief rise in heart rate can be caused by a number of factors, including dehydration. During a fever, it is important to consume plenty of water. A fast or irregular heart beat might cause the following symptoms:

- Rapid or irregular heart beat
- Feeling lightheaded or dizzy
- Discomfort in chest

Post-COVID symptoms include severe weariness, poor stamina, lack of vitamins, thyroid, high blood pressure, and high blood sugar. These symptoms can have several origins.

Type 1 heart attacks are caused by a blood clot blocking any artery in the heart and are uncommon during COVID-19 or after COVID-19 infection. The number of Type 2 heart attacks is going up, which is terrible. Such as a fast heartbeat, low blood oxygen levels, or anemia could cause this: not enough oxygen to reach the heart muscle. During COVID 19, some patients had a high troponin level in their blood, an abnormal EKG, and chest discomfort. These are symptoms of heart tissue damage. A person got sick. Among the long-term effects is damage to the lung and other body parts. You could die as it moves from one lung to another. About 80% of people who have COVID-19 have mild to moderate symptoms due to this. They might have a dry cough, a sore throat, or even pneumonia if they get sick (R.F. Orlikoff,1989).

A lung infection can cause inflamed alveoli. Chest pain, coughing, and shortness of breath are symptoms of pneumonia. Some individuals' breathing issues may become so severe that they necessitate hospitalization with oxygen or a machine. COVID-19 pneumonia usually spreads to both lungs. Shortness of breath, coughing, and other symptoms occur when the lungs' air sacs swell with fluid, decreasing oxygen absorption. While most people recover from pneumonia, COVID-19 pneumonia can be rather dangerous. Even after the illness has passed, lung injuries can cause months-long breathing issues. COVID-19 causes shortness of breath a few days after infection. Some people, however, experience no such symptom. The onset of shortness of breath and abrupt decreases in oxygen saturation may help clinicians recognize COVID-19 from other illnesses. It usually emerges between days 4 and 10. Fever, tiredness, physical discomfort, lethargy, and loss of taste and smell are common symptoms. Other symptoms include:

- 83 to 99 percent of people have a fever.
- coughing: 59–82 percent
- exhaustion: 44 to 70%
- Appetite loss: 40 to 84 percent
- aches and pains in the muscles and body: 11 to 35 percent

Another respiratory system-related illness caused by COVID-19 is Acute Respiratory Distress Syndrome (ARDS). As COVID-19-induced pneumonia progresses, an increasing number of air sacs become clogged with fluid from the lungs' tiny blood veins. Breathing difficulties are a symptom of illness, and they can progress to acute respiratory distress syndrome (ARDS), a type of lung failure. Patients with ARDS frequently lose their ability to breathe independently and may require the assistance of a ventilator to assist in oxygenation of the body. Sepsis is another consequence that may occur in COVID-19 patients with severe instances. It is identified when an infection enters the bloodstream and spreads throughout the body, causing tissue damage. The lungs, heart, and other physiological systems work in unison. Sepsis impairs organ cooperation, and entire organ systems, including the lungs and heart, may begin to shut down sequentially (Bernard T. et.al.,1967).

Psychological Problems Associated with COVID-19

COVID -19 infection causes worry in patients, caregivers, family members, near and dear ones, and healthcare professionals because of the risk of transmission and infective potential. In the social, occupational, and psychological spheres, the government has placed many limitations and taken specific measures to prevent transmission. Fear, nervousness, despair, concern, stress, fear of infecting others, palpitations, chest discomfort, and shortness of breath, among other feelings, contribute to an increase in anxiety in people. In most cases, the mental health word refers to a higher than typical amount of stress or worry. However, during this pandemic, new measures and effects may be implemented, mainly due to quarantine or isolation, disrupting people's everyday activities, habits, and way of life. It causes patients and their dependents to feel lonelier and more depressed. In some circumstances, problematic alcohol consumption, drug use, and self-harm or suicidal behavior are also likely to increase. People who are depressed may experience low mood, weariness, decreased sleep, and appetite, as well as feelings of helplessness, guilt, hopelessness, and a progressive drop in work production. The rapid spread of COVID-19 worldwide has resulted in a significant increase in mental illnesses such as fear, depression, stress, and anxiety, which has become a substantial source of concern. These mental illnesses have been discovered.

HUMAN HEART

The human heart is a muscle pumping station located in the thoracic compartment beneath the sternum in the center of the chest. It circulates blood throughout the body, delivering oxygen and nutrition to all tissues and cells and removing carbon dioxide and other waste products. It comprises four chambers and valves that regulate the blood flow throughout the human body. The atria are two chambers in the top half of the heart, and the ventricles are two chambers in the lower half. The septum is a wall that divides the two halves of the heart.

Figure 1. Standard electrocardiogram peaks

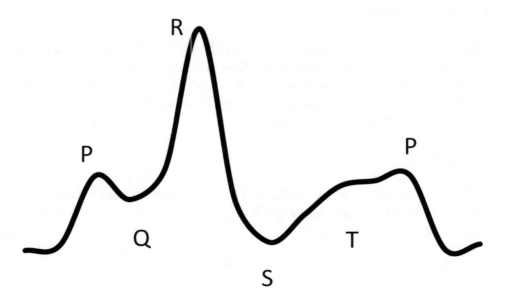

The left atrium receives oxygen-rich blood through arteries, and the right atrium receives oxygen-free blood. The tricuspid valve on the left and the mitral valve on the right make up the atrioventricular valves that separate these chambers. They deliver oxygen-rich blood to all body organs, including the smallest cells. Valves divide the ventricular sections in the same way as the atria. The pulmonary and aortic valves make up the semilunar valves, collectively known as semilunar valves. Any artery obstruction causes a heart attack or injury to the heart muscles. Because the heart is the principal organ in the circulatory system and the blood pumping station, its job of circulating blood and transporting nutrients throughout the body is never-ending. As a result, the heart is a crucial organ whose proper functioning is always necessary. The cardiac cycle ensures that blood is dispersed throughout the body by the heart's blood-pumping process (which comprises one consecutive contraction and expansion of the heart). Each heartbeat produces a consistent electrical activity in the heart. The electrocardiogram can be used to monitor the heart's performance (ECG). Electrodes placed to the outside surface of the skin detect it, and an external device record it. An ECG measures the rate and regularity of heartbeats, chamber size and position, cardiac illness, and the effects of medications or heart-controlling devices like pacemakers. All typical cardiac measurements include the RR-cycle, heart rate, systole and diastole cycles, blood pressure, and pulse pressure. These parameters are calculated using the PR-interval, RR-interval, PQR-duration, QRS complex, ST-segment, P-interval, R-interval, and other key ECG intervals and peaks (A. Deshpande et.al., 2014; K. Charles Friedberg,1966).

Heart Parameters

The RR-cycle, systolic and diastolic cycles, pulse pressure, QRS complex, heart rate, blood pressure, heart rate variability, and other cardiac indicators can all be utilized to determine the physiological status of the heart (K. Charles Friedberg,1966). An electrocardiograph is a critical tool for clinical interpretation since it offers all relevant information about heart function.

- RR-Cycle

The RR cycle is a heart cycle. The ECG is between two R peaks (0.6 to 1 sec). The RR interval is the time between one R wave and the next. In sinus node disorders, RR intervals might be irregular.

- Heart Beat Rate (HBR)

The cardiac cycle is a term used to describe the movement of blood from one heartbeat to the next. The heart rate describes the cycle frequency. One RR-cycle represents one heartbeat. It is calculated by counting RR cycles (60–100 BPM). The RR interval is the period between QRS complexes. Timing two QRS complexes together gives the instantaneous heart rate.

- Blood Pressure (BP)

Blood pressure in the arteries is commonly referred to as arterial blood pressure. It is the pressure placed on the walls of blood arteries by circulating blood. It's one of the most important critical markers. Blood pressure swings between a maximum (systolic) and a lowest (diastolic) pressure with each heartbeat (V. Gemignani et.al., 2008).

- Pulse Pressure

It's the arterial pressure curve throughout a single cardiac cycle. The pulsatile nature of the cardiac output, i.e., the heartbeat, causes the arterial pressure to fluctuate up and down. The interaction of the heart's stroke volume, aorta compliance, and arterial tree resistance to flow determines pulse pressure—the pulse pressure calculated using the difference between the recorded systolic and diastolic pressures.

- Heart Rate Variability

HRV analysis seeks to quantify sinus rhythm variability to assess cardiac autonomic control. Identifying a significant link between the autonomic nervous system and cardiovascular mortality, especially sudden cardiac death, has occurred in the previous two decades (Bernard T. et.al., 1967; D.Kaliyaperumal et.al., 2021; Robert Drury et.al.,2021; V. Gemignani et.al., 2008). A considerable body of research links abnormal heart rate variability (HRV) to death, particularly in arrhythmia-related deaths. HRV has been linked to a worse prognosis following myocardial infarction in several studies (MI or heart attack). As a result, MI survivors routinely use HRV measures to predict future problems and death.

Increased HRV has decreased morbidity and mortality and enhance psychological well-being and quality of life. Heart rate variability, or HRV, is a physiological phenomenon characterized by variations in the time interval between successive heartbeats measured in milliseconds. A typical, healthy heart does not beat uniformly like a metronome; instead, there is continual variance between heartbeats' milliseconds. We are generally unaware of this fluctuation; it is not the same as our pulse rate (beats per minute) rising and falling over our everyday activities. Accurate monitoring of each heartbeat and the period between seconds is required for reliable HRV analysis. HRV is calculated using a variety of methods.

In a typical, healthy scenario, HRV should rise during calming activities like meditation or sleep, when the parasympathetic nervous system takes over. HRV, on the other hand, typically decreases during times of stress, as the sympathetic activity of the body increases to meet the demand. As a result, HRV generally is higher when the heart beats slowly and lower when the heart beats faster, such as during stress or exercise. The HRV level naturally varies daily based on activity and stress levels, such as work-related stress. The natural balance between the two systems can be interrupted if a person is chronically stressed or overworked - physically or psychologically – and the body can become locked in a sympathetically dominated fight state. Even though genetic factors account for around 30% of overall HRV, a person's HRV can be increased by improving their health, exercise, stress management, and recovery skills. High HRV is widely regarded as a marker of a healthy heart. Multiple studies have related it to lower morbidity and mortality and improved psychological well-being and quality of life. Even if some generic reference values are provided, comparing HRV readings to those of other people. The good news is that your lifestyle heavily influences your HRV. We may take proactive steps to improve our habits, increase physical activity, and seek a healthier living.

HRV sheds light on humoral, neuronal, and neurovisceral processes in brain, body, and behavior health and disease, but it hasn't fully matured in the digital age. A synthetic method combines the benefits of the most promising, actionable, and practical aspects to understand how HRV can function as a predictor of COVID19 infection. Longitudinal HRV data collected by a personal device, transferred by a smartphone app, and analyzed by a high-throughput cloud-based machine learning algorithm represents an innovative, low-cost, easily deployable, and scalable method for individual health behavior maintenance as well as communication and decision support with clinical and public health professionals in communities and larger jurisdictions.

HRV is a physiological marker of immunological and inflammatory activity. HRV stands for the instantaneous fluctuation in the electrocardiogram's inter-beat interval (IBI). HRV has been examined and found to link to various illness conditions and human psycho-physiological functioning. More variability in IBI (defined as the time between adjacent R to R peaks in the ECG) in many diseases and circumstances is positively connected with fewer and poorer adverse health or well-being outcomes.

The quantification of sinus rhythm variability is used in HRV studies to determine cardiac autonomic control. Studies conducted over the previous two decades have linked the autonomic nervous system to cardiovascular mortality, especially sudden cardiac death. HRV has been linked to a worse prognosis following myocardial infarction in several studies (MI or heart attack). As a result, HRV measures can be utilized to predict future problems and death in Myocardial infarction patients. The autonomic nervous system (ANS) controls heart rate, HRV, and other involuntary activities like breathing are all controlled by the autonomic nervous system (ANS). HRV reflects the heart rate's complicated autonomic regulation. As a result, HRV measurements provide more information than heart rate measures alone. The autonomic nervous system (ANS) is a part of the peripheral nervous system that controls human body's internal organs (PNS). Nerves connect several organ systems to the central nervous system (CNS), including the brain and spinal cord. It controls body functions such as sweating, digestion, breathing, and heart rate. Because the autonomic control of heart rate can exhibit abnormal abnormalities in physiological functioning, HRV may be valuable in making a diagnostic, prognosis, and therapeutic decisions. There is a range of physiological elements that can influence heart rate variability in healthy people, in addition to pathological (disease) scenarios (HRV). While some of these factors are beyond an individual's control (such as age and genetic composition), others are lifestyle (physical activity, smoking, and other lifestyle choices). As a result, one's lifestyle may influence HRV and its involvement in disease outcomes. The research focuses on the critical link between reduced HRV and death following myocardial infarction. The oscillation between consecutive heartbeats and the fluctuations between straight instantaneous heart rates are also examples of HRV. The phrase "heart rate variability" has come to be used to characterize changes in both fast heart rate and RR intervals (C.Schubert et.al., 2009; J.F.Thayer, 2009; P. Hjemdahl,2007, Pure Appl. Sei. Technol, 2012). Changes in HRV have been connected to particular illnesses. Even though HRV has been the subject of several clinical studies evaluating a variety of cardio-logical and no cardio-logical conditions and clinical states, only two clinical situations have resulted in a consensus on HRV's practical application in adult medicine. HRV deficiency can be employed as a risk predictor and early warning indication of diabetic neuropathy following an acute MI. HRV has been reported to be diminished in several cardio-logical and no cardio-logical illnesses.

Electrocardiography (ECG) is commonly used to evaluate HRV for a specific period. The electrocardiogram (EKG) depicts the heart cycle with four key components: a P wave, a QRS complex, a T wave, and a U wave. HRV is defined as the difference in time between the R peaks on the QRS complexes over several cardiac cycles. HRV is commonly measured using time or frequency domain approaches (Bjorn Schuller et.al.,2013; Frederick Hasty et.al., 2021; Hye-Geum Kim et.al.,2017; Mol MBA et.al., 2021; Lena Sophie et.al.,2021).

TIME-DOMAIN METHODS

The most basic HRV measurements are based on time-domain processes, which determine heart cycle intervals. This is commonly measured as the normal-to-normal (NN or RR) interval between QRS complexes on an ECG recording. It is also possible to determine the instantaneous heart rate. The difference in RR/NN intervals (cycle length) or heart rate is then used to calculate variation. Time-domain approaches, which determine the intervals between cardiac cycles, are the most basic measures of HRV. An ECG recording typically assesses the normal-to-normal (NN or RR) interval between QRS complexes. It's also possible to figure out your current heart rate. The difference between RR/NN intervals (cycle length) or heart rate is then used to calculate variation. Geometric analysis is more accurate than statistical analysis when RR/NN interval measurements are of poor quality. However, because multiple RR/NN intervals are required for conversion into geometric patterns, fractal or geometric approaches typically need 24 hours or more of recording time and are thus unsuitable for analysing shorter recordings (less than 20 minutes). The beat-to-beat or RR/NN intervals are studied in time domain methods to produce variables such as:

- The standard deviation of RR/NN intervals is SDNN.
- SDANN is the standard deviation of average RR/NN intervals determined over short periods, usually 5 minutes. As a result, SDANN is a measure of variations in heart rate caused by cycles lasting longer than 5 minutes. SDNN represents total variability since it reflects all cyclic components that cause variability across the recording period.
- RMSSD stands for the square root of the mean squared difference between successive NNs.
- NN50, the number of consecutive NNs that differ by more than 50 milliseconds.
- pNN50, which is the ratio of NN50 to the total number of NNs.
- NN20, the number of consecutive NNs that differ by more than 20 milliseconds.
- pNN20, which is the proportion of NN20 in the total number of NNs divided by the total number of NNs.

Materials and Methods

Human communication takes the form of speech, which is a vocalized type of communication. The vocal tract is the most physiological feature of the human voice production system. The articulated tract model is shown in figure 2. The vocal tract is divided into five sections:

1. the laryngeal pharynx,
2. the oral pharynx,
3. the oral cavity,
4. the nasal pharynx, and
5. the nasal cavity.

The vocal tract acts as a filter, shaping the excitation sources. From a technological standpoint, thinking about the speech production system in terms of acoustic filtering procedures that affect the air leaving the lungs is more beneficial. The primary acoustic filter is made up of three main cavities. The vocal tract has two speech functions:

1. it can change the spectral distribution of energy in glottal sound waves, and
2. it can help produce obstruent (stop and fricative) sounds. The generation of voice can be seen as airflow, resonance sound, and voice articulation (J. Benesty, 2008); E.Dmitrity et.al., 2009, L.Rabiner et.al., 1978).

Figure 2. Vocal tract model

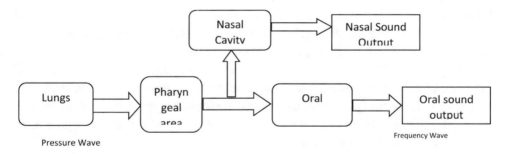

The tongue, lips, velum, jaw, teeth, and palate make up the articulatory system. Because the palate and upper teeth do not move, they are referred to as passive articulators. They provide stable surfaces against which the active articulators (the tongue, lips, jaw, and velum) operate. These regulate the form of the mouth cavity and whether it is connected to the nasal cavity. Hence, the degree to which the excitation signal's various frequencies are amplified or muted. The articulatory system only changes the sound generated by vowel vocal folds, but it also provides excitement for certain consonants, most notably the fricatives in English. Non-pulmonic sounds like clicks produced by the articulatory system rather than the respiratory system are used in several other languages. These regulate the shape of the mouth cavity, whether it is connected to the nasal cavity, and the degree to which the excitation signal's various frequencies are amplified or muted. The articulatory system only changes the sound generated by the vocal folds in the case of vowels. Still, it also provides stimulation in the case of some consonants, most notably the fricatives in English. Non-pulmonic sounds like clicks produced by the articulatory system rather than the respiratory system are found in other languages.

Figure 3. Spectrogram of a speech sample

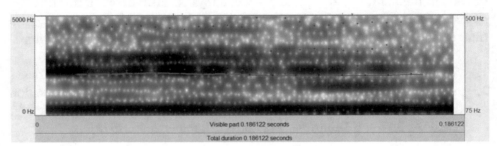

The Short-time Fourier Transform (STFT) is used in voice spectrum analysis. Pitch is calculated using the time-domain spectrum. The format of a speech signal can be established by simulating it as if it were created by a particular source and filter, such as a linear prediction filter. Four or more significant resonances, generally known as "formants," can be found in the human vocal tract. The spectral peaks of the voice's sound spectrum |P(f)| are known as formants. Formant is also a term used in speech science and phonetics to describe the acoustic resonance of the human vocal tract. It's usually measured with a spectrogram, as illustrated in figure 3, as an amplitude peak in the sound's frequency spectrum.

COVID 19 patients' voice samples for their infection days have been gathered. These samples have been digitized to remove noise. The necessary data was taken from these samples and used to plot a vowel triangle for each day of infection using a speech analysis technique.

1. Voice samples of COVID patients (adults) for fourteen days are recorded. Each patient had to recite the 52 alphabets of the Hindi character set.
2. Speech samples are recorded using the Windows Sound Recorder version and a microphone system.
3. Gold wave digital audio editor, a speech signal editing and filtering software, is used.

4. PRAAT, a program that can determine spectrogram and extracts formants from spoken utterances, removes Formant frequencies using spectrogram (Speech Signal Processing with PRAAT, 2012).
5. The acquired speech data were analysed and plotted using MATLAB 2012a for the 64-bit platform.

The System Flow Diagram can be Described using the Steps Below:

Step I: Speech samples from COVID 19 patients were collected.

Step II: Collected speech samples were digitized, and utterances were isolated using gold wave software.

Step III: In MATLAB, formants from the PRAAT spectrogram were extracted and plotted versus days.

Step IV: Vowel triangles were plotted on each patient for each day of infection and an average day following COVID 19 infection.

Figure 4. Flowchart of methodology implemented

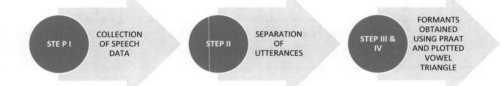

Figure 5, 6 and 7 show the normal ACG, COVID-19 infection day 5 and day 2 ACGs respectively. The figure clears the fact that the RR cycle duration is contracted in the infection day as compared to that of in normal condition.

173

Figure 5. Normal ACG of the sample

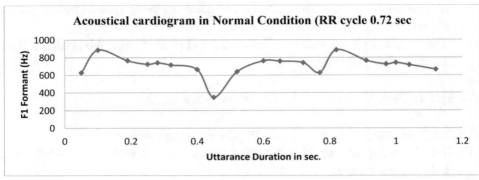

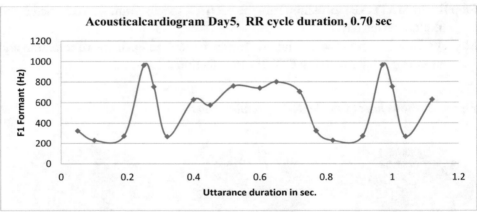

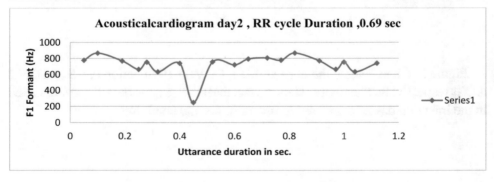

Figure 6. ACG Day 5 of COVID infection

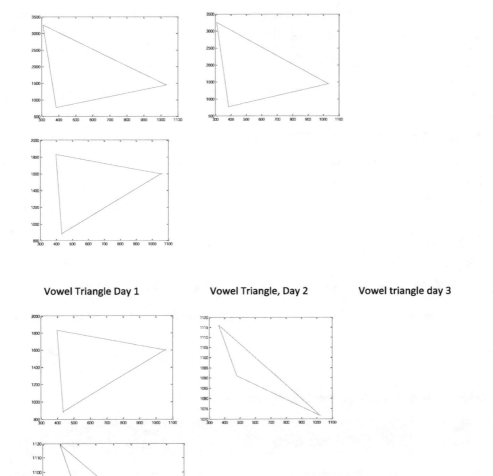

Vowel Triangle Day 1   Vowel Triangle, Day 2   Vowel triangle day 3

Vowel Triangle Day 4   Vowel triangle day5   Vowel Triangle Day 6

Figure 7. ACG, day 2 of COVID infection

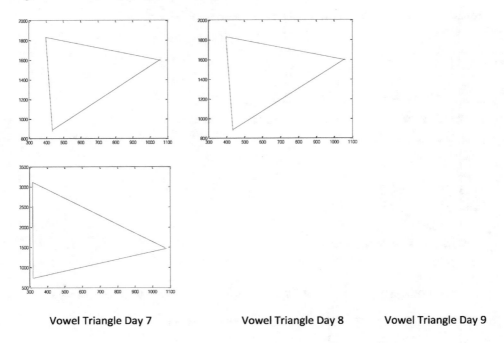

Vowel Triangle Day 7   Vowel Triangle Day 8   Vowel Triangle Day 9

Table 1. Mental condition prediction from speech features

Day of Infection	F1 Formant Hz	F2 Formant Hz	Area of Vowel Triangle in sq.Hz	Euclidean Distance
Day 2				
aa	1060	1291		
ee	342	2044		
oo	383	776	499663	2025
Mean	575	1493		
day 3				
aa	1062	1596		
ee	399	1830		
oo	436	873	312916	1588
Mean	632	1433		
day 4				

Continued on following page

Table 1. Continued

Day of Infection	F1 Formant Hz	F2 Formant Hz	Area of Vowel Triangle in sq.Hz	Euclidean Distance
aa	1062	1696		
ee	400	1430	192409	1279
oo	453	870		
Mean				
Day 5				
aa	1017	1072		
ee	361	1116	5604	973
oo	479	1091		
Mean	619	1093		
Day 6				
aa	1022	1078		
ee	399	1121	29731	932
oo	436	1023		
Mean	619	1074		
Day 7				
aa	1045	1145		
ee	403	1401	114438	1131
oo	487	1011		
Mean	645	1185		
Day 8				
aa	1062	1136		
ee	408	1934	307281	1624
oo	423	976		
Mean	631	1348		
Day 9				
aa	1068	1213		
ee	356	1789	317168	1520
oo	387	873		
Mean	603	1291		
day 10				
aa	1060	1291		
ee	342	2044	439775	1761
oo	383	776		
Mean	595	1370		

Continued on following page

Table 1. Continued

Day of Infection	F1 Formant Hz	F2 Formant Hz	Area of Vowel Triangle in sq.Hz	Euclidean Distance
day 11				
aa	1045	1437		
ee	367	2108	408527	1813
oo	473	798		
Mean	628	1447		
day 12				
aa	1017	1472		
ee	361	2116	460218	1867
oo	312	761		
Mean	563	1449		
post covid				
aa	1072	1479		
ee	317	2112	519939	1886
oo	319	733		
Mean	569	1441		

RESULTS AND DISCUSSION

The samples of the some COVID-19 patients have been collected during the consecutive fourteen days of infection. The regular ECGandspeechsamplesofthepatienthasbeencollectedandanalyzed.
Furtherthepatient's ECG and speech parameters have been compared with that of the normal healthy condition of the same informant. The data has been tabulated in table 1 for plotting of vowel triangle and it's analysis.

Figure 8. Vowel triangles of a COVID-19 patient for 14 days of infection

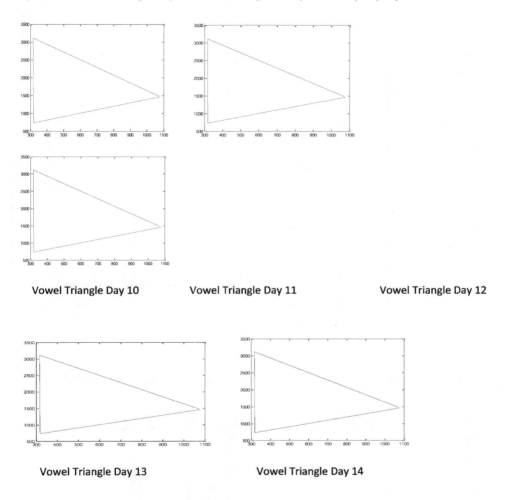

Vowel Triangle Day 10   Vowel Triangle Day 11   Vowel Triangle Day 12

Vowel Triangle Day 13   Vowel Triangle Day 14

Speech samples were recorded through a microphone and subjected to digitization. The required speech segmental have been extracted and analyzed through gold wave software and a speech signal processing tool PRAAT. About five minutes of speech recording is done for each day while resting. The retrieved speech features are based on the recorded speech. HRV was estimated using three methods: HRV (mean), SDNN, SDANN, or RMSSD from the ACG sample.

Table 2. Day wise heart rate variability for days of COVID-19 infection

Day	HRV (ms)	Mean RR in sec	HB in 5 min	BPM
day 1	60	0.71	414	82.8
day 2	57	0.71	430	86
day 3	50	0.69	441	88.2
day 4	43	0.7	440	88
day 5	44	0.71	441	88.2
day 6	43	0.72	422	84.4
day 7	47	0.74	425	85
day 8	46	0.78	403	80.6
day 9	47	0.74	410	82
day 10	53	0.73	435	87
day 11	53	0.72	412	82.4
day 12	56	0.71	412	82.4
day 13	57	0.73	408	81.6
day 14	58	0.72	412	82.4

Figure 9. HRV variations of a COVID-19 patient for the days of infection

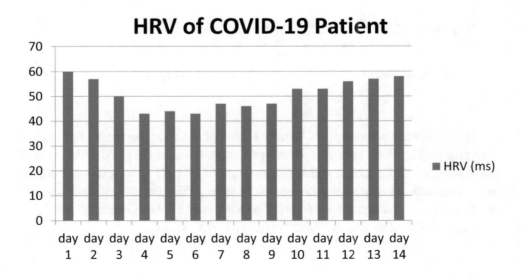

The HRV graph in Figure 9 and data tabulated in table 2 shows that HRV has decreased during severe infection days: day 3, day 4 and day 5 and again started rising from day 6.

Also, the vowel triangles analysis for the day mentioned above states the stressful condition of the patient. The decrease in HRV for these days also indicates stressful mental conditions and increased patient heart rate. One can predict the psychological and heart condition of the patient from speech signal analysis.

CONCLUSION

Acoustic-cardiogram (ACG) analysis is used to forecast a patient's heart rate variability (HRV) using extracted speech data. ACG analysis can be used to predict the patient's heart rate variability (HRV), obtained from extracted speech features. It is concluded that vowel triangle and acoustic-cardiogram analysis techniques provide a straightforward, non-invasive, and risk-free method for monitoring the behavioural and physiological health of COVID 19 patients continuously, benefiting both medical staff and patients.

In this research, study is based on data sets observations and analysis. It is mentioned, that speech of the COVID 19 patient can be used to monitor the patients' physiological and psychological condition. Vowel triangle analysis and Acoustical cardiogram analysis can be a tool to assess the patient's heart rate variability and stressful situation very safely without the involvement of expert medical staff and expensive laboratory setup.

REFERENCES

Benesty. (2008). Springer handbook of speech processing. Springer.

Berstein, A., & Cohen, A. (1985). Speech processing applied for chest diagnosis. *14'th Conv. of Elect. & Electronics Engg.*

Buchhorn, R., Baumann, C., & Willaschek, C. (2020, August). Heart rate variability in a patient with coronavirus disease 2019. *International Cardiovascular Forum Journal, 20.*

Deshpande, A., Thakur, K., & Zadgaonkar, A. S. (2014, April). Assessment of heart rate variability from speech analysis. *The Journal of the Acoustical Society of America, 135*(4), 2427. doi:10.1121/1.4878075

Deshpande, N., Thakur, K., & Zadgaonkar, A. S. (2014, May). Assessment of heart rate variability from speech analysis. In *Proceedings of Meetings on Acoustics 167ASA* (Vol. 21, No. 1, p. 055004). Acoustical Society of America.

Drury, R. L., Jarczok, M., Owens, A., & Thayer, J. F. (2021). Wireless Heart Rate Variability in Assessing Community COVID-19. *Frontiers in Neuroscience*, 15.

Engel, B. T., & Chism, R. A. (1967). Effect of increases and decreases in breathing rate on heart rate and finger pulse volume. *Psychophysiology*, *4*(1), 83–89.

Fant, G. (1960). *Acoustic theory of speech production*. Mouton.

Friedberg Charles, K. (1966). *Diseases of the Heart*. Saunders Pub.

Gang, Y., & Malik, M. (2009). Non-invasive risk stratification for implantable cardioverter-defibrillator placement—heart rate variability. *The American Heart Hospital Journal*, *7*(1), 39–44. https://doi.org/10.15420/ahhj.2009.7.1.39

Gemignani, V., Bianchini, E., Faita, F., Giannoni, M., Pasanisi, E., Picano, E., & Bombardini, T. (2008, September). *Assessment of cardiologic systole and diastole duration in exercise stress tests with a transcutaneous accelerometer sensor. In 2008 Computers in Cardiology*. IEEE.

Hasty, F., García, G., Dávila, H., Wittels, S. H., Hendricks, S., & Chong, S. (2021). Heart rate variability as a possible predictive marker for acute inflammatory response in COVID-19 patients. *Military Medicine*, *186*(1-2), e34–e38.

Heart rate variability: standards of measurement, physiological interpretation and clinical use. Task Force of the European Society of Cardiology and the North American Society of Pacing and Electrophysiology. (1996). *Circulation, 93*(5), 1043–1065.

Hjemdahl, P. (2000). Cardiovascular system and stress. Encyclopedia of Stress, 1, 389-403.

Kaliyaperumal, D., Karthikeyan, R. K., Alagesan, M., & Ramalingam, S. (2021). Characterization of cardiac autonomic function in COVID-19 using heart rate variability: A hospital based preliminary observational study. *Journal of Basic and Clinical Physiology and Pharmacology*, *32*(3), 247–253.

Kamaleswaran, R., Sadan, O., Kandiah, P., Li, Q., Thomas, T., Blum, J., ... Buchman, T. (2021). 227: Altered Heart Rate Variability Predicts Mortality Early Among Critically Ill COVID-19 Patients. *Critical Care Medicine*, *49*(1), 99.

Kim, H. G., Cheon, E. J., Bai, D. S., Lee, Y. H., & Koo, B. H. (2018). Stress and Heart Rate Variability: A Meta-Analysis and Review of the Literature. *Psychiatry Investigation*, *15*(3), 235–245. https://doi.org/10.30773/pi.2017.08.17

Mol, M. B., Strous, M. T., van Osch, F. H., Vogelaar, F. J., Barten, D. G., Farchi, M., ... Gidron, Y. (2021). Heart-rate-variability (HRV), predicts outcomes in COVID-19. *PLoS One*, *16*(10), e0258841.

Orlikoff, R. F., & Baken, R. J. (1989). Fundamental frequency modulation of the human voice by the heartbeat: Preliminary results and possible mechanisms. *The Journal of the Acoustical Society of America*, *85*(2), 888–893.

Pfeifer, L. S., Heyers, K., Ocklenburg, S., & Wolf, O. T. (2021). Stress research during the COVID-19 pandemic and beyond. *Neuroscience and Biobehavioral Reviews*, *131*, 581–596. https://doi.org/10.1016/j.neubiorev.2021.09.045

Rabiner, L. R. (1978). *Digital processing of speech signal*. Academic Press.

Salari, N., Hosseinian-Far, A., Jalali, R., Vaisi-Raygani, A., Rasoulpoor, S., Mohammadi, M., ... Khaledi-Paveh, B. (2020). Prevalence of stress, anxiety, depression among the general population during the COVID-19 pandemic: A systematic review and meta-analysis. *Globalization and Health*, *16*(1), 1–11.

Schubert, C., Lambertz, M., Nelesen, R. A., Bardwell, W., Choi, J. B., & Dimsdale, J. E. (2009). Effects of stress on heart rate complexity—A comparison between short-term and chronic stress. *Biological Psychology*, *80*(3), 325–332.

Schuller, B., Friedmann, F., & Eyben, F. (2013, May). Automatic recognition of physiological parameters in the human voice: Heart rate and skin conductance. In *2013 IEEE International Conference on Acoustics, Speech and Signal Processing* (pp. 7219-7223). IEEE.

Skopin, D., & Baglikov, S. (2009, June). Heartbeat feature extraction from vowel speech signal using 2D spectrum representation. *Proc. the 4th Int. Conf. Information Technology*.

Thayer, J. F. (2009). *Heart rate variability: A neurovisceral integration model*. Academic Press.

Weenink, D. (2014). Speech signal processing with Praat. *Haettu, 16*.

Chapter 9

A Survey on Behavioral Change During the COVID–19 Outbreak in India

Tanu Rizvi
Shri Shankaracharya Technical Campus, Bhilai, India

Devanand Bhonsle
Shri Shankaracharya Technical Campus, Bhilai, India

Roshni Rahangdale
Shri Shankaracharya Technical Campus, Bhilai, India

Jaspal Bagga
Shri Shankaracharya Technical Campus, Bhilai, India

ABSTRACT

This study describes the immediate and long-term effects in behavioral and psychological symptoms due to COVID-19. To handle the situation, the Indian government tried in various levels lockdown, scanning of the patients, social distancing, compulsorily wearing the mask, vaccination, quarantine centers, etc., but in the long-term, all these activities affected social and physiological status. In extreme cases, people suffer from depression, which can be characterized by various factors like tiredness, poor sleep, pessimism, guilt, hopelessness, lack of confidence, low mood, gradual reduction in work output, loss of appetite, feeling helpless, loneliness, etc.

DOI: 10.4018/978-1-7998-9831-3.ch009

BACKGROUND AND INTRODUCTION

Pandemics are the unfortunate consistent facet which affect human life over the centuries. It cause threatening to the lives not only for the human beings but for other creatures also. History is the wittiness of different pandemics viz. Spanish flu in 1918, Asian flu in 1957, Hog kong flu in 1958 and now Covid-19(Zhang et. al, 2019). Although Covid-19 is originated from Wuhan city of China but it have been spread all over the world. Hardly there is a country which is not affected by it. We can say that all the countries are suffering from its bad effects economically. However it does not affect the economics of the world only but it is the reason of various health issues which cause death on large scale. Economically the whole world is categories into three types:

1. **Developed Countries**
2. **Developing Countries**
3. **Undeveloped Countries**

However, according to the Gross National Income (GNI), classification is done in four types:

1. **High income countries**
2. **upper-middle income countries**
3. **lower-middle income countries**
4. **low income countries**

It seems that all the developed countries are capable to handle all the situations of any kind of disasters whether it is natural or manmade but ground reality is totally different from it (Glanz. K. et. al.,2011). According to the present scenario; it is seen that the mostly the developed countries from Europe, America and Asia are severely affected. Ur planet encountered with different viruses in last many years and SARS and MARS viruses are expected in the future (Francisco. R.et. al, 2020). Many economic and health consequences of pandemics are documented very well but their behavioral implications are not well understood. Corona virus disease 2019 in short called COVID-19 refers to an infection (SARS-CoV-2) of the lower respiratory tract. It was firstly detected in Wuhan, a city of China in December 2019(Das. G. et. al,2020). In March 2020, World Health Organization (WHO) declared it a global pandemic. As a result, the government of many countries implemented full or partial lock down for a long duration to reduce the spreading of the virus (Crosta. A. D. et. al,2020). Even the international airlines and ships services were also banned for long duration and time to time many countries restrict their airline services from different countries (West. R. et. al,2020). To study the human behavior academically many articles have been written. This study is done on the basis of various parameters which will be disused in this chapter. Psychology and sociology are two of the branches of studies which study the human behavior (Cassenti. D. et. al,2020). These two branches are very wide and they help the doctors, researchers, thinkers, psychologists and sociologists to understand and analyze various aspects of human behavior with different parameters (Weston. D. et. al,2020). This study describes the effect of immediate and long term effects in behavioral and psychological symptoms due to COVID-19. Whole world in affected very badly and our country India was not the exception (Chopra. S. et. al,2020). This disease affected our country socially, economically, physically and psychologically (Bavel. J. J. V. et. al,2020). To handle the situation our government tried in various levels viz. lockdown, scanning of the patients, social distancing, compulsorily wearing the mask, vaccination, quarantine centers etc (Chatterjee. K. et. al,2020). Some of these are precautionary measures and some are intermediate one. These are for safety of human beings but in the long term all these activities affected our social and physiological status (Matos. A.D. et. al,2021). To understand and compare human behavior; many authors surveyed and reached in a conclusion that COVID-19 affected whole world in such a way that there is a huge gap between behavioral aspects before and during this scenario. We studied various articles, research papers, doctors, psychologists and opinion of intellectuals to understand this change. Although these strict actions became effective to avoid the spreading of the virus but at the other hand it severely affected the global economic system as a result a big economical crisis came into existence (Kollamparambill. et. al, 2021). Many agencies tried to understand the change in the economy of various countries but simultaneously many researchers are trying to understand the behavior change in human being due to the present scenario. Because COVID-19 does not only affects the human body but it also affected our mental health (Singh. K. et. al,2021; WHO,2020). However this mental condition is not directly connected to the virus but it is due to the precautionary measures taken to avoid the spread of the virus (Rawat. D. et. al,2021). Lockdown, curfew, work from home etc. are some of the factors which affected us mentally also. On 24 march 2020, Govt. of India ordered a lockdown all over the country. It was for 3 weeks i. e. for 21 days. For this duration all the companies, organizations, school, colleges, institutions, shops, shopping malls, parks, gardens even public transportations were closed. It stopped the whole moment of entire population of our country. It was a preventive measure against the COVID-19 pandemic in India. Thereafter many restrictions were to be imposed on public and services to reduce the spread of virus. We all are the witness of this lockdown and unlock situations. Time to time state government have taken precautionary measures and it is continue. In 2021, India faced second wave which was more difficult to handle; as a result many casualties have been encountered.

In this chapter; we tried to understand the change in the behavior of the human being with different age group so that its instantaneous as well as long term effects can be widely analyzed among a large population. This study will help the other authors also to understand the direct and indirect impact of virus attack in our society. Since we concentrate on the physical and psychological aspect only; we will not discuss any economical effect. Research articles and paper were studied to the relevant topics entitle with the pandemic, social effects on the behavior, cultural influences on behavior, effects on the physical health, effects on the psychology aspects, effects on decision making etc. From this survey we identified several effective changes in the behavior change during COVID-19 pandemic. However this change does not follow a regular pattern but it is random because the candidates have been selected from different age group. Every individual has different condition viz. gender, locality/area/ surroundings, education, number of family members, responsibilities toward the family, number of family earning family members, economical conditions, job profile/ responsibilities, previous health conditions/ any previous disease history etc. The human behavior depends of various factors which can be understood in the field of behavioral science and psychology (Weston. D. et. al., 2018). In this chapter; we identified several factors which are illustrated in fig. 1. In this figure; we tried to portray the effect of various factors in the human behavior. In general the behavior of a person depends on his/her capabilities, motivation and the most important the opportunities which he/she obtained (Cheng. Y. et. al., 2018). Capability of an individual does not depend on his physic but it is more depended on his/her psychology. For doing something both are equally important. Hence we can say that capability requires self-confidence and physical condition both(Williams. Et. al., 2015). Motivation is another aspect which requires for a person to move towards success. It can be generated either of two ways (David. R. et. al.,2015). First is called self motivation which comes from our own mind while other is generated from our surrounding (Funk. S. et. al., 2015; Michie. S. et. al., 2014). Hence we can broadly divide it into two viz. automatic and reflective. Similarly opportunity is another factor which affects behavior of individual. It may rise from physical or social. These three major factor affects the behavior of every individuals.

Figure 1. Behavior change Aspects

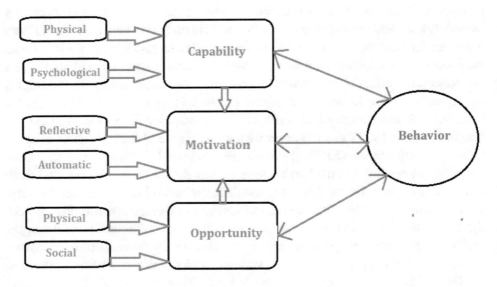

LITERATURE REVIEW

This chapter gives the brief idea about the previous survey done in the field of behavior change in human being during covid-19. Many authors presented their articles for the same. Some of those have been reviewed here to understand the present scenario.

Kavita Singh et.al. (2021) studied on the survey carried out on 1754 Indians with 11% mean with age of 57.8 years out of which nearly the half are men..The rate of response is seventy four percentages. In pandemics lockdown in India nearly 83% faces difficulty in accessing health services,17%in medications,59% people lost their source of income,38% became jobless and 28% of them stopped their intake of healthy stuffs such as fruits and vegetables. The result obtained from regression model shows that 2.30,1.62-3.26 who totally lost their source of income faced a toughest situations in their medications and treatments. The scenario further got worst when the individuals with lost jobs and with diabetes and hypertension faced difficulties in accessing medicines with regression model of 1.90,1.25-2.89. The overall data suggests that most of the participants faced many psychological stress due to low or no source of income in availing the various medical facilities.

Sakshi Chopra et.al (2021). did a survey based on web Questionnaire with life style related behavior was registered with online survey with platform of Google forms. Total nine hundred ninety five responses have been recorded with mean age of 33.4 years and 58.4% of which are males. Usually in youngsters under the age of 30 years. Started to healthy fying their lives by adopting the healthy life styles and discarding the unhealthy habits. About one third of participants that are people with upper socio status gained weight reduced their physical activities and get diverted towards the more screen time accessing the online entertainment platforms and spending a lot of their time on them however some people by using this online activities developed great learning skills using this online platforms only but it depends on individuals. Frequent lockdowns and quarantine increased the stress and anxiety nearly to one fourth of participants affecting their mental health adversely. The negative lifestyle behaviors that spread out during COVID-19 pandemic can be mitigated by understanding the factors which can be helpful to develop interventions.

Gopal Das et.al. (2021) highlighted the characteristics, impacts of COVID-19 scenario with development of a conceptual framework. Four major macro level forces have been identified that highlights the implications of market while characterizing pandemics. The organizing structure 7P's model of marketing are discussed with their implications at a micro level and questionnaires are identified to turn on further inquiry, to generate deeper insights deeply pertaining to marketing implications during pandemics but also to view distantly the new opportunities these scenario. At last authors identified implications for medical education, tourism facilities, healthcare and industry sectors due to unavoidable scene of pandemics.

Alica Delerue Matos et.al. (2021) identified the difference in terms of behaviors between participants aged 50 + with their counterparts and multi morbidity without multi morbidity in twenty five countries of Europe together with Israel. Authors used the pre processed data from the set of questionnaire on the economic biology and socio demographic fromCOVID-19 Share. Wave seven and eight databases were also fully utilized to encounter the individuals with multi morbidity. At last the results showed that when controls included are gender, age, education, financial distress and countries then the precautionary behaviors are exhibited by individuals with multi morbidity than their counterparts as compared without multi morbidity individuals. On the other hand authors observed that the educated individuals, females and those individuals who encountered financial distress adopt more protective behaviors than their counterparts. Italy and Spain shows the higher prevalence of precautionary behaviors in comparison with Finland, Denmark and Sweden. The defensive actions adopted against COVID-19 guarantees that public health must continue to be un concentrated among older aged and middle aged persons with multi morbidity, awareness campaigns should be point the way at men and less educated individuals in countries but also at persons experiencing distress, particularly where people engaged in fewer precautionary behaviors.

Adolfo Di Crosta et.al. (2021) focused on psychological antecedents and individuals behavior. The studies carried out by various authors showed that the

COVID-19 crisis differently affects people willingness to buy primary products such as shopping and secondary products such as headonic shopping. Therefore it may be concluded that changes in individual's behavior changes their level of spending. Authors adopted a line of division between the primary and secondary necessities of consumers. Three thousand eight hundred thirty three peoples are surveyed through online platform with age limit from 18 to 64 during peak of first wave peak Italy. COVID-19 fear and anxiety is the key factor to predict the consumer behavior toward primary necessities. On the other hand depression is used a key factor for consumer behavior toward secondary necessities. Furthermore, personality traits, perceived economic stability, and self-justifications for purchasing were adopted to predict toward primary necessities and secondary necessities present this article presents understanding of consumer behavior changes during the COVID-19 crisis based upon primary and secondary necessities. Psychological factors are considered to develop results that could be helpful to enhance marketing strategies to balance actual consumers' needs and psychological feelings.

Seema Mehta et.al. (2020) focused on a censorious scenario which pushes the behavior of human in different directions with many irreversible aspects of behavior. COVID-19 pandemic is an uncommon crisis, and to control this contagious disease various steps were taken by governments including complete or partial lockdown depending upon the percentage of cases in the area. The elements of the economy are correlated measures of public health frequent shut downs, which resulted in economic vulnerability of the countries hinting towards change in the dynamics of market. The consumers are whole sole drivers of the market competitions, growth and economic assimilation. With this unpredictability of economics, consumers behaviors are transformed in meanwhile the transformation experienced during the crunch will end up a question. The article looked deeply to the behavior of consumers during COVID-19 pandemics, lockdowns when the world becomes still for more than half of year. Further, the article explains the interfolds about consumer behavior in normal times and in crisis times travelling through a maze of literature empowering it with the rapid assessment reports carried out by the consulting organizations during pandemics, substantiates the same with first-conspiring and retelling of experiences by customers and individuals with marketing strategies to bring up a prediction of the pandemic affecting a criteria shift from customers materialistic requirements to customers spiritualism. Further hypothesis are suggested for future researchers to understand the customer. The proposition offers further testable hypotheses for future research to understand consumer sentiments or concerns in buying 'what is sufficient' within the context of market context and how it can be implemented post-COVID-19 crisis in order to ensure a sustained model of marketing. The consumer behavior can be forced and can be related interestingly with other control variables such as nationality, needs, culture, new market segment and age using which new models of customer behavior can be developed.

Rita Francisco et.al. (2020) studied the behavior of adolescents with 52.9% boys with age group from 3 to 18 years ld in three countries namely Italy, Spain and Portugal. The negative impact on psychological behavior based upon social distancing and isolation were scary in case of children and adolescent. Parents of one thousand four hundred eighty children and were a part of this study. A survey using online platform and snowball sampling technique was conducted for 15 consecutive days between the peak periods of pandemic outbreak around the world in April-may 2020. The questionnaires is based upon data, socio, demographic housing conditions and psychological response during quarantine which were made to answered by parents of the above mentioned aged group children based upon behavioral change due to sleeplessness, anxiety, mood, screen time etc as key inputs to study. Results show various changes in psychological behavior, increased screen timing and reduced physical activity. The psychological symptoms were minimal in Italian children as compared to Spanish and Portuguese children. Results from hierarchical multiple regressions show that having an outdoor exit such as gardening, terrace contributes in healthier environment and reduced risking psychological behavior of children. Authors recommended some practice implications for families so as to identify the prediction variables for reduced risk of behavioral change in adolescent and children.

Umakrishnan Kollamparambil et.al. (2020) identified the driver of response behavior using seemingly related regression method and special regressors ranging from probit control using multivariate estimation techniques with bivariate statistics, concentration indices the behavior response to COVID-19 r enhances as shown by findings in this research. The most preventive measures are hand washing, use of face mask, sanitizing. Other measures, includes practicing social distancing, reducing close contact, avoiding crowds. The higher income groups, educated ones and older adolescents. There is increased risk perception nt differ and has risk inperception. The significant drivers of healthy behavior response are health models, self efficacy, awareness and The findings validate the health-belief model, with perceived risk, self-efficacy, perceived awareness and blockade to other traditional socio norms. Usually the higher socio economic groups and educated individuals practice use of sanitizers mostly where as the respondents of lower economic groups are not in favor of practicing such measures. The lower socio economic group suffers from dilemma of adopting the preventive measures and are optimally biased towards several barriers. There urgent need to target such groups in order to incorporate responsive approach to the preventive measure strategies.

Dale Weston et.al. (2020) identified a wide range of more commonly applied strategies with broad framework for their use within an contagious disease and emergency response context. Authors provided a path with the key recommendations to incorporate the disease modelers, researchers, practitioners go ahead. The systematic application of theories has been presented specially for researchers and practitioners as a base to their future research. At last the disease modelers can get a initiative with theories incorporated here to ensure that the full range of relevant factors such as psychological, emotional, physical are incorporated into their models. The consultation of In all behavioral scientists are highly recommended to ensure the proper incorporation of theories.

Nan Zhang et al. (2019) focused on the spread of influenza and COVID-19 infections based upon the reported cases and database on internal surveillance and studied the behavior changes in human due to attack of this viruses based upon telephone survey data and mass transit data from railway authorities. Here authors simulated susceptible exposed infected recovered SEIR model to incorporate the risk reduction of influenza transmission resulting in change of human behavior. The number of passengers as compared to 2019 fell down to fifty two percent. The local residents spent their 33% of time at home engaged in home stuffs only. Each person, on average, came into pandemic periods. Adults, Older aged persons, students and workers daily number close contact gets reduced to 84%,31%,65%,39% respectively. The rate of close contact decreases by 8.2%, 30.7%, 66.2%, 38.4%, 47.6%, 42.0%, and 37.1%, respectively in localities, work surroundings, education hubs, restaurants, shopping market and public transports. The simulation results shows the reduction in reproduction in influenza by 62.9% based upon the adoption of this human behavior. Similarly the spread of COVID-19 viruses reduces to 47.1% due to this behavior of avoidance of human to human close contacts. Thus author concluded that reduction in human to human contact reduces the risk of COVID-19 and influenza infections.

From the above literature survey it may be concluded that behavior change can be categorized into four type's viz. accelerating behavior, sensitive behavior, sustained behavior and transient behavior. Each of these categories affects an individual partially or completely. Accelerating behaviors increase rapidly after the first outbreak and continue in future. Sustain momentum behaviors include use of digital services in a wide range such as use of digital wallets, online videos, use of different applications from play store of mobile phone and other digital media platforms. Due to this behavior; many digital platforms like you tube, netflix, hot star, amazon prime, flipcart, paytm, google pay, phone pay etc. are growing day by day. This behavior change may sustain even after the end of the pandemic situations. Hence we can say that this behavior can sustain even in the post pandemic situation. Sensitive behaviors come into to rise and fall category and it depends on the intensity of the pandemic and associate lockdown.This category includes supermarket chain and online doctor consultation. Before the pandemic situation we Indians prefer to go to the shops and mall to purchase the things and even for a small health issue prefer to visit to the doctor's clinic but in the present scenario many of us use online shopping and even doctors are available online for the consultation. This pattern may sustain even after pandemic but no completely. Transient behavioral change have been seen in the initial stage of pandemic when our country India faced the first lockdown; at this span of time people moved towards the online fitness and hobby classes and maximum of us tried to groom ourselves but as the pandemic situation continues; people did not inclined towards these. Hence it may be easily said that transient behavioral change would not have been sustain in future even in the pandemic situation.

METHODOLOGY

This section deals with the methodology which describes the complete scenario of pandemics, lockdowns and it's after effects. It is practically not possible to analyze all the situation, condition and effect of the present scenario completely even then we have try to understand change in the human behavior in all the age group from 18 to 60 years above. In this span of time, it was very difficult to contact directly to the people and to convince them for their feedback because most of the candidates or their family members were suffering from the disease. Some time situation was panic and at that time condition was worse. So this survey has been done between October 2021 to December 2021 i. e for a span of about three months. The literature used above have many technical terms like accelerating behavior, sensitive behavior, sustained behavior and transient behavior are not to be used because it was again difficult to make the candidates understand (Angus. K. et. al.,2013; Michie. S. et. al., 2011). For the survey, we have prepared questionnaire and distributed among many people who are approachable. Those candidates who stay away from our localities were asked the report telephonically. However it was not easy because some of them are not comfortable to answer. But after a rigorous exercise, we have collected the response from the candidates. In this survey; we included the questions which were very easy to understand. We divided the candidates into five categories viz. 18 to 30 years, 31 to 40 years, 41 to 50 years, 51 to 60 years and above 60. We have chosen 50 members from each group and tried to take 50% men and 50% women. However it was not feasible due to present scenario but all the group consist of men and female both.To better understanding of the behavior change, we have categorized the parameters into two viz. adverse effects and positive aspects(Bush. A. et. al.,2011; Fras.M. E. et.al.,2011). The area is very wide and cannot be completely covered in this chapter. So we have chosen some of the common factors. First of all we have discussed an adverse effect which includes:

1.   Feeling nervous and stressed

2. Lack in physical activities
3. Weight gain
4. Increased screen time
5. Loss of concentration
6. Sleeplessness
7. Unfriendliness

We have chosen these 7 points which are very common for each and every one to understand easily and no need to explain it further. Many candidates were not approachable hence these simple terminologies work to analyze the human behavior efficiently.

Along with these negative aspects we have chosen 5 good habits also which are helpful for all of us and they may sustain even after pandemic. They are:

1. Habit to wash hands
2. Wearing mask
3. Healthier habits
4. Adaption of new technologies
5. Digital payment

The survey done in various stages viz.

Step 1: Selection of people from different groups
Step 2: Distribution of questionnaire to the candidates who were approachable and healthy, those who were neither healthy nor approachable were directly asked the answer telephonically. Those who were not able to give prompt reply due to any reason were sent the Google form.
Step 3: Collection of the response through questionnaire, telephonically or Google form.
Step 4: Check the response according to the age group.
Step 5: Prepare the table and graph to see the change in behavior.
Step 6: Stop the survey.

Below is the results and discussion about the survey done It reflects our results in the form of tables and graphs for five different age groups as discussed earlier.

RESULTS AND DISCUSSIONS

In this part, we have discussed the results of our survey to understand the effect of COVID-19 on our behavior physically and psychologically. For this purpose we chose the people of age group from 18 to 60 above. However to understand more clearly; we have divided age group into 5 subgroups:

1.   18 to 30 years
2.   31 to 40 years
3.   41 to 50 years
4.   51 to 60 years
5.   **Above 60**

All the aforementioned points have been discussed with all the people with different categories of age groups. Below is the discussion of each point related to their change in behavior. Results have been shown in the form of table and graphs.

1.   **Feeling nervous and stressed:** It is obvious for a human being to feel low according to the situation and surrounding but during Covid-19 no one could be escaped from its adverse effect. The causes of nervousness include: worry about his/her and families health, loss of money due to down market, loss in business due to lockdown, insecurities towards the job, deduction in salary, worry about future etc.. According to our survey; no one was exception that didn't face any of at least one problems discussed above. Table 1 shows the numbers of people from different age groups who felt the aforementioned problems. Fig. 2 shows the graph for the table 1 for only the group 18 to 30. From the table it is clear that different age group has different numbers of people who feel nervousness before and during covid-19. However it is found that nos. of candidates who are suffering from this problem is more which shows the adverse effect of present situation.

Table 1. Nervousness verses age group

Age Group		No. of Candidates				
		Never	**Sometimes**	**Often**	**Very often**	**Always**
18-30	Before	9	15	13	9	4
	During	0	8	23	16	3
30-40	Before	10	16	12	10	2
	During	0	12	21	15	2
41-50	Before	8	14	13	10	5
	During	0	14	18	12	6
51-60	Before	5	8	10	12	15
	During	0	5	15	25	5
above 60	Before	2	5	20	13	10
	During	0	1	24	19	6

Figure 2. Nervousness verses age group of 18-30

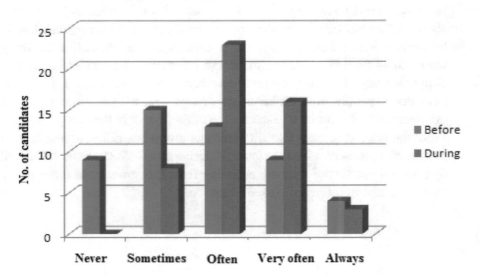

2. **Lack in physical activities:** Due to lockdown; movement stopped in many respects Professional starts doing their work from home, students got their online classes. Schools, colleges, coaching, restaurants, gardens, parks etc. are closed many a times hence many various restrictions in day to day life made our life

very lazy as a result our physical activities become less day by day. Its further effects come in the form of laziness, procrastination, loss of concentration etc. Table 2 shows the numbers of people from different age groups who felt the aforementioned problems. Fig. 3 shows the graph for the table 2 for only the group 18 to 30. This table illustrates that the physical activities have been reduced during covid-19 in all age groups.

Table 2. Physical activities verses age group

Age Group		No. of Candidates				
		Never	Sometimes	Often	Very often	Always
18-30	Before	0	9	8	21	12
	During	2	35	10	3	0
30-40	Before	0	0	44	5	1
	During	0	42	6	2	0
41-50	Before	0	1	35	9	5
	During	2	37	7	4	0
51-60	Before	2	21	15	10	2
	During	8	35	5	2	0
above 60	Before	2	27	13	7	1
	During	30	15	3	2	0

Figure 3. Physical activities verses age group of 18-30

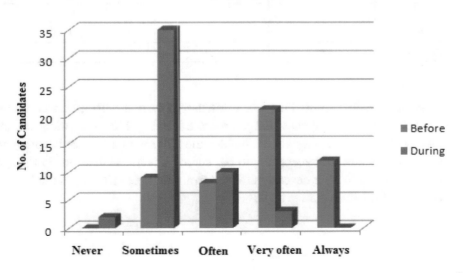

3. **Weight gain:** Since people are residing in their home and not going anywhere unnecessarily hence their physical activities have become very less. Those who are working and doing their professional work from home are also facing the problems of weight gain. This problem increased mostly in the kids as they are not allowed to go outside and they have to be in their home only. Mostly kids play mobile games or video games in their computer or laptop or they spend their time watching television or mobile screen. Hence due to lack of physical activities; weight is increasing almost in all age groups. However it was not easy to get the exact weight. But most of the people reported us that they put on weight from 5 to 10kg and even more during lockdown.

4. **Increased screen time:** This is the biggest problem encountered in all the age group. It may include mobile screen, television, laptop etc. Since kids cannot go outside, parents give them mobile or allow them to see the television. Students attend their classes and giving examination in online mode, professionals are working from home using mobile and laptop, old age people also use these gadgets for communication and entertainment. So we can conclude that this is the general problem and not even a single person would have escape from this problem. Table 3 shows the numbers of people from different age groups who felt the aforementioned problems.

Table 3. Increase screen time verses age group during pandemic

Age Group	No. of Candidates		
	Negligible	1-5 hours	More than 5 hours
18-30	5	10	35
30-40	3	38	9
41-50	2	26	22
51-60	29	12	9
above 60	40	9	1

5. **Loss of concentration:** Due to excess use of virtual world; concentration has become poor in almost all age group. Especially kids and youngster are mostly affected. Since we did not include the kids below 18 hence it cannot be said with a claim. But according to our survey it is found that mostly the age group from 18 to 50 is severely affected from it. Table4 illustrates the loss of concentration among all groups.

Table 4. Loss of concentration verses age group during pandemic

Age Group	No. of Candidates	
	slight	More
18-30	12	38
30-40	7	43
41-50	13	37
51-60	35	15
above 60	40	10

6. **Sleeplessness:** As the schedule of everybody has been massed up hence the biggest problem arises called sleeplessness. Work from home, lockdown etc. directly affected our normal schedule. Most of us are physically inactive which also leads to this problem. Table 5 illustrates the no. of people of different age group who encountered with sleeplessness.

Table 5. Sleeplessness verses age group during pandemic

Age Group	No. of Candidates	
	slight	More
18-30	5	45
30-40	33	17
41-50	29	21
51-60	27	23
above 60	8	42

7. **Unfriendliness:** Due to many lockdowns and restrictions, many of us do not in touch with our friends, neighbors and society. This situation made many people unfriendly and people have become habitual of this lifestyle. Almost all people said yes to the answer.

Along with the above negative points in behavior, we experience some positive aspects also however these positive aspects are not directly connected to the human behavior but we should not forget to be positive to fight against the evil of our whole human being. These habits are:

1. Washing hands and taking care about hygiene.

2.	Wearing mask before going out which help us against air pollution.
3.	Healthier habits like yoga, exercise, consumption of fruits and healthy meals.
4.	Adaption of new technologies which includes use of virtual classroom for study, savvy of computers, mobile and other electronic gadgets.
5.	Digital payment means through digital wallet of various apps like google pay, phone pay, ru pay etc. It is safe because it does not have any physical contact. It is transparent and good for our economy also.

CONCLUSION AND FUTURE RESEARCH DIRECTIONS

From the above discussion it is clear that COVID-19 has led the whole world to its knees and the entire world is struggling to discontinue the chain of the growth of the virus. Many scientists are doing research to finish the cause of the COVID-19. Many companies have introduced vaccines which work as a shield on our body to save life. However it is not easy to finish it hundred percent as virus is producing its mutants and in present many mutants are available in different countries. In became worse that it is not affecting the health of human being but it affected our state of mind in such a way that we should try to overcome from this situation. We all have to be very strong not only physically but mentally also. Sooner or later this virus will become weaker and weaker but human must be strong enough to save our planet and future generation. Few good aspects of the current situations are that we have adopted good habits like, washing hand before eating something. We also avoid touching our nose and eyes by hand again and again. We also wear mask which helps us to protect from the pollution, we avoid going out unnecessarily which save fuels and air pollution, sound pollution and traffic reduces. Now days we care about our health but we should also care about our mental health. We should do yoga or some exercise. We should avoid negative news from news papers, radio, and television or from any media of communication. We also should avoid talking and discussion on this topic because it affects our psychological balance. Hence to imperative to keep balance in our behavior and lifestyle we should be positive in all aspects. For those people who are already affected and there is imbalance in their behavior, some counseling program must be organized. Various health programs have been organized by social workers and government. People should take the advantage of those programs.

REFERENCES

Angus, K., Cairns, G., Purves, R., Bryce, S., MacDonald, L., & Gordon, R. (2013). *Systematic literature Review to Examine the Evidence for The Effectiveness of interventions that use Theories and Models of Behaviour Change: Towards the Prevention and Control of Communicable Diseases*. Stockholm European Centre for Disease Prevention and Control.

Bavel, J. J. V., Baicker, K., Boggio, P. S., Capraro, V., Cichocka, A., Cikara, M., Molly, J., Crockett, A. J., Douglas, K.M., Druckman, J. N., Drury, J., Dube, O., Ellemers, N., Finkel, E.J., Fowler, J. H., Gelfand, M., Han, S., Haslam, S. A., Jetten, J., Kitayama, S., ... Willer, R. (2020). Using Social and Behavioural Science to Support COVID-19 Pandemic Response. *Nature Human Behaviour, 460*(4), 460–471.

Bish, A., & Michie, S. (2011). *Demographic and Attitudinal Determinants of Protective Behaviours during a Pandemic*. Department of Health.

Cassenti. D., & Weston. (2020). Advances in Human Factors in Simulation and Modeling. Advances in intelligent systems and computing. BMC Public Health, *20*.

Chatterjee, K., Shankar, S., Chatterjee, K., & Yadav, A. K. (2020). Corona virus disease 2019 in India: Post-lockdown scenarios and provisioning for health care. *ELSEVIER Medical Journal, Armed Forces India*, *76*(4), 387–394. doi:10.1016/j.mjafi.2020.06.004 PMID:32836711

Cheng, Y., Liu, D., Chen, J., Namilae, S., Thropp, J., & Seong, Y. (2018). Human Behavior Under Emergency And Its Simulation Modeling. *RE:view*.

Chopra, S., Ranjan, P., Singh, V., Kumar, S., Arora, M., Hasan, M. S., Kasiraj, R., Suryansh, Kaur, D., Vikram, N. K., Malhotra, A., Kumari, A., Klanidhi, K. B., & Baitha, U. (2020). Impact of COVID-19 on Lifestyle-Related Behaviours- A Cross-Sectional Audit of Responses from Nine Hundred And Ninety-Five Participants From India. *Diabetes & Metabolic Syndrome*, *14*(6), 2021–2030. doi:10.1016/j.dsx.2020.09.034 PMID:33099144

Crosta, A. D., Ceccato, I., Marchetti, D., Malva, P. L., Maiella, R., Cannito, R., Cip, M., Mammarella, N., Palumbo, N., Verrocchio, M. C., Palumbo, R., & Domenico, A. D. (2020). Psychological Factors and Consumer Behavior during the COVID-19 Pandemic. *PLoS One*, 1–23. PMID:34398916

Das, G., Jain, S. P., Maheswaran, D., Slotegraaf, R. J., & Srinivasan, R. (2021). Pandemics and Marketing: Insights, Impacts, and Research Opportunities. *Journal of the Academy of Marketing Science*, *49*(5), 835–854. doi:10.100711747-021-00786-y PMID:33994600

Davis, R., Campbell, R., Hildon, Z., Hobbs, L., & Michie, S. (2015). Theories of Behaviour and Behaviour Change Across the Social and Behavioural Sciences: A Scoping Review. *Health Psychology Review*, *9*(3), 323–344. doi:10.1080/1743719 9.2014.941722 PMID:25104107

Francisco, R., Pedro, M., Delvecchio, E., Espada, J. P., Morales, A., Mazzeschi, C., & Orgiles, M. (2020). Psychological Symptoms and Behavioral Changes in Children and Adolescents during the Early Phase of COVID-19 Quarantine in Three European Countries. *Frontiers in Psychiatry*, *11*, 1–14. doi:10.3389/fpsyt.2020.570164 PMID:33343415

Frıas, M. E., Williamson, G., & Frıas, M. V. (2011). Agent-Based Modeling of Epidemic Spreading Using Social Networks and Human Mobility Patterns. *Proceedings Third International Conference on Privacy, Security, Risk and Trust and IEEE third international conference on social computing*, 57–64.

Funk, S., Bansal, S., Bauch, C. T., Eames, K. T., Edmunds, W. J., & Galvani, A. P. (2015). Nine challenges in Incorporating the Dynamics of Behaviour in Infectious Diseases Models. *Epidemics, 10*, 21–5.

Glanz, K., & Bishop, D. B. (2010). The Role of Behavioral Science Theory in Development and Implementation of Public Health Interventions. *Annual Review of Public Health*, *31*(1), 399–418. doi:10.1146/annurev.publhealth.012809.103604 PMID:20070207

Kollamparambil, U., & Oyenubi, A. (2021). Behavioural Response to the COVID-19 2021 Pandemic in South Africa. *PLoS One*, 1–19. PMID:33861811

Matos, A. D., Paiva, A. F. D., Cunha, C., & Voss, G. (2021). Precautionary Behaviours of Individuals with Multimorbidity during The COVID-19 Pandemic. *European Journal of Ageing*, 1–9. PMID:35002593

Michie. S., Van. S. M. M., & West. R. (2011). The Behaviour Change Wheel: A New method for Characterising and Designing Behaviour Change Interventions. *SCI Implement, 6*.

Michie, S., West, R., Campbell, R., Brown, J., & Gainforth, H. (2014). *ABC of Behaviour Change Theories*. Silverback Publishing.

Rawat, D., Dixit, V., Gulati, S., Gulati, S., & Gulati, A. (2021). Impact of COVID-19 Outbreak on Lifestyle Behaviour: A Review of Studies Published in India. *Diabetes & metabolic Syndrome*, *15*(1), 331–336.

Singh, K., Raghav, P., Singh, G., Pritish Baskaran, T. B., Bishnoi, A., Gautam, V., Chaudhary, A. K., Kumar, A., Kumar, S., & Sahu, S. (2021). Lifestyle and Behavioral Changes During Nationwide Lockdown in India-A Cross-Sectional Analysis. *Journal of Family Medicine and Primary Care*, 10(7), 2661–2667. doi:10.4103/jfmpc.jfmpc_2464_20 PMID:34568152

West, R., Michie, S., Rubin, G. J., & Amlot, R. (2020). Applying Principles of Behavior Change to Reduce SARS-Cov-2 Transmission. *Nature Human Behaviour*, 4(5), 451–459. doi:10.103841562-020-0887-9 PMID:32377018

Weston, D., Hauck, K., & Amlot, R. (2018). Infection Prevention Behaviour and Infectious Disease Modeling: A Review of The Literature and Recommendations For The Future. *BMC Public Health*, 18(1), 336. doi:10.118612889-018-5223-1 PMID:29523125

Weston, D. I. A., & Amlot, R. (2020). Examining the Application of Behavior Change Theories in the Context of Infectious Disease Outbreaks and Emergency Response: A Review of Reviews. *BMC Public Health*, 20(1), 1–19. doi:10.118612889-020-09519-2 PMID:33004011

Williams, L., Rasmussen, S., Kleczkowski, A., Maharaj, S., & Cairns, N. (2015). Protection Motivation Theory and Social Distancing Behaviour in Response to a Simulated Infectious Disease Epidemic. *Psychology Health and Medicine*, 20(7), 832–837. doi:10.1080/13548506.2015.1028946 PMID:25835044

World Health Organization. (2020). *Middle East respiratory syndrome corona virus*. MERS-CoV.

Zhang, N., Jia, W., Lei, H., Wang, P., Zhao, P., Guo, Y., Dung, C. H., Bu, Z., Xue, P., Xie, J., Zhang, Y., Cheng, R., & Li, Y. (2019). Effects of Human Behavior Changes During the Coronavirus Disease 2019 (COVID-19) Pandemic on Influenza Spread in Hong Kong. Oxford University Press.

Section 3
From Artificial Intelligence to Healthcare: Comparison, IoT, and Cloud

Chapter 10
Smart Healthcare and Intelligent Medical Systems

Neha Dewangan
Pandit Ravishankar Shukla University, Raipur, India

Prafulla Vyas
Disha College, Raipur, India

Ankita
Pandit Ravishankar Shukla University, Raipur, India

Sunandan Mandal
Pandit Ravishankar Shukla University, Raipur, India

ABSTRACT

A smart healthcare system is a need of the present world. Artificial intelligence, the internet of things, big data, etc. are essential technologies that build a smart and intelligent healthcare system. Deployment of a smart healthcare system not only serves diagnosis and treatment to more patients but also reduces the workload on health workers. Some patients face difficulties using the technology, which needs to be simplified. The most important issue in a smart healthcare system is cyber security. In smart healthcare systems, wearable devices and hospital management store patient information in digital format, which is available in cloud storage, which can be hacked, and it needs strong cyber security. With the development of technologies, smart healthcare systems can provide more intelligent and convenient applications and services. It can provide better service, self-health management, timely and appropriate medical service that can be accessed whenever needed, personalized medical service, improve the doctor-patient relationship, and reduce the cost of services.

DOI: 10.4018/978-1-7998-9831-3.ch010

INTRODUCTION

Smart and intelligent technologies are employed in every essential field of today's world. The branch of medicine has also used these technologies to strengthen the medical system. New technologies like the internet of things (IoT), big data analysis, cloud computing, artificial intelligence (AI) help to build up the medical system smart and intelligent (Tian et al., 2019). Healthcare (HLC) systems are becoming more capable, more convenient, and more personalized after the implementation of the available state-of-the-art technologies and the removal of old technologies. To establish the smart HLC system, technological advancement takes place in all the levels of traditional HLC systems and also developed the field of the intelligent medical system. It changes the concept of treatment and management and also helps patients to sustain a healthy lifestyle. These changes in the HLC system are applied based on enhancing the healthcare service experience and the necessity of the patient and the doctor. The intelligent medical system is capable to handle emergencies with AI and machine learning technology which help in decision making. The smart HLC system has reached rural areas where proper medical facilities were not available. It uses smart gadgets to monitor and maintain the patient's condition. This system makes medical services easier and less costly. It also aids every person from children to the elderly to live a healthy lifestyle.

BACKGROUND

Smart health service system uses intelligent technology such as AI and signals processing that helps in diagnosing and treatment of different types of diseases like cancer, epilepsy, autism, schizophrenia, etc. (Singh et al., 2015; Mandal et al., 2021; Shahamiri & Thabtah, 2020; Tikka et al., 2020). It also helps to provide an alternative option to the patients having a physical disability due to a paralysis attack or any accident. There is much research has done and ongoing in the field of biomedical technology, which improves the medical system. In the era of technology, biomedical technology has made biomedical chips and some wearable devices that monitor our health and store the data for future reference, which help to understand our body more deeply (Baker et al., 2017). Smart healthcare and intelligent medical system use intelligent technology such as AI, machine learning, big data, IoT to improve the service. Smart healthcare and intelligent system help users to aware and educated about their medical status as well as keep them healthy by providing suggestions. Smart healthcare assists the user to manage some emergencies by themselves. It improves the quality of service for patients and makes it more convenient at a low cost. Smart healthcare uses the latest technologies to their maximum potential so that it utilizes the available sources. With the cooperation of smart medical systems, doctors can monitor the condition of patients anywhere and provide services to their patients without any geographical barriers. With the increase of smart devices and technology, the HLC system becomes more intelligent and smart that helps every person from children to the elderly to make a living healthy.

The medical facilities in India represent a very complex scenario because of the large population of India. Hence developing country such as India faces a huge population problem that is one of the major reasons for the average quality of HLC facilities. The population is high in India and the financial status of most of the people is low hence affording good quality health care is quite impossible for this larger population. In one survey of the world health organization (WHO), it was found out that in India there are less than 10 doctors per 10 thousand people of India ("World Health," 2021). Because of the workload pressure, the efficiency and performance of HLC workers are affected. There are limited HLC workers and limited medical facilities in developing and poor countries and the number of patients are more, hence the workloads on the medical staff are more. Thus the diagnosing of the diseases for a large population is difficult to handle with the traditional medical system. Smart Medical System helps HLC workers to lower their workload and improve their capabilities in diagnosing diseases. These technologies work in real-time and provide suitable suggestions, which help doctors to diagnose the disease in an early stage and start treatment. These technologies also predict the health issues that can occur in the future using the data analysis and prevent it by suggesting proper medication. In some regional areas, widely there are no medical facilities available. The smart medical system reaches villages and regional areas and provides some medical consultation and services through current communication technology. Smart HLC system uses the internet to access dynamic information and to connect people with materials and institutions intelligently related to healthcare. For example, someone can get an appointment using the internet. There is no requirement to go to the hospital and stand in a line for hours to make an appointment. There are many applications and websites available for consultation and appointment of a doctor. Online appointments, 24/7 online consultation, chat or call with doctors, order medicine online, free home delivery medical service, etc. are the services provided through these applications. Due to the pandemic, the whole world faced medical crises, during this time healthcare workers in developed countries and some regions of developing countries handled it efficiently with the help of an intelligent medical system. Smart HLC systems helped early detection and diagnosis of diseases. It also supports the associate participants to interact, share the resources and make the proper decisions.

Crucial Technologies of Intelligent Medical System

In the last few decades, technologies explicitly artificial intelligence, IoT, machine learning, bio-sensors, wearable technology, big data, mobile computing, cloud computing were developed. The combinations of these advanced technologies are helped to make the medical system smart and intelligent. A brief explanation of these technologies is described in this subsection.

Artificial Intelligence

Artificial intelligence (AI) is the foremost used technology in the medical system. Many types of research have been done and are ongoing in the medical field supported by AI. It is a technology that helped machines to communicate with humans and analyze the data like an expert of that field with higher precision and speed. AI-based decision-making techniques have many advantages over the traditional clinical analytic system. AI helps healthcare workers to diagnose and treatment of the disease. It uses different algorithms and interacts with medical training data, which allows the system to diagnose the disease or make the decision in real-time (Reddy et al., 2019). In the medical field, AI can be used in neurological diseases and trauma because it mostly takes away some patients' abilities to move, speak and interact with people and the environment. Therefore the artificial intelligence-based system helps those patients to interact with people efficiently by using distinct algorithms. The administrative workload of the enormous HLC centers can be reduced by using the state-of-the-art AI system. AI-based prediction and management services can also support the efficient utilization of the available resources. It can help to handle and automate repetitive and routine tasks like patient data entry and automatic review of laboratory data and imaging results. Hence, it can free the time for healthcare workers to provide more time so they can look after patients. The future outcomes of patients suffering from long-term diseases can also be predicted with AI. By using algorithms and computer programming which depends upon the massive scale of clinical data and raw information provided by the healthcare professional, AI systems can make decisions that can help the healthcare professional to make decisions accurately. These types of AI-based healthcare support systems help to lower medical errors as well as increase the efficiency and consistency of the HLC system. With the assistance of AI, HLC workers can deliver better services to patients.

Machine Learning

Machine Learning is one of the most common sub-divisions of artificial intelligence. Its purpose is to train models with data. It plays an important role in the medical field, including the development of the new clinical procedure, the handling of patient data and records (Magoulas & Prentza, 1999). With the assistance of machine learning, many actions can be finished by automatic modes such as automated messaging alert and related target contains that provokes action at important moments. Machine learning offers a variety of ways to personalized and improved the treatment process. Machine learning-based virtual nurse is also one of the applications that make the treatment much easier for patients. It is a voice-controlled healthcare assistant that collects information related to any illness, health disorder, and medicines. It also communicates with the patient and provides positive motivation to the patients that help to improve their health day by day.

This machine learning-based system can give real-time advice to patients on the conditions where reaching hospitals or finding a doctor is difficult. Machine learning-based systems can also be used to educate patients about disease pathways and outcomes of different treatment options. It can impact healthcare workers, healthcare institutes, and HLC systems in improving efficiency while reducing the cost of treatment.

Internet of Things

Internet of Things (IoT) is one of the major technologies that are utilized in the sector of healthcare management systems. This technology is additionally referred to as IoMT (Internet of Medical Things) is extremely popular and has added the element of smartness in the healthcare industry. It assists HLC workers to identify, monitoring, and obtain information about the patient's condition. It also provides information that can aid the HLC workers to identify future health issues, so they can start early treatment for the disease, which results in the better delivery of the HLC system (Catarinucci et al., 2015). The IoT-based devices can collect and transfer health data such as blood pressure, heart rate, oxygen level, glucose level, weight, sleep duration, etc. These data can be shared over a cloud network and regardless of time, location, and device it can be accessed using the authorized credentials by an appointed physician, insurance company, external consultant, and health firm. Combination IoT and other state-of-the-art technologies are enhanced the automation processes in patient care and HLC facilities. Since IoT makes accessible machine-to-machine communication and eases information exchange more effective healthcare services can be delivered to the human being. It also helps to provide cost-effective service as well as better planning of resources allocation. It makes easier data acquisition from multiple sources and faster complex analyses as well. The IoMT based devices enable real-time signal analyses that remove the requirement of large storage for raw data. The advantage of real-time analyses using IoMT based devices reduces the unnecessary load of the cloud networks and servers. Hence, only final analyses reports are required to overcloud on cloud storage. It also reduces susceptible errors in the distinct medical report and helps in quick and right decision making. This can aid the senior citizen to keep a close track of body vitals such as heart rate, blood pressure, glucose level, sleep pattern, etc. It can also monitor and remind the schedule of medications. The portable IoMT devices make it a lot easier for people to conduct or manage their routine health checkups such as routine blood tests. Soon, the IoMT based devices will rule out all the other non-IoMT based medical systems.

Wearable technology

Wearable technology is also named wearables. Wearables are electronic devices that can be worn and used for signal acquisition and vitals measurement of patients. This type of electronic device can also be classified into non-invasive and invasive wearables. Non-invasive wearables are simply embedded in clothing or attached over the skin of the patient and the invasive wearables are implanted into the patient's body. These devices are tiny microprocessor-based wireless enable an embedded system that can able to send or receive data to the cloud server using the smartphones. Wearable technology allows the continuous monitoring of users' physical activity, behavior, physiological and biochemical parameters. These devices are comfortable to wear, consume less power, allow data to be combined with health information, which helps to reduce the risk caused by disease (Sultan, 2015). Fit bands, smartwatches, web-enabled glasses, VR headsets, bodysuits are some examples of wearable devices. The concept of the patient wearable device is to monitor the healthcare data. Wearable devices are small in size and portable so it is possible to monitor the vitals of patients/ users anywhere rather than using old devices to monitor the vitals of patients in hospitals or homes only. Some wearables are also helping in the regular tracking of the physical activity of the patient. That further support disease management as well as patient management. Precise and accurate vital information of patients helps to take impactful clinical decision-making. The fitness band-based wearable devices are the most popular in the medical field. If the fitness band is held in the right place of the body then the inbuilt sensors can detect the vitals of the user and send the collected data to an authorized person, also notifying the user if detect any irregularity. Now a day's most people are aware of health issues and pay attention to their lifestyle and diets, these wearables help user to maintain their fitness and diet plan using the internet. Wearable technology in healthcare has several benefits such as its personal and part of user's lifestyle, its focus on healthy habits, it can track and improve user's goals in healthcare, it is portable and affordable. With the advancement of smart technology that can implant on the body, HLC workers can work with their patients to collect information for their treatment anywhere, along with helping them to practice healthy habits in their lifestyle.

Mobile Computing

Mobile Computing is one of the most important technologies utilized in the medical field as a mobile HLC system (Ma et al., 2018). Advanced wireless, portable and mobile electronic devices like laptops, palmtops, and wearables are utilized the mobile computing technology for information processing and storage. Mobile computing enables communication in a different location and at any time. The number of customers using a smartphone has been increasing day by day thus the new mobile applications has increased in a different field such as education, commercial, medical. There are large numbers of mobile apps which are used for medical services. Medical professionals use these mobile applications for getting information, time management, scheduling appointment, connecting and treatment of patients, etc. Using mobile devices in clinical practices has accelerated the rapid development of the medical profession. It has not only improved the traditional patient monitoring and management but also assist and support clinical decision-making. It is beneficial for HLC professionals to use smartphones and medical mobile applications to give better services to patients and save time as well. The research and development in the application of mobile computing in the HLC system will make the HLC system smarter.

Big data

Big data analysis is a very important segment the data science. As huge amounts of data are generated in the medical field, it is nearly impossible to manage and process the data using traditional data processing system. Hence big data analysis is going to take over the traditional analysis technique. The medical data are in a different format, type, and context hence it is difficult to merge all types of healthcare data into a conventional database, making it enormously challenging to process (Baro et al., 2015). Big data is larger, more complex data sets that are used to manage a huge amount of data. The high volume of data, high velocity, and a large number of variables in the data are three characteristics of big data also known as 3V characteristics. Using big data-based healthcare data analytics, doctors and administrators may get better medical as well as financial decisions. Higher-level analysis and diagnosis of medical data are possible using big data analysis. Therefore it is easy to process and decide large and complex medical data such as on epidemic or pandemic related huge medical data. The HLC systems work at different levels and generate different kinds of information at all levels that can be processed using big data analysis. Patient medical history like diagnosis and prescribed medicine-related data, as well as complex clinical data like electroencephalogram, electrocardiogram, or x-ray, can be handled with big data technology. Traditional medical records were either typed in form or handwritten on paper, as time goes it gets older and difficult to access. With the advancement of technology and computer systems, it is possible to digitalize all types of medical data into a digital format which is known as electronic health records (EHR). Big data can manage and process these digital data. Hence the smart HLC system has become more standard and easy to manage all levels of healthcare data.

Cloud computing

After big data, cloud computing is the dominant technology that made the HLC technologies smarter. Scalability, cost-effectiveness, and system flexibility are the important properties that are achieved by smart HLC systems with the support of cloud computing (Dang et al., 2019). Nowadays, the demand for cloud computing HLC solutions is growing exponentially due to a large number of cloud computing-based medical collaborations. It is an internet-based system that provides a virtual storage system that can store a large amount of data and is accessible anywhere to an authorized person. It works in real-time and manages all types of data. In a traditional health care system, it is very difficult to manage all the records of patients and other documents as well as it is time taking. In smart health care systems, cloud computing plays the role to stores all the records of patients into the cloud server, which is easily accessible and easy to manage. Cloud computing has made everything easy, even small health care centers can gain access to information and store it at a low cost. With the help of cloud computing, at a low cost with effective manner hospitals and health care institutes can now deliver better services to their patients. There are many smart medical applications and services are available online that are utilized to assist medical professionals and patients. These applications and services are using cloud computing, big data, mobile computing, and AI-based integrated technology. Cloud computing makes the HLC system scalable and flexible as per the requirement of organizations. Maintenance of cloud computing technologies like software and hardware updates is not the burden of the organization. Hence, cloud computing provides opportunities to the healthcare organization to improve the entire medical system with new and advanced techniques.

Bio - Sensors

Biosensors are the analytical tools utilized to detect and respond to the biological inputs that come from the part of the human body such as tissue, cell, muscles, or any organ. These tiny devices have a wide range of applications like diagnosis, monitoring, biomedicine, defense, security, etc. (Vigneshvar et al., 2016). Medication monitoring and detection of irregularities in the body can also be detected using biosensors. Biosensors involve biotechnology with electrochemistry, nanotechnology, and bioelectronics to detect the biological elements in our body. Biosensors are made with different materials and work on different principles. These sensors are usually made of optical/visual, polymer, silica, glass, and other nano-materials. Biocompatibilities, abundance, suitable electronic, optical, and mechanical properties are some characteristics used to select and make the biosensor. For advanced applications, silicon nano-materials shows promising characteristics for making bio-sensor device. No toxicity is another important necessity of sensors used in biomedical applications. Bio-imaging, bio-sensing, and treatment of cancer are some examples of the application of bio-sensors. The first electrochemical-based biosensor device is Glucometer. Glucose biosensors are very popular in hospitals to monitor the level of glucose in the blood for diabetic patients. Further, these bio-sensors can be categorized into in-vitro and in-vivo types. In-Vitro type sensors are attached externally to the human body. These types of biosensors reduce the involvement of lab and hospital facilities in healthcare. On the other hand, in-vivo sensors are implantable devices that are placed inside the human body and there is a need to fulfill the regulations and standard of sterilization. There is a variety of biosensors used in the medical field such as heart rate sensor, SPO2 sensor to monitor the oxygen level in the blood, etc. Biosensors are made of highly sensitive materials to provide accurate measurement; it provides a basis to understand technological improvement in biomedical instrumentation. Biosensors are also used in wearable devices.

Few recent research based on the mentioned technologies is tabulated in Table 1. IoT, wearable ECG, and cloud computing-based heart status monitoring system was proposed by Yang et al. (2016). For the secrecy and the security of the medical data of patients, a big data-based distributed framework was reported by Sarkar (2017). Ma et al. (2018) were reported an intelligent HLC architecture for smart HLC environment using big data and cloud computing techniques. A unique deep learning-based HLC recommender system was proposed by Deng and Huangfu (2019). Tikka et al. (2020) were proposed an intelligent model for the identification of schizophrenia disease. Further, an autism disorder screen using a convolution neural network (CNN) was reported by Shahamiri and Thabtah (2020). An epileptic seizure detection model using a majority-vote-based attribute selection and hybrid machine learning model was proposed by Mandal et al. (2021). Blockchain and IoT-based COVID-19 patient tracking system was reported by Alam (2021). Atrey et al. (2021) were reported a computer-aided system (CAS) to segment the breast lesion using both mammography and ultrasound images and the CNN classification approach.

For the COVID-19 virus detection, a two-dimensional (2D) biosensor was developed by Fathi-Hafshejani et al. (2021) using tungsten diselenide (WSe2) and field-effect transistor (FET) design. Roy et al. were reported a hybrid classification model for the segmentation of cancer tumors using a convolution neural network

(CNN) with connected component analysis (CCA). This AI-based model can assist the radiologist during the segmentation of tumors. A speech signal-based hybrid one-dimensional deep learning model for language impairment classification was proposed by Sharma and Singh (2022). From Table 1, it can be observed that data security, computer-aided disease diagnosis tool, and biosensor-based research are currently in the major focus.

Table 1. Brief overview of some recent research on assistive and smart healthcare technique

Author	Issue Addressed	Descriptions	Devices and technologies	Disease diagnosis and HLC support
Yang et al. (2016)	Development of ECG monitoring system from a remote place	Heart status can be monitored from remote places using advanced IoT based techniques	IoT, Wearable, ECG, Cloud computing	Heart status monitoring
Sarkar (2017)	Design a distributed big data framework for HLC data security	Reported a big data framework for secrecy and security of HLC related data	Big data	Support the HLC data security
Ma et al. (2018)	Design architecture of intelligent HLC system	Reported a layer-wise architecture of intelligent HLC system to access and store the HLC data in the cloud	Big data, Cloud and mobile computing	Optimization of HLC system
Deng and Huangfu (2019)	Design a healthcare recommender system (HRS)	Proposed collaborative variational deep learning (CVDL) based HRS for the patient and medical experts	Deep learning	Support the smart HLC system
Tikka et al. (2020)	Design a model for schizophrenia identification	Electro-encephalogram (EEG) and Support vector machine-based schizophrenia detection was proposed	Machine Learning, EEG	Diagnosis of Schizophrenia
Shahamiri and Thabtah (2020)	Developed an AI-based autism screening	Proposed a convolution neural network (CNN) based intelligent screening system for autism patient	AI, CNN	Help in the screening process autism patient
Mandal et al. (2021)	Design a model for epilepsy detection	Majority voting feature selection and support vector neural network (SVNN) were used for epileptic seizure classification	Hybrid machine learning, EEG	Epilepsy detection
Alam (2021)	Design a four-layer IoT and blockchain-based COVID-19 patient monitoring model	Addressed the data security and patient tracking with the help of IoT and blockchain technique	IoT, Blockchain	COVID-19 patient monitoring system

Continued on following page

Table 1. Continued

Author	Issue Addressed	Descriptions	Devices and technologies	Disease diagnosis and HLC support
Atrey et al. (2021)	Design a bimodal breast lesion detection model	Proposed a computer-aided segmentation technique using mammography and ultrasound modality and CNN classifier	Machine learning, Mammography, Ultrasound	Breast lesion detection and diagnosis
Fathi-Hafshejani et al. (2021)	Design and implement a 2D biosensor for COVID-19 virus detection	Reported a two-dimensional tungsten diselenide (WSe_2) and field-effect transistor (FET) based biosensor for virus detection	Biosensor, FET	COVID-19 detection
Roy et al. (2022)	Design a hybrid model for segmenting the malignant tumor from a mammogram	A combination of convolution neural network (CNN) with connected component analysis (CCA) were employed for malignant tumor segmentation	Hybrid machine learning, mammography	Cancer detection and diagnosis
Sharma and Singh (2022)	Design a diagnosis system to classify specific language-impaired children	Reported a hybrid one-dimensional deep learning model for language impairment classification using speech signal	Hybrid deep learning, Speech signal recording unit	Assist in the diagnosis of specific language impairment

Table 2 shows an overview of some recently reported HLC models. Ghosh et al. (2016) were proposed IoT based HLC system for observation of patients from a remote place. The proposed architecture was divided into three modules namely sensing, main and interaction module. The functionality of the system was tested and validated with real-time patient health records. Saha et al. (2017) were also proposed a monitoring system for healthcare. IoT, cloud computing, and biosensors were technologies used in this HLC model. A 24 by 7 patient monitoring system was proposed by Ruman et al. (2020). With this system, patient health data like heart rate, blood pressure, temperature, and Electrocardiography (ECG) were monitored wirelessly. Hameed et al. (2020) were reported IoT and fuzzy neural network-based intelligent HLC systems. The proposed HLC system was also able to decide according to the healthcare data of the patient. An AI-based HLC system for COVID-19 patient screening was proposed by Ahmed et al. (2022). In this system, the patient's chest X-ray images were taken for screening.

Table 2. Overview of some recently reported HLC model

Author	Descriptions	Technologies used	Advantages	Limitation
Ghosh et al. (2016)	Proposed IoT based HLC system for a remote place	IoT, Sensors, Mobile computing	Low cost and less power consuming HLC model	Only ECG and temperature sensors were used.
Saha et al. (2017)	Proposed a patient monitoring model using IoT	Cloud computing, IoT, Sensors	A large number of vital information can be captured	Experimental performance need to verify
Ruman et al. (2020)	Proposed wireless patient monitoring system	IoT, Sensors, Android application, Cloud computing	24 x 7 monitoring system	Only heart rate, pressure, temperature, and ECG can be monitored
Hameed et al. (2020)	Reported IoT and AI-based HLC system	IoT, Fuzzy Neural Network, sensors	The AI-based system can able to decide according to the captured data.	Only temperature, pressure, and pulse rate sensor are used.
Ahmed et al. (2022)	Reported an HLC system for Screening of COVID-19 patient	AI, X-ray, IoT	The AI-based system can detect COVID-19 patients using chest x-ray images	Screening of COVID-19 and pneumonia patient is possible

From Table 2, it can also be seen that most HLC systems are used to monitor body temperature, ECG, blood pressure, and heart rate only. There are many other diseases leftover that required medical imaging of other parts of the body and signal acquisition like computed tomography, Electroencephalography (EEG), Electromyography (EMG). There is a need to do more research in this direction. These recent researches on the medical field and the implementations show that the traditional HLC systems are drastically changed into advanced and smart HLC systems. The crucial technologies based clinical tools for the medical professional, HLC architecture, or HLC applications all of them together enhance the performance of the HLC system.

SMART HEALTHCARE ARCHITECTURE

A typical architecture of a smart HLC system is depicted in Figure 1. The combination of technologies, such as IoT, AI, cloud computing, mobile computing, wearable devices, biosensors, etc. is helped to build the smart HLC system. From Figure 1, the working process of a simple smart HLC system can be understood. Firstly, the patient can schedule the online consultation, create an online database, and payment through the applications and website available. This process can be done by smart hospital staff. According to the disease type, the AI and cloud computing system will recommend the available medical practitioner to the patient. This process helps to reduce the queue of the patient in the hospital. The clinical measurements, such as temperature, blood pressure, pulse rate, respiration rate, etc are recorded using advanced biosensors, and wearable devices. These measurements are also updated into the database with help of IoT devices. Further, the doctor or medical practitioner can access the detailed information of patients such as vital signs, medical history, and present status from the cloud database and also be able to converse with the patient through the cloud network. Doctors can recommend the medicine and pathological test to the patient and that will also be available online in the cloud network. This online information will further help to provide home delivery of medicine and also make available pathological test report for further treatment of the patient. Machine learning-based supervised AI systems will also be available through cloud networks that can help to treatment of the minor problem. From this typical architecture of a smart HLC system, it is clear that the smart HLC system overcome the deficiency of the traditional HLC system. Smart HLC systems make HLC systems easy and make them available for 24 hours and 7 days.

Figure 1. Typical architecture of smart HLC system

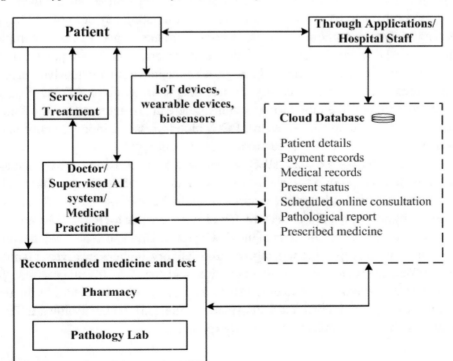

The requirements of smart healthcare can be divided into two categories: functional and non-functional. The former refers to the various requirements that are related to the operation of smart HLC systems. The functional requirements of a smart HLC system vary depending on the application and the hardware component used. Non-functional requirements are often defined by the attributes that can be determined by assessing the quality of an HLC system. These requirements can be classified into ethical requirements and performance requirements. An HLC system that is efficient and reliable should have various features such as low power consumption, portability, reliability, and ease of use.

The components of a smart HLC system are often classified as networking devices, data storage components, computing devices, and sensors or actuators. Networking devices are used to provide a link or path to information from sensors to routers and cloud base stations. Mostly wireless technologies are used as a network component such as Wi-Fi, and Bluetooth. Wireless technology plays an important role in exchanging information and processed data among different elements of a healthcare network that are used in an HLC system. Data storage is the most important part of a smart HLC system. All the information is dependent on these medical data. In a traditional HLC system the data/information was stored in paper files, in a smart HLC system, it is stored in cloud memory so it can be accessed anywhere. Data storage elements within the smart healthcare networks cover a broad range of smart devices from embedded system memory on the sensing device to a big server that can handle big data analytics. Computing devices utilized in this era range from smartphones, tablets, laptops, computers, and PDAs to complex and advanced devices like supercomputers and servers. Sensors are powerful and innovative devices that can detect biological elements with an extensive range of applications, such as drug discovery, disease diagnosis, and biomedicine. Sensors or actuators support the monitoring systems. There are many sensors for different purposes such as temperature sensor, ECG, blood pressure, blood glucose level, SpO2, motion sensor, EMG, accelerometer, gyroscope, etc.

The architecture of the smart HLC system can also be classified into three major categories namely app-oriented, things-oriented, and semantics-oriented. The reliable and secure transmission between the applications in the smartphones and the sensors is ensured by app-oriented architecture. It is also responsible for the establishment of a customized network for the users of the HLC system. Things-oriented architectures help to improve real-time monitoring, on-time delivery, higher sensitivity, maintain higher efficiency with lower power dissipation, and smart intelligent processing of the new HLC system. The semantic-oriented ensure the improvement in the user experience using previous feedback information collected by smart healthcare. These unique capabilities complement the user experience.

APPLICATION

The applications of smart healthcare are described in detail in the further subsections.

Health Management

Health management is very important in the present day. Recently the world is facing new types of viruses and there is a need for an improved system that can manage every type of change and challenge. The traditional hospital and doctor-patient management system are incapable of dealing with an increased number of patients and diseases. The smart HLC system pays more attention to patient self-management (Zhu et al., 2019). It does not always need a healthcare worker to monitor the condition of patients. It monitors the condition of patients using wearable devices such as fit bands in real-time and gives immediate suggestions or feedback. Wearable device uses different type of advanced sensors, processors, and wireless module to continue sensing and monitor the behavior of patient in an intelligent manner. These devices are comfortable to wear, consume less power, allow data to be combined with health information, which helps to reduce the risk caused by disease. It is easier for medical institutes to monitor the condition of the patient, their behavior, and diagnose the disease. Smart bands, smartphones, etc. provide the platform for successfully monitoring. Smart health management can help people to maintain a healthy lifestyle. Which decreases the frequently going hospitals also saves money and time. Smart homes can also help in health management. Smart homes provide home assistants that can help children, the elderly, and disabled people. Smart homes or apartments are integrated with sensors and actuators in infrastructure, which monitor the resident's physical sign and environment. The smart home also improves the living experience and maintains living a healthy lifestyle. The home monitoring system can collect health data of residents and provide some simple health services, helping people who want to reduce their dependency on HLC providers and improve the quality of life at home. Smart HLC technologies either devices or healthcare applications support the patients to handle and self-manage the non-critical medical condition. It helps healthcare workers to reduce their workload and improve health services towards relevant and economical medical services for patients.

Smart Diagnosis

Smart diagnosis is the productive outcomes of application of the IoT, AI-based medical equipment, surgical robots, etc., in the diagnosis and treatment that makes disease diagnosis more intelligent and precise (Chui et al., 2017). AI is a technology that can communicate with computers like a human. AI has many advantages over traditional techniques and makes all the diagnostic techniques smarter. AI assists the HLC workers to diagnose and treatment of the disease. It uses different algorithms and interacts with medical training data, which allows the system to diagnose the disease or make the decision in real-time. AI-based diagnoses improve the thinking and decision-making ability in diagnosis that achieve great results. Smart diagnoses give suggestions based on the data of patients. It is reported that sometimes the accuracy of AI-based systems is more than the experienced doctor, especially in pathology and imaging. For example, the result is more accurate when the surgery is done by a robotic arm as compared to surgery done by a doctor. The use of smart diagnosis reduces the incidence of missed diagnosis, misdiagnosis, malfunctioning during surgeries, and provides good and proper medical treatment to the patients. Using the smart diagnosis system, medical experts can be able to develop a personalized treatment plan as per the condition and disease status of the individual patient very accurately. The applications of AI in the medical field make the development and implementation of the surgical plan easier and also bring changes in medical education, research, communication, and medical treatment.

Virtual Assistant

A virtual assistant is a program that communicates with patients. It is based on techniques such as IoT, speech recognition algorithms, deep learning, that rely on information provided by users. Virtual assistants respond according to the user's preference or needs after calculations (Sharmin et al., 2006). In the smart HLC, virtual assistant plays the key role to communicate with HLC workers and health institutes. Virtual assistants use multiple language understanding technologies, programmed by experts to help users complete different tasks from reminder creation to home automation. It makes communication much easier and more convenient. Virtual assistants break the barrier of language it covert one language into another language that can be understood easily. Doctors can respond automatically to the patient based on their symptoms and medical history which already existed in the system. The implementation of virtual assistants can help medical institutes and research centers to reduce manpower and material resources and respond according to the need with high efficiency. The virtual assistant can also be used to improve the mental health of humans.

Healthcare Mobile Apps

These days technology has become part of our lives. Using the Smartphone for different purposes makes life easier. In the healthcare field, there are various types of mobile applications which provide many services such as:

- Searching doctors
- 24/7 medical consultation from experts
- Easy medicine availability
- A reliable source of information
- Online registration and appointment
- Information in Multilingual
- Remote Medical Assistance

These mobile applications save the time of users, provide good services at low cost, work accurately and also provide security (Boudreaux et al., 2014).

Smart Hospital

Smart HLC system consists of the smart hospital which is based on technology such as IoT, digital devices, and intelligent services. It relies on an information and communication technology-based environment. It personalizes and improves the features related to patient care and health monitoring, also provides services to medical staff. Smart hospitals have integrated system that works on IoT-based digital devices, including multiple digital systems and intelligent building (Sundaravadivel et al., 2017). The technology can also be used for the identification of patients and medical staff using RFID cards. Using RFID cards for individuals make hospital secure and the information can only be accessed by authorized person. In the smart hospital, the patient can use many features such as a human-less information center that provide true information, online appointment, improve doctor-patient relation, etc. The smart hospital makes patients' medical treatment easier and more convenient in short time duration. Smart healthcare also includes the pharmaceutical industry for drug production and research institutes for drug development. It manages the production, circulation, and inventory management, anti-counterfeiting, and other processes. This makes to achieve a safe, reliable, stable, and efficient circulation of materials in hospitals. Smart hospitals can maximize the utilization of medical resources, help hospitals make development decisions, reduce medical costs. In addition, smart hospitals improve the experience of the doctor-patient relationship and service quality of hospital management.

Drug Research

With the use of new technologies such as big data and AI in scientific research, it is more convenient and precise to conduct drug research and developed the drug (Vaishya et al., 2020). Drug development is a long process including target screening, drug discovery, and the number of clinical trials. The traditional drug developments are utilized manual target screening to reach the effective points and it is a time-consuming process. Nowadays, this process is speedup with automated target screening processes. Real-time data can be collected at any time and optimization of the screening process is done with an AI-based system. High throughput-based screening and synthesis for drug research also needs more cost and is also associated with a high-risk factor. AI-based simulated drug screening is an alternative solution to reduce the cost as well as the associated risk. AI-based drug discovery can help to predict the drug molecule's activities precisely and improve the drug discovery efficiency. The new technologies namely IoT, AI, and big data are also involved in the clinical trials. Using these advanced techniques in drug research can facilitate the entire screening process and help to determine suitable target subjects. Hence, these smart technologies can reduce the risk and cost factor as well as the time involved in the drug discovery process and give efficient and accurate results in drug development.

Smart Diagnosis for COVID-19

In the December of 2019, the world has found the first case of the pandemic, and the world health organization (WHO) has declared public health emergency (Hosseinifard et al., 2021). The cause of the pandemic situation is the global spreading of the severe acute respiratory syndrome coronavirus 2 (SARS-CoV-2) that also known as a novel coronavirus (COVID-19). Novel coronavirus or COVID-19 spread fast, transmitted from human to human. To control the pandemic, a lockdown has been imposed to prevent the spread of the coronavirus. Billions of people worldwide are affected with COVID-19 and create not only health issues in them but also weaken them economically and socially. Within a few months, many people lost their lives and faced health-related issues, which has symptoms like COVID-19. The pandemic has raised the issue of healthcare facilities. There was a panic situation for every country that how to control and stop spreading the virus, how to cure or diagnose the coronavirus because there were no medicine or treatment. Health centers were open only for emergency services or for coronavirus-related problems. For other health-related issues, health centers were closed to prevent the spreading of the coronavirus. At that time smart services helped doctors in the detection and diagnosis of the patients. The main problem was to detect the coronavirus in real-time; the early diagnosis was the most effective way to manage the spread of infections. The incubation period of the COVID-19 is very long approximately 2 to 14 days. During this period no symptoms of inflection appear clearly. The symptoms are appearing very late approximately from 8 to 16 days after infection. Since the incubation period is very long therefore it is supported the virus to spread out and infect the human in multiple. "Fever, cough, fatigue, sore throat, headache" are the reported symptoms of COVID-19. These were similar to cold/flu-like symptoms. Hence, there is a need for a specific COVID-19 test. An enzyme-linked immune-sorbent assay (ELISA), RTPCR (Reverse Transcription-Polymerase Chain Reaction), rapid antigen test (RAT), computed tomography scan, and a variety of biosensors are utilized to detect the coronavirus. Testing strategy, test duration, equipment utilized are some important factors that affect the sensitivity of the COVID-19 tests. In the current pandemic situation, health workers have preferred AI, IoT, and mobile computing-based remote monitoring devices for patients' diagnostic and treatment. These types of advanced devices are provided real-time feedback that helps to take a necessary and fast decision on disease treatment. Smart healthcare can also able to track the suspected subject (infected or non-infected patient) with advanced technologies and help to make a better plan to break the transmission chain and stop the widespread of COVID-19 type diseases.

ISSUES AND CHALLENGES

The smart HLC system has many advantages over the traditional HLC system, but there are still some issues that need to be solved. Smart HLC system uses smart and intelligent technologies such as AI, big data, IoT. In the future, there will be more challenges in the medical field and it needs the development of technologies. Currently, the smart HLC system needed more macro guidance, advanced research on the integration of technologies and programmatic documents, which will help to improve the performance and reduce waste of resources. Lack of uniformity and standardization in medical institutions are important issues for data integrity. The data generated in the medical field is very large and complex. Therefore, data sharing and communication have faced high difficulties. The smart HLC system also lacks compatibility between different platforms and devices, which can be solved by improving the ability to analyze information using big data. Some patients face difficulties using the technology which needs to be simplified. Some technologies that are used in this smart system are still in the stage of investigation and maintenance and up-gradation are still required. There is always an unknown risk factor attached with this technology if the safety and security precautions will not be used properly. The most important issue in a smart system is cyber security. In this system, wearable devices and hospital management store the patient's information in digital format, which is available in cloud storage, that can be hacked and it needs strong security. This system is connected via the internet, the patient can contact the doctor online, but when there is a network issue it was difficult to access services. In some rural areas where people always face network issues, it is problematic to use smart healthcare services.

CONCLUSION

The smart HLC system is a very useful and vast application in the HLC system. The technological advancement in applied technologies makes the smart HLC systems more intelligent and convenient for the supply of applications and services. This HLC system can provide better service, self-heath management, timely and proper medical service that can be accessed whenever needed, personalized medical service, improve the doctor-patient relationship, reduce the cost of services, etc. In medical institutes, a smart HLC system can reduce the stress of healthcare workers, manage the patient's information and record efficiently and in a smarter way, improve the patient's experience while reducing the service cost. This system is also beneficial for the institutions conducting research. Smart and intelligent technologies can reduce the cost and time of research, improve research experience, and also reduce the risk factor attached to the research. This HLC system is accomplished to manage and decide in real-time emergencies. Smart healthcare can also reduce the insufficiency of medical resources. It helps to promote the implementation of clinical reform and prevention strategies. Advanced decision-making capabilities also assist in the utilization of medical resources and provide economic medical facilities. Overall the smart and intelligent medical system provides better services and helps to maintain a healthy lifestyle. Some issues need to be solved. There is still a need for more research in AI-based clinical tools based on a larger dataset. These generalized clinical tools will assist the medical expert during the diagnosis and treatment of a specific disease. Data security is another key issue of a smart HLC system. There is a need for the design and implementation of an advanced data security model based on blockchain that can be the future of data security. The solution depends on the development process of technology, as the technology develops the problems will be solved, but it also needs the joint efforts of the doctor, patients, healthcare, and technology development institutes.

REFERENCES

Ahmed, I., Jeon, G., & Chehri, A. (2022). An IoT-enabled smart health care system for screening of COVID-19 with multi layers features fusion and selection. *Computing*, 1–18. doi:10.100700607-021-00992-0

AlamT. (2021). *Blockchain-Enabled Mobile Healthcare System Architecture for the Real-Time Monitoring of the COVID-19 Patients*. doi:10.2139/ssrn.3772643

Atrey, K., Singh, B. K., Roy, A., & Bodhey, N. K. (2021). Real-time automated segmentation of breast lesions using CNN-based deep learning paradigm: Investigation on mammogram and ultrasound. *International Journal of Imaging Systems and Technology*, ima.22690. doi:10.1002/ima.22690

Baker, S. B., Xiang, W., & Atkinson, I. (2017). Internet of things for smart healthcare: Technologies, challenges, and opportunities. *IEEE Access: Practical Innovations, Open Solutions*, 5, 26521–26544. doi:10.1109/ACCESS.2017.2775180

Baro, E., Degoul, S., Beuscart, R., & Chazard, E. (2015). Toward a literature-driven definition of big data in healthcare. *BioMed Research International*, *2015*, 2015. doi:10.1155/2015/639021 PMID:26137488

Boudreaux, E. D., Waring, M. E., Hayes, R. B., Sadasivam, R. S., Mullen, S., & Pagoto, S. (2014). Evaluating and selecting mobile health apps: Strategies for healthcare providers and healthcare organizations. *Translational Behavioral Medicine*, *4*(4), 363–371. doi:10.100713142-014-0293-9 PMID:25584085

Catarinucci, L., De Donno, D., Mainetti, L., Palano, L., Patrono, L., Stefanizzi, M. L., & Tarricone, L. (2015). An IoT-aware architecture for smart HLC systems. *IEEE Internet of Things Journal*, 2(6), 515–526. doi:10.1109/JIOT.2015.2417684

Chui, K. T., Alhalabi, W., Pang, S. S. H., Pablos, P. O. D., Liu, R. W., & Zhao, M. (2017). Disease diagnosis in smart healthcare: Innovation, technologies and applications. *Sustainability*, *9*(12), 2309. doi:10.3390u9122309

Dang, L. M., Piran, M., Han, D., Min, K., & Moon, H. (2019). A survey on internet of things and cloud computing for healthcare. *Electronics (Basel)*, *8*(7), 768. doi:10.3390/electronics8070768

Deng, X., & Huangfu, F. (2019). Collaborative variational deep learning for healthcare recommendation. *IEEE Access: Practical Innovations, Open Solutions*, 7, 55679–55688. doi:10.1109/ACCESS.2019.2913468

Fathi-Hafshejani, P., Azam, N., Wang, L., Kuroda, M. A., Hamilton, M. C., Hasim, S., & Mahjouri-Samani, M. (2021). Two-dimensional-material-based field-effect transistor biosensor for detecting COVID-19 Virus (SARS-CoV-2). *ACS Nano*, *15*(7), 11461–11469. doi:10.1021/acsnano.1c01188 PMID:34181385

Ghosh, A. M., Halder, D., & Hossain, S. A. (2016, May). Remote health monitoring system through IoT. In *2016 5th International Conference on Informatics, Electronics and Vision (ICIEV)* (pp. 921-926). IEEE. 10.1109/ICIEV.2016.7760135

Hameed, K., Bajwa, I. S., Ramzan, S., Anwar, W., & Khan, A. (2020). An intelligent IoT based healthcare system using fuzzy neural networks. *Scientific Programming*, *2020*, 2020. doi:10.1155/2020/8836927

Hosseinifard, M., Naghdi, T., Morales-Narváez, E., & Golmohammadi, H. (2021). Toward Smart Diagnostics in a Pandemic Scenario: COVID-19. *Frontiers in Bioengineering and Biotechnology*, *9*, 510. doi:10.3389/fbioe.2021.637203 PMID:34222208

Ma, X., Wang, Z., Zhou, S., Wen, H., & Zhang, Y. (2018, June). Intelligent HLC systems assisted by data analytics and mobile computing. In 2018 14th International Wireless Communications & Mobile Computing Conference (IWCMC) (pp. 1317-1322). IEEE.

Magoulas, G. D., & Prentza, A. (1999, July). Machine learning in medical applications. In *Advanced course on artificial intelligence* (pp. 300–307). Springer.

Mandal, S., Singh, B. K., & Thakur, K. (2021). Majority voting-based hybrid feature selection in machine learning paradigm for epilepsy detection using EEG. *International Journal of Computational Vision and Robotics*, *11*(4), 385–400. doi:10.1504/IJCVR.2021.116558

Reddy, S., Fox, J., & Purohit, M. P. (2019). Artificial intelligence-enabled healthcare delivery. *Journal of the Royal Society of Medicine*, *112*(1), 22–28. doi:10.1177/0141076818815510 PMID:30507284

Roy, A., Singh, B. K., Banchhor, S. K., & Verma, K. (2022). Segmentation of malignant tumours in mammogram images: A hybrid approach using convolutional neural networks and connected component analysis. *Expert Systems: International Journal of Knowledge Engineering and Neural Networks*, *39*(1), e12826. doi:10.1111/exsy.12826

Ruman, M. R., Barua, A., Rahman, W., Jahan, K. R., Roni, M. J., & Rahman, M. F. (2020, February). IoT based emergency health monitoring system. In *2020 International Conference on Industry 4.0 Technology (I4Tech)* (pp. 159-162). IEEE. 10.1109/I4Tech48345.2020.9102647

Saha, H. N., Auddy, S., Pal, S., Kumar, S., Pandey, S., Singh, R., Singh, A. K., Sharan, P., Ghosh, D., & Saha, S. (2017, August). Health monitoring using internet of things (IoT). In *2017 8th Annual Industrial Automation and Electromechanical Engineering Conference (IEMECON)* (pp. 69-73). IEEE.

Sarkar, B. K. (2017). Big data for secure healthcare system: A conceptual design. *Complex & Intelligent Systems*, *3*(2), 133–151. doi:10.100740747-017-0040-1

Shahamiri, S. R., & Thabtah, F. (2020). Autism AI: A new autism screening system based on Artificial Intelligence. *Cognitive Computation*, *12*(4), 766–777. doi:10.100712559-020-09743-3

Sharma, Y., & Singh, B. K. (2022). One-dimensional convolutional neural network and hybrid deep-learning paradigm for classification of specific language impaired children using their speech. *Computer Methods and Programs in Biomedicine*, *213*, 106487. doi:10.1016/j.cmpb.2021.106487 PMID:34763173

Sharmin, M., Ahmed, S., Ahamed, S. I., Haque, M. M., & Khan, A. J. (2006, March). Healthcare aide: towards a virtual assistant for doctors using pervasive middleware. In *Fourth Annual IEEE International Conference on Pervasive Computing and Communications Workshops (PERCOMW'06)*. IEEE. 10.1109/PERCOMW.2006.63

Singh, B. K., Verma, K., & Thoke, A. S. (2015). Investigations on impact of feature normalization techniques on classifier's performance in breast tumor classification. *International Journal of Computers and Applications*, *116*(19).

Sultan, N. (2015). Reflective thoughts on the potential and challenges of wearable technology for healthcare provision and medical education. *International Journal of Information Management*, *35*(5), 521–526. doi:10.1016/j.ijinfomgt.2015.04.010

Sundaravadivel, P., Kougianos, E., Mohanty, S. P., & Ganapathiraju, M. K. (2017). Everything you wanted to know about smart health care: Evaluating the different technologies and components of the internet of things for better health. *IEEE Consumer Electronics Magazine*, *7*(1), 18–28. doi:10.1109/MCE.2017.2755378

Tian, S., Yang, W., Le Grange, J. M., Wang, P., Huang, W., & Ye, Z. (2019). Smart healthcare: Making medical care more intelligent. *Global Health Journal*, *3*(3), 62–65. doi:10.1016/j.glohj.2019.07.001

Tikka, S. K., Singh, B. K., Nizamie, S. H., Garg, S., Mandal, S., Thakur, K., & Singh, L. K. (2020). Artificial intelligence-based classification of schizophrenia: A high density electroencephalographic and support vector machine study. *Indian Journal of Psychiatry*, *62*(3), 273. doi:10.4103/psychiatry.IndianJPsychiatry_91_20 PMID:32773870

Vaishya, R., Javaid, M., Khan, I. H., & Haleem, A. (2020). Artificial Intelligence (AI) applications for COVID-19 pandemic. *Diabetes & Metabolic Syndrome*, *14*(4), 337–339. doi:10.1016/j.dsx.2020.04.012 PMID:32305024

Vigneshvar, S., Sudhakumari, C. C., Senthilkumaran, B., & Prakash, H. (2016). Recent advances in biosensor technology for potential applications–an overview. *Frontiers in Bioengineering and Biotechnology, 4*, 11. doi:10.3389/fbioe.2016.00011 PMID:26909346

World Health Organization. (2021). *Medical doctors (per 10,000).* Retrieved from https://www.who.int/data/gho/data/indicators/indicator-details/GHO/medical-doctors-(per-10-000-population)

Yang, Z., Zhou, Q., Lei, L., Zheng, K., & Xiang, W. (2016). An IoT-cloud based wearable ECG monitoring system for smart healthcare. *Journal of Medical Systems, 40*(12), 1–11. doi:10.100710916-016-0644-9 PMID:27796840

Zhu, H., Wu, C. K., Koo, C. H., Tsang, Y. T., Liu, Y., Chi, H. R., & Tsang, K. F. (2019). Smart healthcare in the era of internet-of-things. *IEEE Consumer Electronics Magazine, 8*(5), 26–30. doi:10.1109/MCE.2019.2923929

Chapter 11
A Real-Time Cloud-Based Healthcare Monitoring System

Manjushree Nayak
National Institute of Science and Technology, India

Anjli Barman
Aadarsh College, Raipur, India

ABSTRACT

Health is a basic necessity, and access to high-quality healthcare is a human right. Cloud computing provides a base for better reliable and cost-efficient business applications for corporate purposes. Cloud computing provides a good structure and a good cost for the organization with reduced administration. Recent advances in sensor communication, sensor sensing, and microelectronics are focused on monitoring and managing chronic diseases and potential emergencies. Health monitoring can be managed by one or both: the cost of main challenges and citizen-centered care. This likewise permits a specialist to make electronic visits, including no transportation with full correspondence from the specialist to the patient. They can see one another, which permits the specialist to see the wounds. The authors discussed home hospitalization frameworks on the IoT and cloud-based healthcare monitoring systems in this chapter.

INTRODUCTION

Many primary healthcare clinics in rural areas do not have any computerized systems and rely only on paper-based systems, which require patients to keep their records. It is difficult and expensive to compile a nationwide overview of patient statistics using

DOI: 10.4018/978-1-7998-9831-3.ch011

several methodologies. On a more fundamental level, sharing information within the healthcare industry is difficult for individual organizations. Mobile & wireless technology offer some intriguing potential for a low-cost, high-reach service, with alternatives open to the government to improve the efficiency& effectiveness of its primary health care delivery process. There is substantial evidence that mobile technology could be useful in correcting the existing system's slow response rates in rural areas. The study presents a method for retrieving a patient's health status and delivering health-promoting messages in a non-intrusive manner via a wireless body-area network; they can connect. We conclude Cloud computing is the arising popular expression on the Internet. It is rising step by step because of its wealthy features of services. Cloud computing refers to applications and services on distributed networks utilizing virtualized resources and regular web and systems administration guidelines. Cloud computing is another kind of computing where our patterns of using the Internet change. The term: Cloud is analogical to the Internet. The term: Cloud Computing is used to calculate the Internet and the capacity to run a program or application on many associated PCs over the network simultaneously. It is the future of the Internet. It is additionally called the fifth era of computing after the Mainframe, Personal Computer, client-server computer, and the web. Cloud computing has changed the methods of utilizing computing resources. It's referring to a genuine change in outlook. The huge scope construction of cloud computing was upheld by the commercialization of the Internet and the development of numerous administration organizations. Cloud computing is the web's future. Numerous firms are attempting to decrease their IT expenditures and, as a result. IT organizations and virtualization technology facilitate their usage. Cloud computing enables a business to have a strong structure and a low cost while also reducing administration. The application or cloud framework type is specified. Cloud computing raises safety and security concerns for many number of enterprises and organizations. They share resources with unknown firms, have discrepancies in cloud storage management, lack crucial encryption and data integrity, and are subject to government rules, licenses, and information regarding the cloud computing domain of Internet security. It will liberate resources for customers; anybody will be able to use high-performance computing on a need-to-know basis and at any suitable time and from any part or location. Cloud computing enables the long-held ideal of utility computing to become a reality, with pay-as-you-go, generally available computer resources.

The primary benefit of cloud innovation is the accessibility and availability of information and applications from any place, and whenever. Cloud diminishes the expenses and intricacy identified with acquiring and dealing with the data innovation framework. The element ——On-Demand Service reduced software, hardware, and dispatching time. With the upside of cloud technologies, software labs, and applications as well as equipment-based labs, for example, network research centers would now be able to be changed to cloud environments. Not always and all administrations, applications get advantage from the cloud organization prospects. Issues like idleness, personal time, and transaction control, and specific protections are of significant concern. Cloud computing is network-based; innovation service blackouts are conceivable and can happen under any circumstance.

In the medical field, the widespread usage of medical devices and their connectivity to sophisticated networks or/and the Internet has opened up new possibilities for human medical diagnosis, treatment, and monitoring, as well as wireless body area networks (WBAN) and remote patient monitoring. The omnipresent gadgets, also known as clinical sensors, are affixed to specific parts of patients' bodies to measure clinical data such as blood pressure, sugar level, pulse rate, and other medical indicators. The collected medical data is communicated to the medical aid or medical counsel via remote media, such as cellular networks, for further analysis. In this case, the medical data obtained is reviewed to make different judgments. Medical data assessments can also be performed with robotized medical logical equipment, such as electrocardiogram analyzers, which are accounted for as part of the telemonitoring framework (A. Neloy, 2019). Telemonitoring systems are not new novel solutions in the field of observation (B. Xu, 2014) Conveyed to monitor the health state of indoor or remote patients to survive emergencies and combat and analyses important diseases before they deteriorate. For today's networks, cloud computing frameworks provide a powerful and adaptive solution.

Additionally, they have played a significant role in medical care frameworks in data monitoring, procurement, and capacity. By utilizing and distributing public cloud registration technology for medical services, the whole preparation of medical service frameworks becomes considerably more efficient and manageable. As we can see in fig 1, this implies that hospitals can easily leverage public cloud administrations to support the continuum of medical services and handle the administration. The connected IT requirements enable hospitals to recover continuous patient data quickly while keeping it securely divided between frameworks (and clients), adaptable in times of responsibility, and consistently available when required. Taking this into account, a health association that utilizes a cloud computing framework is prepared to control its overall organizational structure as an understandable optimum medical care framework emerges as a solution.

Figure 1. Typical cloud computing structure for healthcare system

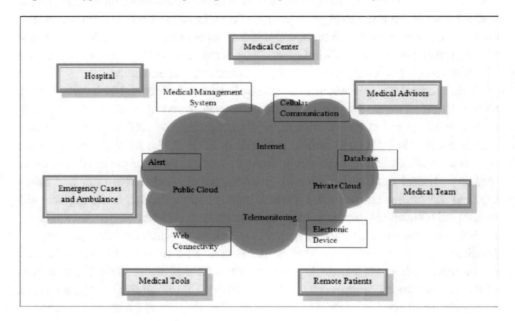

Additionally, the public cloud is useful for monitoring data and administering services in cloud computing, and it may be acceptable for flexibility and security in universal medical care frameworks. Medical data recovery is important, and it must be protected while being transmitted over the Internet. Due to security concerns and the need to maintain a high level of protection during data transfers, a few medical organizations have avoided adopting public cloud platforms. In summary, public cloud services are efficient and secure, yet due to their open nature, they have some potential weaknesses. Private cloud computing is a necessary and credible arrangement for medical data exchanges, ensuring data privacy and authorized access; moreover, medical associations may use their other substantial resources.

LITERATURE REVIEW

"Machine Learning-based Health Prediction System Using IBM Cloud as PaaS," A. A. Neloy, S. Alam, R. A. Bindu, and N. J. Moni, 2019. This project aims to develop a system that will enable hospitals to deliver real-time feedback to critical patients. The purpose of this study is to provide the standard structure, associated terminology, and differential model for monitoring crucial patient health status by utilizing a study device and IBM cloud computing services such as Platform as a Service (PaaS). The study's primary objective is to predict patient health using machine learning (ML). This study will take place on IBM Cloud, namely IBM Watson Studio, hosting and storing our data and machine learning models. As fundamental predictions for our machine learning models, we employed Naive Bayes, Logistic Regression, K-Neighbors Classifier, Decision Tree Classifier, Random Forest Classifier, Gradient Boosting Classifier, and MLP Classifier. The collaborative learning bag insertion approach was applied to increase the model's accuracy. The following algorithms are used to collaborate on learning: Additional Tree Planting, Random Forest Planting (A. Neloy, 2019).

According to Xu, L., and Cai, H., and Jiang, L., "Architecture of an M-Health Monitoring System Using Cloud Computing for Elderly Home Applications," 2014. This work aims to develop and implement a structure for mobile health monitoring systems based on cloud computing (Could-MHMS) for typical healthcare applications. The cloud-based module, data management module, and resource allocation and assignment component are incorporated in the framework's features. Monitoring data is stored in the distributed database module across many tenancy areas. The data management unit uses domain expertise to assess the well-being of the observed persons. This web service architecture is intended to allocate and distribute publicly funded healthcare resources dynamically. These three modules work in tandem to conduct critical health monitoring functions such as data gathering, storage, analysis, and resource allocation. Finally, we demonstrate how our technique and architecture may be applied to senior homes (B. Xu, 2014).

U.Dhanaliya and A. Devani, "E-Health Care System Implementation Using Web Services and Cloud Computing," In 2016, developing a healthcare system takes a large number of workers, mainly if a patient requires ongoing monitoring. The strength of technological tools allowed the medical system to become more productive and convenient. Any condition of a patient could be tracked and managed virtually by using IoT devices. We describe an E-Healthcare system provided by cloud computing and online services in this paper. The uses of cloud computing enabled remote monitoring and controlling. It updates the patient's measured parameters automatically and sends alert emails through SMTP (Simple Mail Transfer Protocol) (Devani, 2016).

R, Mr. Dilip. (2020), the Author suggests about Cloud Computing is being used to develop a graphical system for patient monitoring. Speech Recognition Technology has made it possible for computers to understand and follow human speech commands. By merging the Virtual Instrumentation Technology and Speech Recognition Techniques, things such as physique parameters are frequently checked. This can be accomplished with the help of the LabVIEW Platform. The electro-acoustic transducer device is used to obtain voice instructions from humans and to carry out signal processing operations for surveillance and dominance of the interfaced devices. At the side of the devices, the electro-acoustic transducer signals are interfaced with the LabVIEW Platform. The LabVIEW code can provide a good management signal to keep an eye on the body's parameters. The entire project was completed on the LabVIEW platform (Dilip., 2020).

H. B. Aziz, S. Sharmin, and T. Ahammad, "Cloud Based Remote Healthcare Monitoring System Using IoT," 2019. The major purpose of this study is to use the Internet of Things to construct a cloud-based remote healthcare monitoring system. The suggested architecture uses sensor nodes to collect and transmit patient health data to the cloud. The information will be processed further and analyzed in the cloud. A smart device can examine the data remotely at any time and from any location. In addition, any aberrant data will be reported to the appropriate authorities. Finally, IoT devices are used to construct the system, which efficiently offers us health-related data (H. B. Aziz, 2019).

E.A. Karajah and I. Ishaq, "Health part for Arduino for Online Monitoring on the Go Heart Give Monitor System", 2020, Author suggest Vital signs are checked via the health station system. The Heart Rate Monitor is a device that measures a patient's heart rate and temperature range and uploads it to the cloud. Medical workers can then use real-time cloud services to check the patient's health from any place and any time. This module is interfaced with a Smartphone, which notifies a notification if heart rate data change. After 5 unusual results, this would instantly contact the Doctor or the Patient whose contact is saved in the database. This technology is put to the test and measured against ECG equipment. The results are quite accurate, with a 97.4 percent accuracy rate (Ishaq, 2020).

J. J. Jijesh, Shivashankar, L. Rashmi, S. Jayashree, S. Kiran A, and S. Shreyas, "Design and Development of Intuitive Environment with Health Monitoring System Using Internet of Things," 2018 These smart devices collect data such as temperature, heart rate, and eye movements to assess the patient's well-being. The testing undertaking in the IoT is passing the gathered data to the expert, making the correct conclusion based on the data gathered, and advising the patient. The construction of a patient health monitoring framework utilizing IoT devices is provided in this proposed work to gather the relevant parameters and analyses the data obtained from the IoT gadgets. The patient health monitoring system (PHMS) also advises the patient of any possible precautions they should take. The PHMS framework provides medical care to the patient as well as the next steps to take if a basic scenario arises. The PHMS framework is evaluated for certain criteria, and the decisions based on the information obtained from the source are accepted (J. J. Jijesh, 2018).

J. Wang, J. Yang, and Z. Zhang, "Design of Accurate Measurement for Structure Monitoring Using Fiber Bragg Grating Sensors Using a Cloud Computing Platform," 2021 Scaling up enough servers to handle real-time data collection, transmission, and storage is challenging. The cloud platform for Fiber Bragg Grating Sensors employs an erbium-doped fiber cascaded Bragg grating structure, configures the FBG demodulator acquisition and analysis software appropriately, deploys the health monitoring system in the cloud, establishes a cloud platform for a high-efficiency health monitoring optical fiber sensor network, increases system scalability, enables flexible application and service deployment, and ensures security and reliability. It can satisfy the needs of some specialized or broad application domains for interdisciplinary practical, comprehensive beneficial application research in automation technology, structural mechanics, computer technology, Internet architecture, cloud deployment, and multidisciplinary practice, thorough valuable application research (J. Wang, 2021).

S. Joshi and S. Joshi, "A Sensor-based Secured Health Monitoring and Alerting Technique Using Internet of Things," 2019. This work develops a sensory-based health monitoring system with acceptable safety characteristics using Huffman compression coding and Rivest Shamir Adleman (RSA) encryption technology. Additionally, the alarm system is constructed utilizing embedded software and the Internet of Things and is based on the prediction approach. This suggested system is a more sophisticated version of existing systems that may benefit mobility patients or those in the intensive care unit (Joshi, 2019).

"Developing an e-Health System Based on IoT, Fog, and Cloud Computing," K. Monteiro, É. Rocha, É. Silva, G. L. Santos, W. Santos, and P. T. Endo. 2018, Numerous attempts have been made by educational institutions and businesses to develop new applications that improve this part of the population's quality of life; utilities like vital sign monitoring, fall alarm systems, and heart attacks are becoming increasingly prevalent. The most of these e-health solutions use IoT (Internet of Things) technology. However, due to technological constraints, the Internet of Things cannot handle, store, or ensure the quality of these services. As a result, to deliver high-quality e-health services, IoT relies on two primary partners: fog and cloud computing. This article discusses the e-health architecture currently being developed, which incorporates IoT for data collecting, a fog for data processing and storage, and a cloud for data processing, analysis, and long-term storage. Additionally, we have overcome significant obstacles in producing high-quality, highly efficient e-health applications (K. Monteiro, 2018).

L. Lakshmi, A. N. Kalyani, G. N. Satish, D. Swapna, and M. P. Reddy, "Fog Computing and IoT-enabled Cloud Systems in Health Care," 2021 they will protect them in a variety of dangerous situations. Various sensor devices are distributed over the globe in various locations. Every day, a vast amount of information is gathered. The most significant obstacles in healthcare systems include processing, storing in a safe environment, executing various computations involving sensitive data, and rapid responses. Fog computing and IoT-enabled cloud computing, according to scientists, are the greatest ways to overcome the issues of traditional health care. People can also use wearable IoT devices to check their health issues such as frequent pulse rate monitoring, blood pressure monitoring, oxygen levels, ECGs, and sugar levels. The use of deep and machine learning algorithms to forecast a person's health condition using data acquired from wearable IoT is a potential undertaking currently. As a result, the response time is crucial (L. Lakshmi, 2021).

M. R. Ruman, A. Barua, W. Rahman, K. R. Jahan, M. Jamil Roni, and M. F. Rahman, "IoT Based Emergency Health Monitoring System," 2020 This paper depicts a system that uses IoT to monitor a patient's body whole day means 24 hours a day, seven days a week. Patient monitoring systems are gaining in popularity among researchers and patient guardians these days. Every 15 seconds, this system may measure physiological parameters from the patient's body. This system is in charge of collecting the patient's pulse, body temperature, and heart rate and sending the data to an IoT Cloud platform through WiFi-Module, where the patient's health status is maintained. It allows a medical specialist or approved person to keep track of a patient's health on a cloud server, where the specialist or authorized person may keep track of the patient's status at all times. The research's proposed outcome is to provide patients with appropriate and effective health care (M. R. Ruman, 2020).

M. S. Uddin, J. B. Alam, and S. Banu, "Real time patient monitoring system based on Internet of Things," 2017 Monitoring of vehicles or assets, children/pets, fleet management, parking management, water, and oil leaks, and energy grid monitoring, and so on are all examples of remote monitoring systems. In this study, we propose an intelligent patient monitoring system that uses sensor-based connected networks to automatically monitor patients' health. The biological behaviors of a patient are collected using a variety of sensors. The relevant biological data is subsequently sent to the Internet of Things cloud. The system is more sophisticated in that it can detect a patient's serious state by analyzing sensor data and sending push notifications to doctors, nurses, and In charge of the hospital. Doctors And Nurses gain from this method since they may monitor their patients without having to visit them in person. With limited access, patients' families can also profit from this method (M. S. Uddin, 2017).

S. Mekid, "Iot for Health and Usage Monitoring Systems: Mitigating Consequences in Manufacturing under Cbm," 2021 An IoT-based condition monitoring system is built by collecting enormous data and applying true prognostics in the cloud server to predict likely danger. The features that are necessary for IoT applications in manufacturing are outlined in this article. The HUMS structural application is explained, as well as the usage of sensors affixed to the insert of a cutting tool to measure wear. The IoT will be connected to the Thing speak Cloud for data processing using a Wi-Fi-based microcontroller. The entire system may be used to swiftly examine the information gathered. The proposed system's experimental values are dependable, user-friendly, and cost-effective (Mekid, 2021).

N. Axak, M. Korablyov, and M. Ushakov, "Cloud Architecture for Remote Medical Monitoring," 2020, Due to remote cloud health monitoring, patients registered in a medical institution will be able to obtain medical care on time if they use the remote cloud monitoring model. The interaction of the web interface, the intelligent data processing layer, the agent unit, the accumulation and analysis of experience, and the adaptation of neural network data processing for high-performance computing systems allows for the provision of services and emergency decisions of various levels of complexity (N. Axak, 2020).

S. Chinchole and S. Patel, "Cloud and sensors-based obesity monitoring system," 2017 The demand for developing a smart system to address this problem has been gradually increasing, according to the International Conference On Intelligent Sustainable Systems (ICISS), 2017. To monitor the user's lifestyle, the real-time system proposed in the study employs cloud computing, data analytics, and sensors. The system monitors the user's BMI, sets up smart alarms, and gives recommendations for a healthier diet and exercise routine. The system also has the qualities of being user-friendly, cost-effective, and efficient (Patel, 2017).

V.Tripathi and F. Shakeel, "Monitoring HealthCare System using IoT- An immaculate paring," 2017, The structure is linked healthcare module and smart medical equipment has immense promise not only for businesses but also for people's overall well-being. IoT-driven monitoring can be used to keep track of hospitalized patients whose physiological status necessitates constant attention. This sort of solution uses sensors to gather extensive data, then analyses and stores the data using gateways and the cloud, before sending the studied data remotely for additional evaluation and feedback. It simplifies the process of obtaining a medical specialist come by at frequent intervals to ensure the patient's condition, instead of having a medical specialist come by at periodic intervals. The main objective of the paper is to get a comprehensive overview of such a research field, emphasizing the sensors used in health monitoring, how smart health monitoring devices work, how data are collected, and how reports can be generated based on several parameters (Shakeel, 2017).

K. Plathong and B. Surakratanasakul, "A Case Study of Using Cloud Computing to Integrate the Internet of Things with the Health Level 7 Protocol for Real-Time Healthcare Monitoring" 2017, one of them is the Internet of Things, which enables the connection of gadgets. Numerous medical equipment, including wearables, digital blood pressure monitors, and glucose meters, are now available via the Internet of Things. The data collected from these devices has been utilized to deliver accurate therapy to patients and adapted from prior research reports. The researcher is aware of the critical nature of secure medical data transfer and can handle large amounts of data. This article describes a conceptual architecture for combining the Internet of Things with the Health Level 7 protocol to enable cloud-based real-time healthcare monitoring. The conceptual framework's objective is to aid elderly or isolated folks in monitoring their health remotely at any time using an Internet of Things medical device. These data are recorded in real-time and transmitted to the cloud using JSON. Consequently, public health and hospitals may use web-based information to diagnose and treat patients and provide health recommendations (Surakratanasakul, 2017).

Suresh, R & Robin, Rene. (2021). by author Cloud Computing is used to create an efficient VOIP-enabled health monitoring system. This study describes an integrated framework consisting of a series of sensor nodes that uses cloud computing technologies to monitor human health and activities. The most sophisticated sensors, such as a web camera, gyroscope, and accelerometer, are employed to sense the patient's actions. Sensors track human activity, and the data is sent to the cloud, where doctors, caregivers, clinics, and pharmacies may access it in the event of an emergency (Suresh, 2021).

"Health Monitoring System Using Internet of Things," through V. Patil, S. S. Thakur, and V. Kshirsagar This work suggests using the IoT devices to monitor and maintain a patient's condition, even if the patient is busy with his daily routine, and to assess the patient's health state for specialists. This article focuses on a non-biomedical sensor-based health monitoring system that measures five parameters: ECG, heartbeat, oxygen, temperature, and pulse rate. The proposed method makes use of an Arduino Mega Controller, which is linked to non-invasive biological sensors. Using Arduino Mega, the information is presented on any digital monitoring system. The data collected by the sensors is sent to the ThingSpeak cloud, which allows doctors and persons concerned to store and access patient real-time information. The Internet of Things (IoT) is a strong domain in which sensors can interact and data can be seen over the Internet (V. Patil, 2018).

Tamilselvi, S. Sribalaji, P. Vigneshwaran, P. Vinu, and J. GeethaRamani, "IoT Based Health Monitoring System," 2020 The Internet of Things (IoT) plays a critical role in coma patient health monitoring. Continuous fitness monitoring can save up to 60% of human lives by prompt detection. The technologies are sparsely designed for real-time monitoring of coma patients' vital signs. It is more acceptable to identify a patient's state of health via GSM and IoT. This suggested system uses a variety of intelligent sensors, including temperature, heart rate, eye blink, and SPO2 (Peripheral Capillary Oxygen Saturation) sensors, to acquire data on the patient's body temperature and coronary heart rate, eye movement, and oxygen saturation percentage. The ARDUINO-UNO board serves as the microcontroller, taking advantage of the cloud computing idea. The accelerometer sensor was used to visualize the bodily movement of coma sufferers. The patient's vital parameters are sent to the legal individual's smartphones and laptops through a cloud server (V. Tamilselvi, 2020).

Y. Xiong, Z. Jiang, H. Fang, and H. Fan, "Research on Health Condition Assessment Method for Spacecraft Power Control System Based on SVM and Cloud Model," 2019To address the problems of health level classification and uncertainty mapping in the health assessment application of the spacecraft power control system, a combination of support vector machine (SVM) and cloud model is proposed to realize the spacecraft power control system's health status measurement. The algorithm's basic methods and implementation approach are then outlined. Finally, utilizing historical in-orbit operational data from a spacecraft's power management system, the health condition of the spacecraft's power control system is evaluated using SVM and a cloud model, as well as the method's performance. The results demonstrate that the approach can correctly analyze the performance and health of critical components of the spacecraft's power system. It is used to aid in the online health assessment and operational decision-making processes for essential components of the spacecraft power supply (Y. Xiong, 2019).

METHODOLOGY

Cloud Computing

The term Cloud Computing is becoming increasingly prevalent on the internet. It is steadily rising as a result of its extensive and diverse service offerings. Cloud computing refers to applications and services that run on remote networks and are accessed using standard web and system administration procedures. Cloud Computing is a type of computing in which our Internet usage patterns alter. Cloud is a phrase that is analogous to the Internet. The phrase "cloud computing" refers to the ability to perform calculations through the Internet and to execute a software or application on multiple PCs connected to a network at the same time. It is the Internet's future. After the mainframe, personal computer, client-server computing, and the Web, it is sometimes known as the fifth era of computing.

Cloud computing has changed the methods of utilizing computing resources. It's referring to a genuine change in outlook. The huge scope construction of cloud computing was upheld by the commercialization of the Internet and the development of numerous administration organizations. Cloud computing is the upcoming age of the web. It will make resources free for clients; anybody can utilize the high computing based on need and any time anyplace. Cloud computing makes the since a long time ago held dream of utility computing possible with pay-more only as costs arise, universally available computing resources.

The main advantage of cloud technology is the accessibility and availability of data and applications from anywhere, and at any time. Cloud decreases the costs and complexity related to obtaining and managing the information technology infrastructure. The feature ——On-Demand Services reduced software, hardware, and launching time. Not only software labs and apps but also hardware-based labs like network laboratories can now be moved to cloud settings thanks to cloud technology. Not always and all services, applications get benefit from the cloud deployment possibilities. Issues like latency, downtime, and transaction control, and in particular securities are of major concern. Cloud computing is network-based; technology service outages are a possibility and can occur for any reason.

1. Service Models

Software-As-A-Service (SAAS), Platform-As-A-Service (PAAS), And Infrastructure-As-A-Service (IAAS) these three are well-known service models connected with Cloud Computing.

- Software as a Service (SaaS): The customer may access the provider's applications through cloud architecture. A thin client interface, such as a Web browser (e.g., web-based email), or a programmed interface is used to access the apps from several client devices. With the possible exception of limited user-specific application configuration choices, the customer does not manage or control the underlying cloud infrastructure, including the network, servers, operating systems, storage, or even particular programmed capabilities.
- Platform as a Service (PaaS): The customer is given the option of putting self-developed or purchased applications into the cloud infrastructure using the provider's programming languages and tools. The consumer has no control or administration over the cloud infrastructure's core components, including the network, servers, operating systems, and storage.
- Infrastructure as a Service (IaaS): The capability provided to the consumer is to provide processing, storage, networks, and other fundamental computing resources where the consumer is able to deploy and run arbitrary software, which can include operating systems and applications. The consumer does not manage or control the underlying cloud infrastructure but has control over operating systems, storage, deployed applications; and possibly limited control of select networking components (e.g., host firewalls).

Figure 2. Cloud Computing Structure

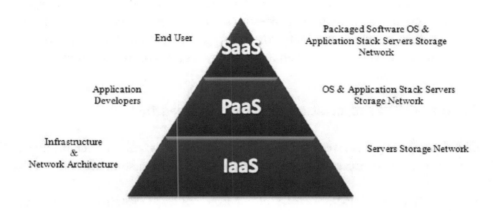

In the Fig. 2 the cost of using public clouds is typically low for the end-user, and there is no capital investment required. Due to private clouds' greater level of consolidation and resource pooling, capital expenditure is still lower than the cost of owning and operating infrastructure. In addition, compared to public clouds, private clouds provide more security and compliance support. As a result, some businesses may prefer to use private clouds for mission-critical and secure applications while using public clouds for routine tasks like application development and testing environments and e-mail.

2. Deployment Models

In particular, there are 04 types of distribution types namely Private Cloud, Hybrid Cloud, Public Cloud, and Community Cloud.

- Private Cloud: The above cloud structure is designed specifically for the needs of a single enterprise with several clients (e.g., business units). It may be yours, a company, or a third party, and it could be on or off the premises.
- Public Cloud: This public cloud is entirely open for use by the entire public. It might be a corporation, educational institution, or government entity that owns, operates, and manages it, or a combination of the three. It resides on the cloud service provider's premises.
- Hybrid Cloud: This cloud structure consists of two or more distinct cloud infrastructures (private, public, or hybrid) that are kept separate yet interconnected to manage data and applications using standard or comparable technologies (e.g., cloud compression to load.)

- Community Cloud: A community cloud in computing is a collaborative effort in which infrastructure is shared between several organizations from a specific community with common concerns (security, compliance, jurisdiction, etc.), whether managed internally or by a third-party and hosted internally or externally. This is controlled and used by a group of organizations that have shared interest.

Essential Characteristics of Cloud Computing

Cloud computing has five distinguishing characteristics: self-service on-demand, broadband network access, seamless integration, rapid expansion, and rating services.

- On-Demand Self-Service: A cloud user may use computer resources on-demand, such as server time and network storage, without interacting with each service provider separately.
- Integration Services: with the multi-employer model, provider computer resources are integrated to serve many consumers, with a range of visual and visual resources dynamically assigned and redistributed in response to customer demands. While the customer is frequently unable to control or get information about the precise location, they can specify a location with a high output level, so establishing a sense of local authenticity (e.g., country, region, or data center). Applications include storage, computation, memory, and network bandwidth.
- Broad Network Access: Skills may be acquired in several ways over the network, which supports the use of tiny or thin client platforms (e.g., cell phones, tablets, laptops, and workstations).
- Rapid Elasticity: Skills may be given fast and flexibly, and in some cases automatically, in response to external and internal demand. To the customer, accessible energy looks boundless and is available at any time and at any price.
- Rated Service: Cloud-based solutions leverage rating capabilities at a given level appropriate for the kind of service to automate the management and improvement of app usage (e.g., storage, processing, bandwidth, and active user accounts). Both the service provider and the service consumer can monitor, track, and report on the service's usage.

Some Major Cloud Computing Service Providers

Cloud computing has great benefits for organizations. So private cloud providers also provide cloud services with larger substandard services

- Google (Google App Engine): Google App is suitable for all types of applications such as Business, Consumers, Marketing, Mobile, and Website.
- Microsoft Windows Azure: Microsoft windows azure is an open cloud platform that allows the user to build and manage applications. Users can create applications using multilingual, tools or framework.net, node.js, JAVA, PHP.
- Amazon EC2 (aws.amazon.com) Computer: Amazon has the ability to meet the needs of a user program whether it is a single server or a large collection. AEC is a web service that provides computing capacity that can be expanded in the cloud. Amazon EC2 web service allows 27 users to find and build with minimal conflict. Amazon EC2 provides complete control over its computer users and allows them to operate the Amazon computer.
- Machine learning and data mining: Clinical assistance apps are often built around the concept of comparing gathered data to a patient's normal range and producing warnings when an aberrant condition is discovered. Notifications should be used as a last choice in clinical support applications, as they may create an excessive demand on emergency systems in the event of false alarms. Other measures, such as surveys, should reduce false warnings after identifying an abnormal value in the monitored parameter. On the other hand, current healthcare applications are enhanced by using data mining and machine learning techniques to provide effective clinical decision support for patients.

Predicting changes in conjunction with decision assistance will reduce clinician engagement. Without the aid of a professional, feedback such as advice regarding medication, health care, medical centre, medical team, and exercise can be delivered to individual patients.

Figure 3. Worldwide market share of leading cloud infrastructure service providers in 2019

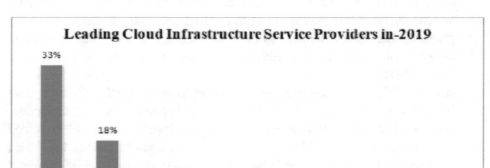

As shown in Fig. 3, cloud computing has the greatest impact on how IT infrastructure and platforms are set up, deployed, and provisioned from the perspective of end-users. Cloud based applications should be able to interact with the cloud ecosystem, including other cloud based and non-cloud-based applications.

CONCLUSION

As technological demands increase, medical systems have been updated with new innovative materials (i.e., intelligent health systems); however, many challenges remain, including the transportation of remotely located information and remote connectivity issues, particularly prevalent in healthcare systems. Along with this, the cost is a significant factor, increasing when current approaches are updated to include innovations. As a result, the cloud computing platform is one of the most excellent alternatives available in the modern era for resolving challenges.

This study discussed the health concerns confronting traditional healthcare models in our aging society, such as the growth in chronic illnesses and the rising expenses of hospital and clinical services. Effective and efficient medical systems are required to alleviate strain on hospital systems and healthcare professionals, enhance the quality of service, and lower healthcare costs. The potential for remote healthcare monitoring systems based on cloud technology is enormous. The review's findings indicate that the next generation of cloud apps for healthcare should prioritize self-care, data mining, and machine learning. The future work will concentrate on data collecting and processing to construct a cloud-based falls detection and prevention system.

REFERENCES

Axak, N. M. K. (2020). Cloud Architecture for Remote Medical Monitoring. *IEEE 15th International Conference on Computer Sciences and Information Technologies (CSIT)*, 1-4.

Aziz, H. B., & S. S. (2019). Cloud Based Remote Healthcare Monitoring System Using IoT. *International Conference on Sustainable Technologies for Industry 4.0 (STI)*, 1-5. 10.1109/STI47673.2019.9068029

Devani, U. D. (2016). Implementation of E-health care system using web services and cloud computing. *International Conference on Communication and Signal Processing (ICCSP)*, 1034-1036.

Dilip., R. (2020). Development of Graphical System for Patient Monitoring using Cloud Computing. *International Journal of Advanced Science and Technology*, 29.

Ishaq, E. A.-A. (2020). Online Monitoring Health Station Using Arduino Mobile Connected to Cloud service: "Heart Monitor" System. *International Conference on Promising Electronic Technologies (ICPET)*, 38-43.

Jijesh, J. J., & S. L. (2018). Design and Development of Intuitive Environment with Health Monitoring System Using Internet of Things. *IEEE International Conference on Recent Trends in Electronics,Information Technology & Communication Technology (RTEICT)*, 1351-1355. 10.1109/RTEICT42901.2018.9012157

Joshi, S. J. (2019). A Sensor based Secured Health Monitoring and Alert Technique using IoMT. *International Conference on Intelligent Communication and Computational Techniques (ICCT)*, 152-156. 10.1109/ICCT46177.2019.8969047

Lakshmi, L., & A. N. (2021). The preeminence of Fog Computing and IoT enabled Cloud Systems in Health care. *International Conference on Intelligent Communication Technologies and Virtual Mobile Network (ICICV)*, 365-375. 10.1109/ICICV50876.2021.9388408

Mekid, S. (2021). IoT for health and usage monitoring systems: mitigating consequences in manufacturing under CBM. *International Multi-Conference on Systems, Signals & Devices (SSD)*, 569-574.

Monteiro, K., É. R. (2018). Developing an e-Health System Based on IoT, Fog and Cloud Computing. *IEEE/ACM International Conference on Utility and Cloud Computing Companion (UCC Companion)*, 17-18. 10.1109/UCC-Companion.2018.00024

Neloy, A., S. A. (2019). Machine Learning based Health Prediction System using IBM Cloud as PaaS. *International Conference on Trends in Electronics and Informatics (ICOEI)*, 444-450. 10.1109/ICOEI.2019.8862754

Patel, S. C. (2017). Cloud and sensors based obesity monitoring system. *International Conference on Intelligent Sustainable Systems (ICISS)*, 153-156.

Patil, V., & S. S. (2018). Health Monitoring System Using Internet of Things. *International Conference on Intelligent Computing and Control Systems (ICICCS)*, 1523-1525. 10.1109/ICCONS.2018.8662915

Ruman, M. R., & A. B. (2020). IoT Based Emergency Health Monitoring System. *International Conference on Industry 4.0 Technology (I4Tech)*, 159-162.

Shakeel, V. T. (2017). Monitoring Health Care System Using Internet of Things - An Immaculate Pairing. *International Conference on Next Generation Computing and Information Systems (ICNGCIS)*, 153-158.

Surakratanasakul, K. P. (2017). A study of integration Internet of Things with health level 7 protocol for real-time healthcare monitoring by using cloud computing. *10th Biomedical Engineering International Conference (BMEiCON)*, 1-5.

Tamilselvi, V., & S. S. (2020). IoT Based Health Monitoring System. *International Conference on Advanced Computing and Communication Systems (ICACCS)*, 385-389.

Uddin, M. S., & J. B. (2017). Real time patient monitoring system based on Internet of Things. *International Conference on Advances in Electrical Engineering (ICAEE)*, 516-521. 10.1109/ICAEE.2017.8255410

Wang, J. J. Y. (2021). Design of Cloud Computing Platform Based Accurate Measurement for Structure Monitoring Using Fiber Bragg Grating Sensors. *IEEE 2nd International Conference on Big Data, Artificial Intelligence and Internet of Things Engineering (ICBAIE)*, 807-811.

Xiong, Y., & Z. J. (2019). Research on Health Condition Assessment Method for Spacecraft Power Control System Based on SVM and Cloud Model. *Prognostics and System Health Management Conference (PHM-Paris)*, 143-149. 10.1109/PHM-Paris.2019.00032

Xu, B., & L. X. (2014). Architecture of M-Health Monitoring System Based on Cloud Computing for Elderly Homes Application. *Enterprise Systems Conference*, 45-50. 10.1109/ES.2014.11

Chapter 12
Analysis and Comparison of Psychological Constraints Among Various Countries During COVID–19

Tanu Rizvi
Shri Shankaracharya Technical Campus, Bhilai, India

Devanand Bhonsle
Shri Shankaracharya Technical Campus, Bhilai, India

Ruhi Uzma
Anjuman College of Engineering and Technology, India

ABSTRACT

Behavior of any human is mostly permanent as per their personality, but it gets influenced by a variety of factors originating psychologically and socially. However, some temporary factors such as attitude, surroundings, instant mood, culture, etc. may hamper behavior severely. Researchers have published many articles depending upon human behavior and its approach. This study is aimed to describe the effect of external parameters on human behavior in Indians as well as Europeans due to COVID-19 outbreak globally. This study is a survey made on online platform in Indian premises and studies carried by researchers in four European countries: UK, France, the Netherlands, and Denmark. Comparisons have been done with different levels and parameters between India and European countries. This chapter not only concludes the psychological constraints but also the good habits adopted by peoples during COVID-19 pandemic to have a safer future.

DOI: 10.4018/978-1-7998-9831-3.ch012

BACKGROUND AND INTRODUCTION

As referred to the world's history pandemics are consistent part of human life over hundreds of years. These pandemics weather it may be Spanish flu or yellow fever, they are life threatening for humans as well as for other biological creatures (Michie, S. et al, 2014). Globally the world has witnessed many pandemics due to spread of viruses such as Ebola, Nipah etc. Likewise other pandemics COVID-19 was identified to emerge from bats. When dead bats came in contact with humans, they transmitted SARS virus or COVID-19 virus, since the first case was traced in Wuhan China in 2019 and so it was named as Corona virus disease 2019 that is COVID-19(Matos, A. D. et al, 2021). Soon this disease became pandemic globally and thus was the major concern as declared by the World Health Organization (WHO) in 2019. COVID-19 touched the boundaries of almost all the countries of the world (Crosta, A. D. et al, 2020). This strategic pandemic is also responsible for declination in economics globally. It is responsible for millions of causalities around the world harnessing the mental status of individuals to the worst (Cassenti, D. et al, 2020). The world is suffering from last one and a half years till yet with this pandemic. The overall world is grouped to be either developed or developing; in this study four countries stands on the side of developed nations where as the fifth country India stands still as a developing nation.

During COVID-19 outbreak, the governments globally initiated various health safety measurements. This study aimed to highlight the significant similarities and dissimilarities in psychological aspects as an indicator between the great European countries and India; the mental wellness of whose outcomes during the pandemic outbreak around 2020 are identified. We Surveyed data for 300 individuals in India under different parameters using online platforms and telephone method. Usually we tried to balance the individuals in equal numbers of males and females but at some point it's not clearly possible but at least males and females both participated in this survey. However for European countries we surfed the data based upon the research of researchers, doctors, thinkers, scientists and various psychologists around the world (Varga, T. V. et al, 2020). We came to know that being a developing country and lot of other social and economic challenges India withstand the pandemic as a great warrior as compared to the great developed European countries. The major challenge in front of India was its concern for population which is around 138 Crores and that is approximately 250 times as compared to population of any European country. In spite of this situations India survived almost 3 waves with somewhat causalities accounting for less than 1% of its total population. The impacts of lockdowns, quarantines, and unfriendliness as described above have been analyzed. All analysis focuses on the initial stages of lockdowns and quarantines in early march and April

2020 whose main outcomes are anxiety, loneliness, depression, worries, fear and other precautionary behaviors (Basu, S. et al, 2020).

Figure 1. COVID-19 attack and its impact

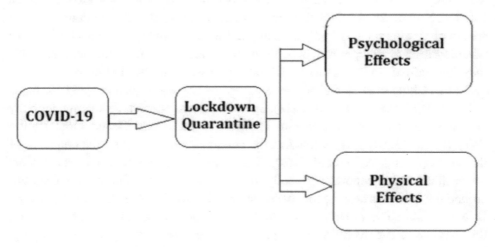

The worries globally are high at start of pandemics whereas there seems a gradual declination on reopening phases as per steps taken by governments of respective nation. Figure 1 shows a general layout of COVID-19 attack which affects the mankind both physically and psychologically.

To handle the overall situation; countries made join efforts with guidelines. International Air routes were completely stopped to prevent the spread of these viruses, various quarantine centers have been prepared for the peoples who were travelling from distance, and several screening has been done to trace the COVID-19 carriers (Kollamparambil, U. et al, 2021). Government of various countries has launched various mobile apps like Arogyasetu in India to trace the people nearby with symptoms. To a great extent this precautionary approaches were very relevant in fight against the transmission of virus but on the other hand the world became halt for months which gives rise to various economic crises and psychological factors. Quarantine and pandemic lockdowns plays a vital role and thus psychologically affecting the individuals of each country (Rawal D. et al, 2021). These conditions are already being monitored and various health policies have been issued to compensate its negative and future consequences. Individuals from European countries and India have thus responded somewhat psychologically in similar ways in spite of difference in actions by individual governments to pandemic concerns. This SARS and MARS induced viruses are greatly to affect the future generations also in very undesirable manners. The theories and science behind these diseases are very well studied and factified but the human behavioral approach is still to be explored (Singh, K. et al, 2021). There is variety of behavioral approach which needs to be discovered soon or later since the mental state of a person is very important factor and which is responsible to ones contribution in nation's economic as well as social responsibilities (Nagarathna, R. et al, 2021).

Ones mental state is not at all directly connected with the virus transfer rather it is an indirect side effects created by the precautionary steps taken by the various agencies and governments (Chhatterjee, K. et al,2020 and Chopra. S. et al,2020). Indian government announced lockdown all over country on 24th March 2020 which was for three weeks in starting. For the same government ordered complete shutdown of school, colleges, coaching, organizations, offices, shops, markets, parks, gardens, temple, mosques, churches, all public transportations etc. the whole mankind moments was stopped at once and people are requested to reside be at same place following all the protocols of pandemics. It was a mandatory preventive measure as ordered by government of India. This lockdown continues with change in limitations from state to state (Bavel, J. J. V. et al, 2020 and Weston, D. et al,2020). Finally from July 2020 onwards government ordered unlocks with various policies depending upon affected area and its population. Presently India has crossed two three waves of this pandemic. Governments of Denmark, France, Netherlands and United Kingdom (UK) also ordered time to time locks and unlocks. The peak period of pandemic varies from country to country but more or less all the countries get severely affected in first wave of pandemic which is from March 2020 to June 2020 mostly.

This article explains the behavioral change in India as surveyed as well as 4 countries of Europe as mentioned above and documented by researchers. This

Figure 2. Psychological aspects of behavior change

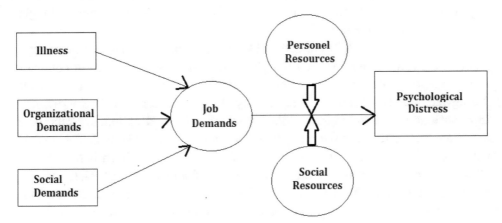

analysis may help in further on term analysis of behavioral approach towards mankind globally. This article purely aimed to focus on psychological aspects of virus attack in various host countries and not any other factor or economic issues. Researchers observed relevant topics with pandemics, its social effects on behavior and cultural effects, its psychological aspects and decision making approaches (Francisco, R. et al,2020 and Zhang, N. et al, 2019). Figure 2 shows that the psychological distress is mostly due to the worries associated with the personnel and social resources of which the various demands acts as input.

LITERATURE REVIEW

This chapter gives idea about the survey done in psychological behavioral change during COVID-19 pandemics across the world. Researchers, thinkers, authors, scientists, doctors and psychologists presented many articles for the same and some of them are studied to get through the behavioral change aspects related to these pandemics to understand the present status globally.

(Nagarathna, R. et al, 2021) identified that Yoga is a well known practice to release stress, anxiety during this pandemic. Yoga is also a immunity simulating act as adopted by many people's during this pandemics. Author further divided their study into parts. In one part the identified the effectiveness of yoga in physical and mental health when adopted on daily basis whereas in second part they evaluated the lifestyle of yoga trainers who are well trained to cope up with psychological distress associated with pandemics. Three health experts from Delhi designed a scale foe rating health assessments and this survey was done using online digital platforms with twenty three thousand seven hundred sixty respondents from India. Peoples were divided into two categories of yoga and non yoga and author found various results for each group.The yoga group were found to be in good mental stability and improved immunity as compared to non yoga group who generally found entangled in unhealthy life style habits

(Varga, T. V. et al, 2021) aimed to identify the similarities and differences in mental health measures between the Northern and Western European countries. Author identified the groups with the condition of lowest or poorest mental health during the COVID-19 attack. They surveyed the data from 205,083 individuals from various European countries like Denmark, United Kingdom's, Netherlands and France so as to study the impacts of this pandemic virus spread. The analysis have been done in the prior time of this pandemic attack that is in early March April 2020 and author found that anxiety, loneliness and all COVID-19 related worries are at peak together with the fear of adopted precautionary behaviors. They found that the worries declined at gradual reopening in the countries however only 7.1%

individuals are found with high level of loneliness in Netherlands basically but this percentage further increase to 13.2-18.1% in other three countries as described above. The adolescents' individuals experience a high level og mental stability which is common in all four countries. people got affected with frequent lockdowns and quarantines. The overall responses of all four countries are same in spite of differences in the governing authorities and their policies.

(Singh, K. et.al. 2021) studied on the survey carried out on 1754 Indians with 11% mean with age of 57.8 years out of which nearly the half are men..The rate of response is seventy four percentages. In pandemics lockdown in India nearly 83% faces difficulty in accessing health services,17%in medications,59% people lost their source of income,38% became jobless and 28% of them stopped their intake of healthy stuffs such as fruits and vegetables. The result obtained from regression model shows that 2.30,1.62-3.26 who totally lost their source of income faced a toughest situations in their medications and treatments. The scenario further got worst when the individuals with lost jobs and with diabetes and hypertension faced difficulties in accessing medicines with regression model of 1.90,1.25-2.89. The overall data suggests that most of the participants faced many psychological stress due to low or no source of income in availing the various medical facilities.

(Chopra, S.et al, 2021) did a survey based on web. Questionnaire with life style related behavior was registered with online survey with platform of Google forms. Total nine hundred ninety five responses have been recorded with mean age of 33.4 years and 58.4% of which are males.Usually in youngsters under the age of 30 years. Started to healthy flying their lives by adopting the healthy life styles and discarding the unhealthy habits. About one third of participants that are people with upper socio status gained weight reduced their physical activities and get diverted towards the more screen time accessing the online entertainment platforms and spending a lot of their time on them however some people by using this online activities developed great learning skills using this online platforms only but it depends on individuals. Frequent lockdowns and quarantine increased the stress and anxiety nearly to one fourth of participants affecting their mental health adversely. The negative lifestyle behaviors that spread out during COVID-19 pandemic can be mitigated by understanding the factors which can be helpful to develop interventions.

(Matos, A. D. et al, 2021) identified the difference in terms of behaviors between participants aged 50 + with their counterparts and multi morbidity without multi morbidity in twenty five countries of Europe together with Israel. Authors used the pre processed data from the set of questionnaire on the economic biology and socio demographic fromCOVID-19 Share. Wave seven and eight databases were also fully utilized to encounter the individuals with multi morbidity. At last the results showed that when controls included are gender, age, education, financial distress and countries then the precautionary behaviors are exhibited by individuals with multi morbidity than their counterparts as compared without multi morbidity individuals. On the other hand authors observed that the educated individuals, females and those individuals who encountered financial distress adopt more protective behaviors than their counterparts. Italy and Spain shows the higher prevalence of precautionary behaviors in comparison with Finland, Denmark and Sweden. The defensive actions adopted against COVID-19 guarantees that public health must continue to be un concentrated among older aged and middle aged persons with multi morbidity, awareness campaigns should be point the way at men and less educated individuals in countries but also at persons experiencing distress, particularly where people engaged in fewer precautionary behaviors.

(Crosta, A. D. et al, 2021) focused on psychological antecedents and individuals behavior. The studies carried out by various authors showed that the COVID-19 crisis differently affects people willingness to buy primary products such as shopping and secondary products such as headonic shopping. Therefore it may be concluded that changes in individual's behavior changes their level of spending. Authors adopted a line of division between the primary and secondary necessities of consumers. Three thousand eight hundred thirty three peoples are surveyed through online platform with age limit from 18 to 64 during peak of first wave peak Italy. COVID-19 fear and anxiety is the key factor to predict the consumer behavior toward primary necessities. On the other hand depression is used a key factor for consumer behavior toward secondary necessities. Furthermore, personality traits, perceived economic stability, and self-justifications for purchasing were adopted to predict toward primary necessities and secondary necessities present this article presents understanding of consumer behavior changes during the COVID-19 crisis based upon primary and secondary necessities. Psychological factors are considered to develop results that could be helpful to enhance marketing strategies to balance actual consumers' needs and psychological feelings.

(Mehta, S. et al, 2020) focused on a censorious scenario which pushes the behavior of human in different directions with many irreversible aspects of behavior. COVID-19 pandemic is an uncommon crisis, and to control this contagious disease various steps were taken by governments including complete or partial lockdown depending upon the percentage of cases in the area. The elements of the economy are correlated measures of public health frequent shut downs, which resulted in economic vulnerability of the countries hinting towards change in the dynamics of market. The consumers are whole sole drivers of the market competitions, growth and economic assimilation. With this unpredictability of economics, consumers behaviors are transformed in meanwhile the transformation experienced during the crunch will end up a question. The article looked deeply to the behavior of consumers during COVID-19 pandemics, lockdowns when the world becomes still for more than half of year. Further, the article explains the interfolds about consumer behavior in normal times and in crisis times travelling through a maze of literature empowering it with the rapid assessment reports carried out by the consulting organizations during pandemics, substantiates the same with first-conspiring and retelling of experiences by customers and individuals with marketing strategies to bring up a prediction of the pandemic affecting a criteria shift from customers materialistic requirements to customers spiritualism. Further hypothesis are suggested for future researchers to understand the customer. The proposition offers further testable hypotheses for future research to understand consumer sentiments or concerns in buying 'what is sufficient' within the context of market context and how it can be implemented post-COVID-19 crisis in order to ensure a sustained model of marketing. The consumer behavior can be forced and can be related interestingly with other control variables such as nationality, needs, culture, new market segment and age using which new models of customer behavior can be developed.

(Francisco, R. et al, 2020) studied the behavior of adolescents with 52.9% boys with age group from 3 to 18 years ld in three countries namely Italy, Spain and Portugal. The negative impact on psychological behavior based upon social distancing and isolation were scary in case of children and adolescent. Parents of one thousand four hundred eighty children and were a part of this study. A survey using online platform and snowball sampling technique was conducted for 15 consecutive days between the peak periods of pandemic outbreak around the world in April-may 2020. The questionnaires is based upon data, socio, demographic housing conditions and psychological response during quarantine which were made to answered by parents of the above mentioned aged group children based upon behavioral change due to sleeplessness, anxiety, mood, screen time etc as key inputs to study. Results show various changes in psychological behavior, increased screen timing and reduced physical activity. The psychological symptoms were minimal in Italian children as compared to Spanish and Portuguese children. Results from hierarchical multiple regressions show that having an outdoor exit such as gardening, terrace contributes in healthier environment and reduced risking psychological behavior of children. Authors recommended some practice implications for families so as to identify the prediction variables for reduced risk of behavioral change in adolescent and children.

(Kollamparambil, U. et al, 2020) identified the driver of response behavior using seemingly related regression method and special regressors ranging from probit control using multivariate estimation techniques with bivariate statistics, concentration indices the behavior response to COVID-19 r enhances as shown by findings in this research. The most preventive measures are hand washing, use of face mask, sanitizing. Other measures, includes practicing social distancing, reducing close contact, avoiding crowds. The higher income groups, educated ones and older adolescents. There is increased risk perception not differ and has risk in perception. The significant drivers of healthy behavior response are health models, self efficacy, awareness and the findings validate the health-belief model, with perceived risk, self-efficacy, perceived awareness and blockade to other traditional socio norms. Usually the higher socio economic groups and educated individuals practice use of sanitizers mostly where as the respondents of lower economic groups are not in favor of practicing such measures. The lower socio economic group suffers from dilemma of adopting the preventive measures and is optimally biased towards several barriers. There urgent need to target such groups in order to incorporate responsive approach to the preventive measure strategies.

(Basu, S. et al, 2020) aimed to highlight the after effects of lockdown on socio and environmental constraints with analysis of changes in individual's life style. This study is an online survey with pre planned questionnaires with over one thousand respondents in India. author figured the changes in society post lockdown to stop the spread of this deadly viruses. Some changes like use of online platforms for teaching, digital payments, work from home options for employees, digital shopping and societal behavior change became permanent part of our life since this pandemic attacks.

(Chhatterjee, K. et al, 2019) studied the post lockdown impacts in Indians. Author evaluated all the factors for post lockdown parameter. they identified the conditions of health care prospects. a compartmental SEIR model was used to calculate the cases with imposed precautionary schemes for further viruses transmission. The parameters for health care have been evaluated using Delphy study tools. author developed a matrix named as "q" to evaluate this pandemic scenario and it as found that the frequent lockdowns till August by Indian government is effective in overall sense and is helpful in ending this pandemic. Trainings have been provide to operate ventilators in emergency conditions. Author simulated the post lockdown conditions and trained medical professionals with their medical devices were found to be a key factor in healthcare constraints though some common community preventive measurements are still required after unlocking the country in various stages.

(Zhang, N. et al, 2019) focused on the spread of influenza and COVID-19 infections based upon the reported cases and database on internal surveillance and studied the behavior changes in human due to attack of this viruses based upon telephone survey data and mass transit data from railway authorities. Here authors simulated susceptible exposed infected recovered SEIR model to incorporate the risk reduction of influenza transmission resulting in change of human behavior. The number of passengers as compared to 2019 fell down to fifty two percent. The local residents spent their 33% of time at home engaged in home stuffs only. Each person, on average, came into pandemic periods. Adults, Older aged persons, students and workers daily number close contact gets reduced to 84%,31%,65%,39% respectively. The rate of close contact decreases by 8.2%, 30.7%, 66.2%, 38.4%, 47.6%, 42.0%, and 37.1%, respectively in localities, work surroundings, education hubs, restaurants, shopping market and public transports. The simulation results show the reduction in reproduction in influenza by 62.9% based upon the adoption of this human behavior. Similarly the spread of COVID-19 viruses reduces to 47.1% due to this behavior of avoidance of human to human close contacts. Thus author concluded that reduction in human to human contact reduces the risk of COVID-19 and influenza infections.

From above studies it is clear that person to person bonding is very important factor to make a person psychologically fit. To understand the human behavior perfectly no system or software has been designed yet since behavior depends upon both the permanent and temporary factors. This disease completely affected social status, economics, psychological parameters etc. and finally the socio thinkers and scientist came to know the after effects like anxiety, depression, loneliness etc from this outbreak which is completely irreplaceable.

METHODOLOGY

This section deals with the methodology which describes the complete scenario of pandemics, lockdowns and it's after effects. It is practically not possible to analyze all the situation, condition and effect of the present scenario completely even then we have tried to understand change in the human behavior in India and other four different European countries namely Denmark, France, Netherlands and UK with people of all the age group. In this span of time, it was very difficult to contact directly to the people and to convince them for their feedback because most of the candidates or their family members were suffering from the disease (Zhang, N. et al, 2019). Some time situation was panic and at that time condition was worse. So this survey has been done between March 2020 to June 2020 i. e for a span of about four months in India and similarly the research for the same period from Denmark, France, Netherlands and UK is analyzed for comparison. For the survey, we have prepared questionnaire and distributed among many people who are approachable. Those candidates who stay away from our localities were asked the report telephonically. However it was not easy because some of them are not comfortable to answer. But after a rigorous exercise, we have collected the response from the candidates. In this survey; we included the questions which were very easy to understand. We divided the candidates into male females and with age group under 30 years, 30-60 Years and above 60 years. We have chosen 50 members from each group and tried to take 50% men and 50% women. However it was not feasible due to present scenario but all the group consist of men and female both. To better understanding of the behavior change, we have categorized the parameters into two viz. adverse disorders and good habits developed. The area is very wide and cannot be completely covered in this chapter. So we have chosen some of the common factors. First of all we have discussed the negative effects of lockdowns which includes:

1. Anxiety
2. Worries
3. Loneliness

We have chosen these 20 points which are very common for each and every one to understand easily and no need to explain it further. Many candidates were not approachable hence these simple terminologies work to analyze the human behavior efficiently. Along with these negative aspects we have chosen adopted good habits which are helpful for all and they may sustain even after pandemic. The adopted good habits like increased hand washing, use of hand disinfectants, wearing mask, physical distancing and avoiding public transportations are summed up to get common results in one criteria. The survey done in India includes:

Stage 1: Selection of people from different groups
Stage 2: Distribution of questionnaire to the candidates who were approachable and healthy, those who were neither healthy nor approachable were directly asked the answer telephonically. Those who were not able to give prompt reply due to any reason were sent the Google form.
Stage 3: Collection of the response through questionnaire, telephonically or Google form.
Stage 4: Check the response according to the age group.
Stage 5: Prepare the table and graph to see the change in behavior.
Stage 6: Stop the survey.

Below is the results and discussion about the survey done in India and analysis of various surveys done by various authors globally. It reflects results in the form of table and graph for different European countries and India as discussed earlier.

RESULTS AND DISCUSSION

In this part, we have discussed the results of our survey in India and compared it with the survey done by the researchers in the four European countries Denmark, France Netherlands and UK to understand the effect of COVID-19 on our behavior due to adopted habits and other precautionary measures. For this purpose in India we chose the people of age group from 18 to 60 above with mix of both male and females. The total respondents in our study are 300. However we compared the results identified by foreign researchers and to make it understand more clearly we grouped the research into following parameters:

1. Anxiety
2. Worries
3. Loneliness

However some good habits also developed during this time which has also been included here in results. All the aforementioned points have been discussed with all the individuals under research. Below is the discussion of each point related to their change in behavior due to frequent lockdowns and adopted habits. Results have been shown in the form of table and graphs.

1. **Anxiety:** It is very normal for mankind to feel low during ups and downs and get affected by the surroundings. COVID-19 spread made these situations to the worst. A very common emotion among in such scenario is anxiety which is generally due to day by day stress and problems. The consistent excessive and irrational presence of these emotions causes anxiety and it hampers the efficiency of a person and soon gets converted into a disorder. The known emotions which are directly or indirectly related to anxiety are phobias, panic and several stress disorders. The common symptoms are confusion, a sense of helplessness; continue negative thoughts, respiratory problems specially breathing, tension, palpitations etc. People dealing with anxiety needs an expert medical help, a psychiatrist and some simple relaxation strategies such as yoga, regular exercise, company of good people, positive news, positive surroundings etc. According to our survey; no one was exception in all five defined countries that didn't face any of at least one problems discussed above. Table 1 shows the percentage of people from different age groups who felt the aforementioned problems and figure 3 is its graphical form. From the table it is clear that different age group has different numbers of people who encountered anxiety during COVID-19 outbreak. Here data for UK and India is compared for lockdown periods which may differ in countries. The peak level of anxiety is experienced between 4 to 17 May in UK whereas in India the peak level occurs from 18 to 31st May since COVID-19 was at peak during this durations of April May 2020. However as compared to UK the anxiety level are much lower in case of India as it is one of the populated country in world so people have many options to have therapy with their family and friends

Table 1. Sleeplessness verses age group during pandemic

ANXIETY (%)	United Kingdom	India
23 March-5 April, 2020	47	22
6 April -19 April, 2020	43	28
20 April -3May, 2020	41	38
4 May-17 May, 2020	40	40
18 May-31 May, 2020	38	42
1June-14 June, 2020	37	37
15 June-21 June, 2020	18	23

Figure 3. Anxiety level developed during lockdowns

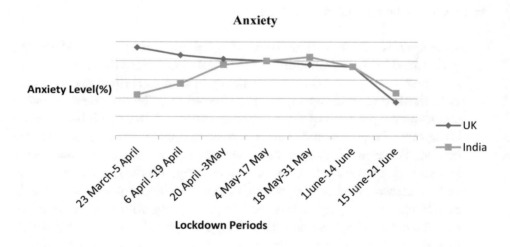

2.   **Worries:** Due to lockdown; movement stopped in many respects Professional starts doing their work from home, students got their online classes. Schools, colleges, coaching, restaurants, gardens, parks etc. are closed many a times hence many various restrictions in day to day life provide a lot of factors for worries. Some factors like job satisfaction, job loss, worries for family, relatives and friends, physical distancing and loss of near and dear ones created a lot of worries during the lockdowns in different countries. Some worried just about the bread and butter, some about medical conditions where as the worst situation started with fear of life in this virus spread. Table 2 shows the percentage of people from different age groups who felt the aforementioned problems. Figure 4 shows the graph for the table 2. The concern parameters used to collect data are:

Table 2. Worries developed in different countries

Worries developed	Denmark (%)	Netherlands (%)	France (%)	India (%)
Becoming Seriously Ill	30	10	40	40
Someone Closed to You Becoming Seriously ill	80	27	80	30
You and Your Family Experiencing Serious Financial Problems	28	05	24	30
Losing Job	5	02	10	50
Long Time Before Resuming Regular Life	52	23	42	20
Not Being Able to See Family Friends	68	25	50	20
Not Concerned About Crisis	02	05	05	05

Figure 4. Worries developed in different countries

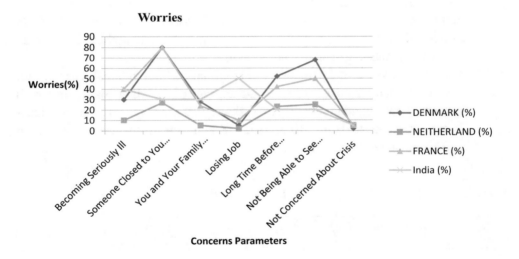

1. Becoming seriously ill
2. Someone closed to you becoming seriously ill
3. You and your family experiencing serious financial problems
4. Losing job
5. Long time before resuming normal life
6. Not being able to see family friends
7. Not concerned about crisis

Here data for Denmark, Netherlands, France and India is compared. The average peak level of common for all countries is worry of becoming seriously ill.

However in India the threat of losing job is very common among people as in every organization people experienced some insecurity towards job. Many factories, plants, companies totally shut down in this lockdowns due to several parameters and many people lost their jobs. So losing your job is important factor in India whereas the important factor common for Denmark, Netherlands and France is someone closed to you becoming seriously ill.

3. **Loneliness:** Since people are residing in their home and not going anywhere unnecessarily their outside interaction have become very less. Those who are working and doing their professional work from home are also facing the problems of loneliness. This problem increased mostly in the adults and males as categorized in Table 3 and Table 4 as they are not allowed to go outside and they have to be in their home only. Mostly people increases newsfeed minimized social contacts but on the other hand the screen time increases with social media, newsfeeds, Netflix, Amazon Prime etc. Though these mediums are useful to an extent but at last absence of people nearby due to social distancing creates loneliness. Kids got engaged in online classes and activities, their parents got engaged in daily household chores and work from home options so a great majority of old aged peoples have nothing to do which creates loneliness primarily among them.

Figure 5 shows that the percentage of loneliness is high in females as they got bored with daily household chores and absence of spending quality time with other then family members. Figure 6 shows that the percentage of loneliness is high in age group below 30 years in UK and Denmark whereas it is high in age group above 60years in India.

Table 3. Loneliness developed in male and female

% of Population with High Loneliness	Denmark	France	Netherlands	UK	India
Male	14	12	5	22	22
Female	15	15	10	25	10

Table 4. Loneliness developed in different age groups

% of Population with High Loneliness	Denmark	France	Netherlands	UK	India
Under 30	25	15	15	30	22
30-60	08	13	8	25	18
Above 60	13	12	05	18	27

Figure 5. Loneliness developed in male and female

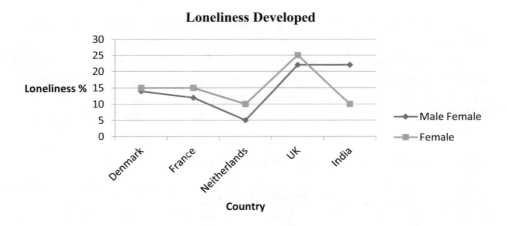

Figure 6. Loneliness developed in different age groups

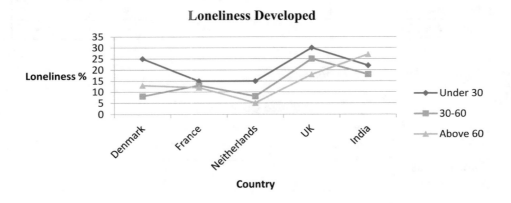

Adopted Good Habits

COVID-19 is responsible for several negative psychological and behavioral effects developed in peoples but in spite of that there are some good habits too which soon or later became a part of everyday essentials. The habits developed which are incorporated as good habits are:

1. Increased hand washing
2. Use of hand disinfectants
3. Physical distancing
4. Wearing Mask

5.   Avoiding public transportation

    Table 5 shows the percentage of people from different age groups in all four
different countries who developed the aforementioned good habits during this virus
spread. Figure 7 shows the graphical representations for the same developed habits.
It has been observed that majority of people in India, France and Netherlands in
survey started the good habit of hand washing whereas use of hand disinfectants is
high in Denmark. The least bothered good habit is wearing mask in Netherlands.

Table 5. Loneliness developed in different age groups

Adopted Good Habits	Denmark (%)	Netherlands (%)	France (%)	India (%)
Increased Hand washing	97	94	96	78
Use of Hand Disinfectants	98	50	93	63
Physical Distancing	80	97	60	48
Wearing Mask	78	5	20	45
Avoiding Public Transportation	80	52	55	37

Figure 7. Adopted good habits

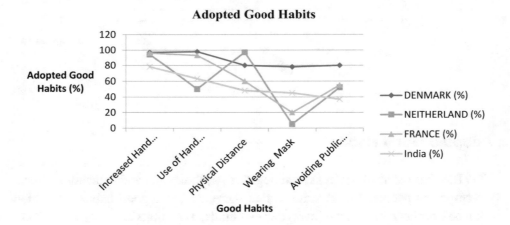

CONCLUSION AND FUTURE RESEARCH DIRECTIONS

From the above discussion it is clear that COVID-19 has led the whole world to its knees and the entire world is struggling to discontinue the chain of the growth of the virus. Many scientists are doing research to finish the cause of the COVID-19. Many companies have introduced vaccines such as Covishield, Covaxine, Pfizer, Jnsenn, Moderna, Sinopharm, Nuvaxovid etc which work as a shield on our body to save life. However it is not easy to finish it hundred percent as virus is producing its mutants and in present many mutants like Alpha, Beta, Delta, Omicron etc. are available in different countries. It is not only affecting the health of human being but also the state of mind in such a way that we should try to overcome from this situation. We all have to be very strong not only physically but mentally also. India, Denmark, France, Netherlands and UK is greatly affected by anxiety due to loss of job and financial threats, due to loss of social terms, illness of loved ones etc. Sooner or later this virus will become weaker and weaker but human must be strong enough to save our planet and future generation. Few good aspects of the current situations are that we have adopted good habits like, washing hand before eating something. We also avoid touching our nose and eyes by hand again and again. We also wear mask which helps us to protect from the pollution, we avoid going out unnecessarily which save fuels and air pollution, sound pollution and traffic reduces. Now days we care about our health but we should also care about our mental health. We should do yoga or some exercise. We should avoid negative newsfeeds from news papers, radio, and television or from any media of communication. We also should avoid talking and discussion on this topic because it affects our psychological balance. Hence to imperative to keep balance in our behavior and lifestyle we should be positive in all aspects. For those people who are already affected and there is imbalance in their behavior, some counseling program must be organized. Various health programs have been organized by social workers and government. People should take the advantage of those programs.

REFERENCES

Basu, S., Karmakar, A., Bidhan, V., Kumar, H., Brar, K., Pandit, M., & Latha, N. (2021). *Impact of Lockdown Due to COVID-19 Outbreak: Lifestyle Changes and Public Health Concerns in India.* Academic Press.

Bavel, J. J. V., Baicker, K., Boggio, P. S., Capraro, V., Cichocka, A., Cikara, M., Molly, J., Crum, A. J., Douglas, K.M., Druckman, J. N., Drury, J., Dube, O., Ellemers, N., Finkel, E.J., Fowler, J. H., Gelfand, M., Han, S., Haslam, S. A., Jetten, J., Kitayama, S., … Willer, R. (2020). Using Social and Behavioural Science to Support COVID-19 Pandemic Response. *Nature Human Behaviour, 460*(4), 460–471.

Cassenti, D., & Weston. (2020). Advances in Human Factors in Simulation and Modeling. *BMC Public Health, 20.*

Chatterjee, K., Shankar, S., Chatterjee, K., & Yadav, A. K. (2020). Corona virus disease 2019 in India: Post-lockdown scenarios and provisioning for health care. Elsevier. *Medical Journal, Armed Forces India, 76*(4), 387–394. doi:10.1016/j.mjafi.2020.06.004 PMID:32836711

Cheng, Y., Liu, D., Chen, J., Namilae, S., Thropp, J., & Seong, Y. (2018). Human Behavior Under Emergency And Its Simulation Modeling. *RE:view.*

Chopra, S., Ranjan, P., Singh, V., Kumar, S., Arora, M., Hasan, M. S., Kasiraj, R., Suryansh, Kaur, D., Vikram, N. K., Malhotra, A., Kumari, A., Klanidhi, K. B., & Baitha, U. (2020). Impact of COVID-19 on Lifestyle-Related Behaviours- A Cross-Sectional Audit of Responses From Nine Hundred And Ninety-Five Participants From India. Elsevier. *Diabetes & Metabolic Syndrome, 14*(6), 2021–2030. doi:10.1016/j.dsx.2020.09.034 PMID:33099144

Crosta, A. D., Ceccato, I., Marchetti, D., Malva, P. L., Maiella, R., Cannito, R., Cip, M., Mammarella, N., Palumbo, N., Verrocchio, M. C., Palumbo, R., & Domenico, A. D. (2020). Psychological Factors and Consumer Behavior during the COVID-19 Pandemic. *PLoS One*, 1–23. PMID:34398916

Davis, R., Campbell, R., Hildon, Z., Hobbs, L., & Michie, S. (2015). Theories of Behaviour and Behaviour Change Across the Social and Behavioural Sciences: A Scoping Review. *Health Psychology Review, 9*(3), 323–344. doi:10.1080/1743719 9.2014.941722 PMID:25104107

Francisco, R., Pedro, M., Delvecchio, E., Espada, J. P., Morales, A., Mazzeschi, C., & Orgiles, M. (2020). Psychological Symptoms and Behavioral Changes in Children and Adolescents during the Early Phase of COVID-19 Quarantine in Three European Countries. *Frontiers in Psychiatry, 11*, 1–14. doi:10.3389/fpsyt.2020.570164 PMID:33343415

Funk, S., Bansal, S., Bauch, C. T., Eames, K. T., Edmunds, W. J., & Galvani. (2015). Nine challenges in Incorporating the Dynamics of Behaviour in Infectious Diseases Models. *Epidemics, 10*, 21–5.

Kollamparambil, U., & Oyenubi, A. (2021). Behavioural Response to the COVID-19. Pandemic in South Africa. *PLoS One*, 1–19. PMID:33861811

Matos, A. D., Paiva, A. F. D., Cunha, C., & Voss, G. (2021). Precautionary Behaviours of Individuals with Multimorbidity during The COVID-19 Pandemic. *European Journal of Ageing*, 1–9. PMID:35002593

Michie, S., West, R., Campbell, R., Brown, J., & Gainforth, H. (2014). *ABC of Behaviour Change Theories*. Silverback Publishing.

Nagarathna, R., Anand, A., Rain, M., Srivastava, V., Sivapuram, M. S., Kulkarni, R., Ilavarasu, J., Sharma, M. N. K., Singh, A., & Nagendra, H. R. (2021). Yoga Practice Is Beneficial for Maintaining Healthy Lifestyle and Endurance Under Restrictions and Stress Imposed by Lockdown During COVID-19 Pandemic. *Frontiers in Psychiatry*, *12*, 1–20. doi:10.3389/fpsyt.2021.613762 PMID:34239456

Rawat, D., Dixit, V., Gulati, S., Gulati, S., & Gulati, A. (2021). Impact of COVID-19 Outbreak on Lifestyle Behaviour: A Review of Studies Published in India. *Diabetes & Metabolic Syndrome, 15*(1), 331–336.

Singh, K., Raghav, P., Singh, G., Pritish Baskaran, T. B., Bishnoi, A., Gautam, V., Chaudhary, A. K., Kumar, A., Kumar, S., & Sahu, S. (2021). Lifestyle and Behavioral Changes During Nationwide Lockdown in India-A Cross-Sectional Analysis. *Journal of Family Medicine and Primary Care*, *10*(7), 2661–2667. doi:10.4103/jfmpc.jfmpc_2464_20 PMID:34568152

Tibor, V., Varga, T. V., Bu, F., Dissin, A. S., Elsenburg, L. K., Bustamante, J. J. H., Matta, J., Zon, S. K. R. V., Brouwer, S., Beultmann, U., Fancourt, D., Hoeyer, K., Goldberg, M., Melchior, M., Larsen, K. S., Zins, M., Clotworthy, A., & Rod, N. H. (2021). Loneliness, worries, anxiety, and precautionary behaviors in response to the COVID-19 pandemic: A longitudinal analysis of 200,000 Western and Northern Europeans. *The Lancet Regional Health - Europe, 2*, 1–9.

Weston, D., Ip, A., & Amlot, R. (2020). Examining the Application of Behavior Change Theories in the Context of Infectious Disease Outbreaks and Emergency Response: A Review of Reviews BMC. *Public Health*, *20*, 1–19. PMID:33004011

Williams, L., Rasmussen, S., Kleczkowski, A., Maharaj, S., & Cairns, N. (2015). Protection Motivation Theory and Social Distancing Behaviour in Response to a Simulated Infectious Disease Epidemic. *Psychology Health and Medicine*, *20*(7), 832–837. doi:10.1080/13548506.2015.1028946 PMID:25835044

Zhang, N., Jia, W., Lei, H., Wang, P., Zhao, P., Guo, Y., Dung, C. H., Bu, Z., Xue, P., Xie, J., Zhang, Y., Cheng, R., & Li, Y. (2019). *Effects of Human Behavior Changes During the Coronavirus Disease 2019 (COVID-19) Pandemic on Influenza Spread in Hong Kong*. Oxford University Press.

Chapter 13
Discriminating Significant Morphological Attributes of Photoplethysmograph Signal for Cuffless Blood Pressure Measurement

Arun Kumar
Bhilai Institute of Technology, India

Padmini Sharma
Chhatrapatishivaji Institute of Technology, India

Mukesh Kumar Chandrakar
Bhilai Institute of Technology, India

ABSTRACT

Photoplethysmograph signal carries very useful cardiac information such heart rate, oxygen saturation level, blood pressure, and diabetic condition. Blood pressure is one such cardiac information that can be estimated by extracting features of PPG signal. Cuff-less blood pressure measurement using photoplethysmograph (PPG) signal is one of non-invasive methods. It allows continuous monitoring of blood pressure in simple, rapid, and low-cost mode. This chapter segregates PPG features and re-investigates their effectiveness in terms of BP measurement. Machine learning algorithm based on K-nearest neighbour is applied for classification of samples. MIMIC II multi-parameter database of ECG and finger PPG is applied on the KNN classifiers. Classification accuracy comes to 92%, and correlation between predicted and observed SBP and DSB are 0.89 and 0.85, respectively.

DOI: 10.4018/978-1-7998-9831-3.ch013

INTRODUCTION

Photoplethysmograph (PPG) is measure of blood volume in unit interval of time it also represents a measure of arterial oxygenation versus time. PPG signal is consisting of systolic, diastolic peak and notch, systolic peak is caused by propelling of blood from heart and secondary peak is caused by reflection of blood in vessel PPG is obtained using optical method by radiating and receiving the infrared light beam on the body organs such as fingertips, forehead or earlobes (Hasanzadeh, Ahmadi, and Mohammadzade 2020). PPG measurement technology is versatile and extended to the different aspects of the cardiovascular surveillance like heart rate, cardiac output oxygen saturation of blood, respiration, anatomic function, micro vascular blood flow, endothelial control, atrial ageing and blood pressure. Association of different PPG signals with cardiac condition and ageing are well proved. PPG signals are recorded from exterior body location such as forehead, earlobe, toe and fingers. Arteries, veins and numerous capillaries are the coverage area of the PPG signal extraction process during the measurement. Tissue penetration of the infrared light and red light is 2.5mm underneath which is more than tissue penetration of green light therefore infrared light is usually preferred for acquiring the PPG signal. Few key points of the PPG signal such as systolic peak, diastolic peak and notch, maximum slop points, inflection point etc. above key points are used to extract some of the morphological features of the PPG signal such as heart rate (HR), Systemic Vascular Resistance (SVR), Reflection Index (RI), Large Artery Stiffness Index (LASI), Inflection Point Area IPA, mNPA, Crest Time (CT) Mean Atrial Pressure (MAP) etc. these morphological features carries vital cardiac information and plays very important role in measuring same.

As already specified that PPG can reveal significant information about different cardiac deceases like blood pressure, blood volume, pre-diabetic condition etc. No mathematical expressions are available which correlates the Blood Pressure (BP) with PPG but some machine learning models are reported by different authors which effectively estimate BP by using PPG and ECG signal. Some features such as Pulse Transit Time (PTT), Pulse arrival Time (PAT), pulse wave velocity (PWT), modified normalized pulse volume (mNPV), heart rate (HR), HR*mNPV vascular transit time (VTT) were used significantly. Some researchers reported that the pulse area, rising time and pulse width, systolic peak also illustrates significant outcomes in BP measurement. Fig. 1 showing the PPG signal and blood pressure signal between cardiac cycles and also depicts the measure of PTT in between the ECG, R wave and Systolic peak of PPG signal (He, Goubran, and Liu 2014).

Figure 1. Simultaneous record of PPG and ECG signal

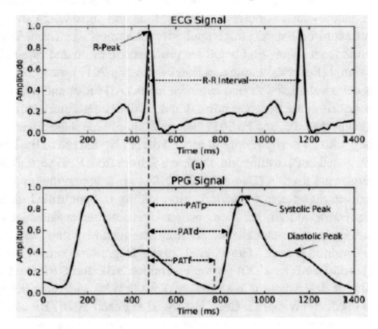

Cuff less BP measurement have several advantages over conventional method such as continuous & real time monitoring, riddance of irritation and pain due to cuff inflammation normal smart phone or portable electronics devices allow BP effortless. In (He, Goubran, and Liu 2014) authors investigated on three different methods to detect diastolic peak and notch which are buried and invisible in PPG signal due to poor reflection of blood in the vessels, such a invisibility leading to shift the main peak of the PPG signal which gives inaccurate PTT and arterial blood pressure ABP. Authors in (Chowdhury et al. 2020) implemented a method of estimating the Systolic Blood Pressure (SBP), Systolic Blood Pressure (DBP) using PPG signal with help of machine learning algorithm. This cuff less pressure measurement system make use of 107 features extracted in different domain such as time domain, frequency domain, statistical and demographic data etc. Three different feature selection method is used to reduce the computation complexity. GPR ML algorithm along with the Relief feature selection method provided effective outcomes on this investigation. A mathematical expression relating SBP and DBP with PTT is proposed by researchers in (Park et al. 2019) and investigated the effectiveness of the same. The relationship between PAT with PTT and PEP is conferred to examine effectiveness of PTT over PAT in terms of BP measurement. Authors in (Khalid et al. 2018) (Esmaili, Kachuee, and Shabany 2017) inspected the efficacy of the regression tree ML algorithm with acceptable measurement accuracy. PPG pulse width features such as pulse area, rising time and pulse width are applied in investigation. Multi-collinearity test is applied to select most significant feature. PPG signal acquired from acquisition board are processed to evaluated using UWT and DWT PPG signal (Bereksi-Reguig and Bereksi-Reguig 2017) second derivative of the PPG signal is calculated to find augment index (AI) index and b/a ratio which are used to discriminate between normal and cardiac condition. Neural network classifier used in (Liu, Po, and Fu 2017) where 21 amplitude related feature of time domain along with 14 newly proposed second derivative feature of the PPG signal are effectively used in BP estimation. Different feature from PPG second derivative contour analysis are used in (Usman et al. 2019) to investigate the type 2 diabetic condition but no significance discrimination among the controlled diabetic and healthy patient are found. Authors demonstrated and obtained reasonable agreement between automatic and manual method from the feature points with improved accuracy and minimal error (Fan P. et.al 2015). Regression model proposed in (Tjajjadi, H. and Ramli,K. 2020) for the estimation SBP and DBP used KNN for the clustering of data where pulse wave velocity (PWV) and some demographic features are used. In (Wang, H. Chao Huang, Hang chen 2016) BP estimation is done by using noninvasive wearable device through BP based model and KNN using PPG and ECG features combined. Researchers demonstrated a calibration free BP measurement method through HR as significant feature and KNN based regression model evaluation (Sanuki, H. et.al 2017). Authors in (Peihao, Meriem and kirati, L. 2021) demonstrated a method to estimate SBP and DBP using semi classical signal analysis (SCSA) of PPG wave, tried to compare the performance using SCSA feature sets in various learning algorithms such as SVM, MLR and decision tree, outcome of the support vector machine is comparatively good in terms of mean absolute error and standard deviation. U-net deep learning architecture is used to estimate arterial BP (ABP) waveform non-invasively using fingertip PPG signal (Athaya, T. and Choi S. 2021). Correlation between predicted ABP waveforms reference waveforms is obtained in terms of average Pearson's correlation coefficient of 0.993 and demonstrated an efficient process to estimate ABP waveform directly using fingertip PPG. Novel method of BP measurements on a smartphone case using Cardio QVARK single-channel ECG monitor with PPG pulse wave recording without cuff has been proposed by the researchers in (Sagirova, Z. et.al 2021) and successfully estimated BP. Investigators proposed a LTSM based auto-encoder model for translating PPG in to atrial blood pressure (Harfiya, L.N. Chang, C. Li, Y H. 2021). proposed model provides an accurate and promising estimation result over a very large number of subject sample.

This paper inspects on potential and efficacy of morphological features of PPG signal to measure BP, also puts an effort to select and identify significant features by the means of feature selection algorithm. effective features in terms of BP estimation are segregated and then send to classifier. A machine learning algorithm KNN is applied for the classification by using morphological features of the PPG signal for BP measurement.

FEATURES USED IN BP MEASUREMENT

There are 24-time domain features, 17-pulse width related features, 16-first and second derivative features, 16-frequency domain features, 18-demographic, 10-statistical features are used in (Chowdhury et al. 2020) for BP estimation. Using large number of features without knowing their significance leads to over fitting in machine learning thus it is essential to eliminate fewer effective features from data set, feature selection plays important role in verifying the effectiveness of the features and reduces computation complexity of machine learning. Researchers investigated on different feature selection method to check suitability of features in terms of BP estimation. although 107 features of different domain are used but features such as PTT, PAT, PEP, PWV, VTT, mNPV, HR, second derivative PPG features are excluded from investigation by the researchers.

Some morphological features of PPG like pulse width 25%, width 50%/t_{pi}, width 75% some frequency domain features like maximum frequency, ratio of first and second frequency and ratio of signal energy, features extracted from second derivative of PPG (14 features) signal, demographic feature such as weight, Body mass index (BMI), height and statistical features kurtosis, spectral entropy, mean and Standard deviation. Instantaneous frequency calculated from the Ensemble empirical mode decomposition (EEMD) gives promising result of estimation (Wei, Hai Cheng et al. 2018) similarly features like PTT, PAT, PEP, PWV, VTT as shown in table 1 These features are good indicator of BP but needs simultaneous record of ECG and PPG signal both. Clinical instrument allows simultaneous recording of ECG & PPG but portable instrument like smart wrist watches, pulse oximeter (finger plethysmograph) does not allow simultaneous recording of signals, morphological features of the PPG play important role in such situation. This paper puts an effort to segregates morphological features of PPG apart from features of simultaneous record of ECG and PPG. It re-investigates to check effectiveness of morphological features collectively in terms of BP measurement, such segregated features are shown in table 2.

Table 1. Features from simultaneous record of ECG & PPG

Features	Description
PTT	It is time difference between R peak of ECG & systolic peak of PPG
PAT	Pulse arrival time
VTT	Vascular transit time
PEP	Projection point
PWV	Shows stiffness of blood vessels, ratio of distance of heart to finger and PTT
HR	Heart Rate

Table 2. Morphological features extracted from PPG signal

PPG Features	Description
HRV	Heart rate variability
SVR	Systemic vascular resistance is resistance of blood flow in total vascular system.
RI	Dicrotic notch reflection index is ratio of amplitude of inflation point and systolic pulse
LASI	Large artery stiffness index is ratio of height and time between systolic peak and inflection of point of PPG
IPA	Ratio of PPG systolic & diastolic pulse area
CT	Crest Time is time to reach up to maximum of systolic peak
mNPV	Modified normalized pulse volume is ratio of peak to peak amplitude of PPG and DC value
Ln HR	Logarithm of HR
Ln mNPV	Logarithm of Modified normalized pulse volume
Ln HR*mNPV	Logarithm of product value of HR and mNPV
TPR	Total peripheral resistance (Mean atrial pressure = Cardiac output * TPR)
A0-2	Area under 0-2 hz of PPG spectra
A2-5	Area under 2-5 hz of PPG spectra
MSTT	Mean slop transit time of systolic curve of PPG
SDPPG	Five Second derivative feature points(a,b,c,d,e)
Kurtosis	Define Sharpness of the peak
Entropy	Measure of degree of randomness in data
Pulse Width	Pulse width at 25% and 75% amplitude of PPG wave.
Skewness	Lack of symmetry from mean of database

Some of this features are solely used by some researchers for BP measurement such as Ln HR and Ln mNPV are used with their linear polynomial equation and accuracy of 70 are also achieved similarly some of the second derivative PPG signal features (SDPPG) combined with the amplitude feature of PPG signal promisingly improved the accuracy as compare to the conventional techniques. In some research CT, LASI and Augmented Index (AI) are also increase the accuracy of the BP measurement whereas HR is only effective to estimate SBP. PPG signal Contour angle α, β and ratio b/a does not show any significant discrimination in between healthy and unhealthy diabetic situation but here it is used to test the discrimination of BP.

PROPOSED METHODOLOGY

In this research some amplitude related features as illustrated in Fig 2(a), and table 2, some second derivative features of PPG signal (SDPPG) (Liu, Po, and Fu 2017): illustrated in Fig 2(b), Pulse width related features: width 25% width 25%/ t_1 width 50%, width 50%/t_{pi}, width 75%, width 75%/tpi, features from PPG contour analysis α,

Figure 2. (a) amplitude features of PPG (b) second derivative feature points (Liu, Po, and Fu 2017)

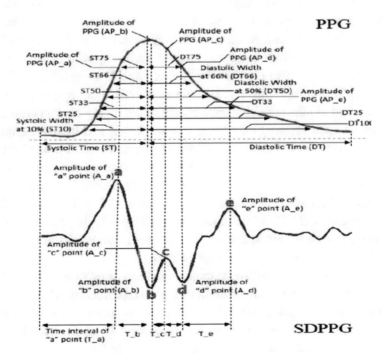

Figure 3. PPG signal contour angles
(Usman et al. 2019)

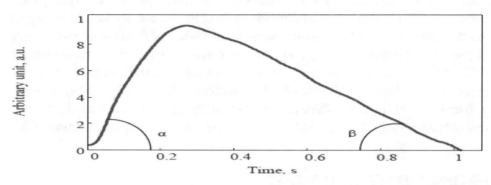

β as shown in from Fig 3 and Pulse area frequency domain features: Peak1 and Peak 2 ratio of peaks, maximum frequency of PPG ($f_{max,}$) amplitude of $f_{max.}$ Statistical data: skewness, Kurtosis, spectral entropy, Shannon's entropy, few time domain features like SVR RI LASI IPA, CT, MSTT, mNP (Matsumura, Kenta, Peter Rolfe, Sogo Toda, and Takehiro Yamakoshi. 2018), HR, Pulse area A0-2, A2-5. rising time and pulse width are extracted from PPG signal are collectively used in investigation but demographic features are excluded because portable measuring device such as smart wrist watch and finger plethysmograph does not allow to feed such information in it.

Efficacy of some significant features reported by different researchers are re-investigated. Matlab^R inbuilt function of feature selection method ReliefF is used in feature selection. ReliefF selection method randomly selects an instance and adjusts weight of respective element depending upon close neighbor (Chowdhury et al. 2020). Multi-co linearity test (Khalid et al. 2018) is applied before feature selection method to eliminate the features which are highly correlated with others because use of such features may leads to over fitting and increase computation complexity of classifier (Khalid et al. 2018). A presence of multi-collinearity among the features affects the generalizability of the method or model applied on the BP estimation in terms of high mean square error between actual value and estimated value. Variance Implantation Factor (VIF) is diagnostic tool of multicollinearity between the features, if VIF > 10 then feature variable is highly collinear with other feature, they must be eliminated from the data set to improve the efficacy of the estimation and minimize the computation effort.

In this paper MIMIC II multi-parameter data base of ECG and finger PPG each record is of 10 second are used, from this data base sample records of 510 are extracted which include DBP & SBP, 80% which are used for training and remaining 20% (110 samples) are used in testing purpose (Waveform Database MIMIC II: 2012). Complete procedure adapted in this work is depicted in fig 4.

Figure 4. Block diagram of the proposed method

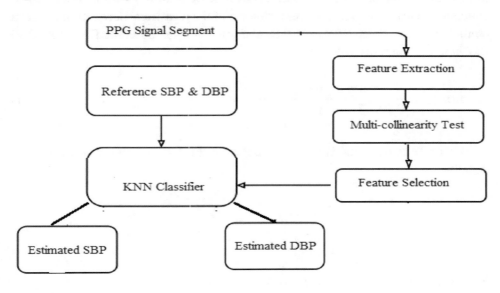

Machine Learning: K- Nearest Neighbor (KNN)

Supervised machine learning method based on K- nearest neighbor (KNN) must be the suitable classifier for the sample type of features used. KNN looks at the data point and classify them with respect to its neighbor's characteristics. KNN with K=1 is the simplest method of classification because it based on the concept that if sample close to each other will depict similar characteristics thus the classification is done on the basis of closeness of the samples. Euclidean distance is used to define the closeness of the request point sample with its nearest neighboring sample of the reference data point.

RESULT AND DISCUSSION

Predictor features which are useful and selected by the ReliefF (Matlab inbuilt function) selection method are SVR RI LASI IPA, CT, MSTT, mNPV, HR, HRV, MAP, Pulse width 25% width 50%, width, IPA, ratio of peaks, skewness, Kurtosis, rising time Ln Hr* mNPV are morphological signal collected from the PPG signal, are selected as significant features by feature selection method. Segregated or selected features are fed to KNN classifiers, where 80% of data sample are used in training and remaining 20% of data samples are used in the testing the accuracy of the classifier. Classification result is evaluated by the classification accuracy using

Eq. 1 with the help of confusion matrix shown in Fig 5 accuracy comes out 92% and confusion matrix visualizes the performance of the classifier. Correlation between predicted and observed SBP is r= 0.89 and predicted and observed DBP is r= 0.85 shown in the Fig 6 (a), (b)

$$\text{Accuracy} = \frac{Tp + Fp}{Tp + Tn + Fp + Fn} \qquad (1)$$

Where *Tp* is true positive, *Tn* true negative, *Fp* false positive and *Fn* is false negative

Figure 5. Confusion matrices of predicted features

	DBP	SBP
DBP	94	16
SBP	19	91

Figure 6. Correlation between a) observed and Predicted SBP b) observed and Predicted DBP

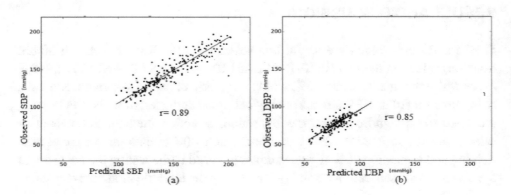

(a) (b)

CONCLUSION

This paper investigated and highlighted the features used in BP measurement such as SVR, RI, LASI, IPA, CT, MSTT, mNPV, HR. effectiveness of such features are re-investigated along with other features such as pulse width features, second derive features etc. The ReleifF feature selection method and multi collinearity test are applied to select suitable features for the BP measurement, features which are suitable for estimation of SBP and DBP are highlighted in result section. Feature selection method eliminated some features are width 75%, CT, amplitude features Ln HR, TPR, A0-2, spectral entropy, remaining features are used by machine learning algorithm for the classification of SBP and DBP. Correlation between predicted and observed SBP and DBP are also evaluated in result section. Although the demographic features are not in use but still correlation between predicted and observed SBP and DBP seems satisfactory. Accuracy and correlation might be increased if demographic features are included.

REFERENCES

Athaya, T., & Choi, S. (2021). An Estimation method of continuous non-invasive arterial blood pressure waveform using photoplethysmography. A U-Net Architecture-Based Approach. *Sensors (Basel)*, *21*(5), 1867. doi:10.339021051867 PMID:33800106

Bereksi-Reguig, M. A., & Bereksi-Reguig, F. (2017). Photoplethysmogram Signal Processing and Analysis in Evaluating Arterial Stiffness. *International Journal of Biomedical Engineering and Technology*, *23*(2–4), 363–378. doi:10.1504/IJBET.2017.10003507

Chowdhury, M. H. (2020). Estimating Blood Pressure from the Photoplethysmogram Signal and Demographic Features Using Machine Learning Techniques. Sensors, 20(11). doi:10.339020113127

Esmaili, A., Kachuee, M., & Shabany, M. (2017). Nonlinear Cuffless Blood Pressure Estimation of Healthy Subjects Using Pulse Transit Time and Arrival Time. *IEEE Transactions on Instrumentation and Measurement*, 66(12), 3299–3308. doi:10.1109/TIM.2017.2745081

Fan, P., Peiyu, H., Shangwen, L., & Wenfeng, D. (2015). *Feature extraction of photoplethysmography signal using wavelet approach*. doi:10.1109/ICDSP.2015.7251876

Harfiya, L. N., Chang, C., & Li, Y. H. (2021). Continuous blood pressur estimation using exclusively photopletysmography by LSTM based signal-to-signal translation. *Sensors (Basel)*, *21*(9), 2952. doi:10.339021092952 PMID:33922447

Hasanzadeh, N., Ahmadi, M. M., & Mohammadzade, H. (2020). Blood Pressure Estimation Using Photoplethysmogram Signal and Its Morphological Features. *IEEE Sensors Journal*, *20*(8), 4300–4310. doi:10.1109/JSEN.2019.2961411

He, X., Goubran, R. A., & Liu, X. P. (2014). Secondary Peak Detection of PPG Signal for Continuous Cuffless Arterial Blood Pressure Measurement. *IEEE Transactions on Instrumentation and Measurement*, *63*(6), 1431–1439. doi:10.1109/TIM.2014.2299524

Khalid, S. G., Zhang, J., Chen, F., & Zheng, D. (2018). Blood Pressure Estimation Using Photoplethysmography Only: Comparison between Different Machine Learning Approaches. *Journal of Healthcare Engineering*, *2018*, 2018. doi:10.1155/2018/1548647 PMID:30425819

Liu, M., Po, L.-M., & Fu, H. (2017). Cuffless Blood Pressure Estimation Based on Photoplethysmography Signal and Its Second Derivative. *International Journal of Computer Theory and Engineering*, *9*(3), 202–206. doi:10.7763/IJCTE.2017.V9.1138

Matsumura, K., Rolfe, P., Toda, S., & Yamakoshi, T. (2018). Cuffless Blood Pressure Estimation Using Only a Smartphone. *Scientific Reports*, *8*(1), 1–9. doi:10.103841598-018-25681-5 PMID:29740088

Park, J., Yang, S., Sohn, J., Lee, J., Lee, S., Ku, Y., & Kim, H. C. (2019). Cuffless and Continuous Blood Pressure Monitoring Using a Single Chest-Worn Device. *IEEE Access: Practical Innovations, Open Solutions*, *7*, 135231–135246. doi:10.1109/ACCESS.2019.2942184

Peihao, M., & Kirati, L. (2021). Central blood pressure estimation from distal ppg measurement using semiclassical signal analysis features. *IEEE Access*. doi:10.1109/ACCESS.2021.3065576

Sagirova, Z., Kuznetsova, N., Gogiberidze, N., Gognieva, D., Suvorov, A., Chomakhidze, P., Omboni, S., Saner, H., & Kopylov, P. (2021). Cuffless blood pressure measurement using a smartphone-case based ecg monitor with photoplethysmography in hypertensive patients. *Sensors*, *21*, 3525. doi:10.3390/s21103525

Sanuki, H., Rui Fukui, T., & Warisawa, S. (2017). Cuffless calibration free blood pressure estimation under ambulatory environment using pulse wave velocity and photoplethysmogram signal. *Proceedings of 10ᵗʰ International conference on biomedical engineering system and technology and application (BIOESTEC 2017)*. 10.5220/0006112500420048

Tjajjadi, H., & Ramli, K. (2020). Noninvasive blood pressure classification based on photoplethysmography using K-nearest neighbors algorithm: A feasible study. *Information, 11*(93). . doi:10.3390/info11020093

Usman, S. (2019). Second Derivative and Contour Analysis of PPG for Diabetic Patients. *2018 IEEE EMBS Conference on Biomedical Engineering and Sciences, IECBES 2018 – Proceedings*, 59–62.

Wang, Huang, & Chen. (2016). Preprocessing of PPG and ECG Signal to estimate blood pressure based on noninvasive wearable device. *Proceeding of International conference on engineering technology and application (ICETA 2016)*.

Waveform DatabaseMIMICII. (2012). https://physionet.org/mimic2/mimic2_ waveform_overview. shtml

Wei, H. C., Xiao, M.-X., Chen, H.-Y., Li, Y.-Q., Wu, H.-T., & Sun, C.-K. (2018). Instantaneous Frequency from Hilbert-Huang Transformation of Digital Volume Pulse as Indicator of Diabetes and Arterial Stiffness in Upper-Middle-Aged Subjects. *Scientific Reports, 8*(1), 1–8. doi:10.103841598-018-34091-6 PMID:30361528

Chapter 14
Survey of Recent Studies on Healthcare Technologies and Computational Intelligence Approaches and Their Applications

Lokesh Kumar Sahu
Pt. Ravishankar Shukla University, India

Vaishali Soni
Pt. Ravishankar Shukla University, India

Prafulla Kumar Vyas
Disha College, India

Anjali Deshpande
M. M. College of Technology, India

ABSTRACT

Digitized healthcare technologies provide healthcare enhancements in the field of medical digital technologies and they also provide better accessibility. The research study indicates that digital healthcare is combining or involving more than one academic discipline like biology science, cognitive science, medical science, biochemistry neuroscience, etc. The complete healthcare technologies are based on computational intelligence, artificial intelligence, etc. This chapter gives an overview of the current and future of healthcare technologies and up-to-date research in the area of digital healthcare intelligence. For artificial intelligence or computational intelligence, healthcare is one of the most promising application areas. This review highlights all about applications of artificial intelligence, telemedicine, blockchain technologies, the internet of things, and big data for solving the problems in medical education and healthcare technologies.

DOI: 10.4018/978-1-7998-9831-3.ch014

INTRODUCTION

Several studies highlight the effect of computational intelligence on healthcare facilities which may improve prognosis, diagnostics and care planning. Nowadays computational Intelligence system are becoming an integral part of healthcare services and soon in the future, it will be incorporated into various aspects of clinical care. Computational intelligence is the study of intelligent systems which includes intelligent synthetic characters, man and machine interface, picture archiving, communication systems that have flexibility towards changing environments and objectives.

In the last few years, various Computational Intelligence based technologies introduced by the researchers for the medical and healthcare act to increase digital knowledge-based systems (DKBS). This examination discusses the latest movements and success in the zone of digital health skills. It completely includes the use of AI, Big Data, BlockChain technology and Telemedicine for clear problems in the healthcare structure. The writing search shows that digital health skills are on extremely required because of pandemic situations as well as covid-19 and the extent of covid-19 through all. The recent trend of healthcare technologies includes the use of 3D printing equipment for the production of organ models, everlasting implants, medical equipment testing, modified 3D drug printing, and medical learning.

Computational Intelligence for Healthcare: Computational Intelligence theory and research of smart computer systems that expand repeatedly by practice. In the previous few years, many CI methods are proposed by researchers to develop the smart system in the area of a health monitoring system. Applications of computational intelligence in multiple areas like discovering new diseases, finding predictive biomarkers and treatments. Artificial Intelligent Systems (AIS) offers great improvements in the area of healthcare assists with machine learning, wireless communication, data analysis, computing computer, mobile computer, etc. In computational intelligence multiple paradigms have to discuss like bio-inspired computing, in this field we will discuss about various technologies in this chapter:

- Artificial Neutral Network (ANN)
- Support Vector Machine (SVM)
- Deep Learning (DL)
- Genetic Algorithms (GA)
- Evolutionary Computing (EC)
- DNA Computing,
- Artificial Intelligence and Analytics(AIA)

The above are increasingly changing the healthcare system and medical system in a remarkable method of using functional procedures from countless branches of information technology (IT).

Artificial Intelligence for Healthcare: Artificial Intelligence helps to save lives and helps to grow technologies used for Digital Healthcare. It even now affects multiple human accomplishments at all social stages. Artificial Intelligence is more expanding worldwide. Applications related to Artificial Intelligence in healthcare and medicine for the public perception are extended personalized medicine, replacement or enhancement etc. In this following topic will be covered-

- Data Mining
- Ontology and Semantic Reasoning
- Clinical Decision Support Systems
- Smart Homes
- Medical Big Data etc

These are the recent technological trends in the field of computational intelligence.

Radiology is one of the main areas of artificial intelligence in healthcare applications. With self-training of digital imaging machines and rapid analysis, increasing the efficiency of medical practice skills. This is based on learning algorithms that can integrate and interact with MRI equipment to improve image reshaping. without any disturbance. Some of Artificial Intelligence applications will be discussed in this chapter

- Ultrasound imaging
- CT imaging
- MRI
- Cancer Diagnosis
- Drug development
- Genomics etc.

In the present time tasks related to covid-19 epidemics, Platforms centered on Artificial Intelligence can help classify and ease epidemiologic risks.

Big Data and E-Health: In the last few years, Big Data analysis has been increasing and improving and also increase management, analysis, and prediction in health care. The use of big data schemes has the prospective to expand the standard, the cost is low of care and the efficiency of the facility and the number of medical faults. There is a trend in fixed worldwide for the use of big data as a stage that accelerates and facilitates the biomedical research and it also delivers the multiple prospects to discover new explanations in biology, remedy, genetics, and pharmacy and it can also help the shorting and analytics of the growing capacity of medical specifics.

The term **Digital Healthcare** or **E-Health** covers a lot of theory, perspective and skills like genomics big data, AI, smart devices, wearable, telemedicine and various types of applications for mobile. In the last few decades, digital health technologies are broadly used in the medical healthcare organization and studied about it and use in biomedicine, research, and health training. The preparation and improvement of the treatment and diagnosis of various issues, it includes the application of digital health standards. The pandemic by the covid-19 for all the countries prompted the need for instant and effective solutions and Artificial Intelligence, Computational Intelligence and many other digital healthcare systems are helping to get out of this pandemic situation. The new technological trends in the digital healthcare systems facilitate the medical experts and assistants with these technologies and reduce the burden on doctors and national health care systems. These platforms can make it easier to diagnose, make appointments and treat an infected patient and digital technology has already had a major impression on the existing digital health care system. E.g., the use of telemedicine has helped to decrease hospitalization and death rates among patients with coronary heart disease and diabetes.

This research study concludes that computational intelligence technologies are upcoming with a technological revolution in the healthcare sector due to its portability, low cost and an important factor of risk prevention on the basis of data-driven decision-making ability.

Healthcare is recognizing individual favorable application regions for computational intelligence and multiple studies highlight the effect of computational intelligence in the field of healthcare facilities which may in improve various types of diagnostics, prognosis, and care planning. In the current days, computational intelligence systems are becoming a part of the healthcare service and soon in the future, it will completely depend on it in the area of healthcare. Digital technologies can encompass the supply of open records on the remedy, fitness, headaches and current progress on bio-scientific studies. In recent years, several CI methods and techniques have been offered by investigators to advance digital knowledge-based systems (DKBS) for different tasks in the field of medical and healthcare schemes. The purpose of the research is to debate and examine the development these days in the use of smart data processing technology, telemedicine, smart devices in the area of block-chain health platforms and medical education. The review highlights the application of artificial intelligence, telemedicine, the internet of thing (smart devices) and medical education. In this paper, we will also discuss about artificial intelligence and a complete system which is based on artificial intelligence concepts and theories. The objective of this paper is present complete knowledge and up to date with research in the field of healthcare artificial intelligence is a brand new area of science. Artificial Intelligence in medical healthcare is completely changing the perspective. Yet, due to lack of rules guidelines and references including private and government administrations (Azzi, 2020).

Healthcare technology is commonly used as "healthcare". We use healthcare technology to develop technology in the field of the healthcare system and improve medical science. Healthcare technology is improving the live of patients by treatment and making the medical process more potential. We can use healthcare technology like artificial intelligence in surgery, drug development, fitness, diagnostics and error reduction, mental health etc. The model of standard healthcare is completely built on supplying medical facilities by the structures of hospitals and clinics. Factors that depends of the healthcare service superiority is the hospital facilities and the accessibility of apparatus. And the model changes from country to country. In recent years some platforms experience new challenges because of the growth of new technologies and call of high-quality medical facilities (Bennett & Chen, 2017).

The execution of digital technologies in medicine can provide. On the additional side diagnostic and medical facilities are available in low-income countries. One of the most promising and rising area is computational intelligence. So, computational intelligence is the kind of procedure that increases through experience. Computer intelligence makes improvements program without any dependence on command. In recent ages, computational intelligence methods give us smart systems in the area of health and health monitoring systems, computational intelligence and artificial offer robust, smart method and intelligent algorithms that can help to solve the problem of health and life science area. There are multiple samples of successful uses of computational intelligence in the area of the healthcare system like diagnosis and prevention, therapeutic decision making, and prognosis also. Following tasks that computational intelligence are used like discovering new diseases and finding therapeutic and predictive biomarkers etc. Also, we discuss challenges as well as ongoing research in the areas of digital health schemes (Buchanan, 2005).

Another most promising and rising area is the use of artificial intelligence in medical healthcare systems like biomedicine and medical training. Artificial intelligence is related to philosophy, possibilities, demonstrations, imaginations, and thoughts. Artificial Intelligence is merged with analytics that improvement in many sectors like healthcare application and technologies. In artificial intelligence, research started in the field of the healthcare system in 20th century and also developed in the application and gives it to clinicians for practice. This review tells about the latest research, trends, and breakthroughs in the area of digital health technology. It also includes the use of artificial intelligence, "big data", block-chain technologies and telemedicine.

Computational Intelligence for Healthcare

In the last few multiple computational intelligence techniques are proposed by researchers to develop smart systems and technology in the area of health monitoring systems. This chapter discusses the complete role of computational intelligence approaches and Techniques that are used in developing intelligent health techniques and smart systems Cook (2006). Computational intelligence applications are in multiple areas of health monitoring systems like discovering new diseases, finding biomarkers for prediction and treatment. There are multiple diseases are present like cancer, brain tumor, heart, thrombosis diseases, diabetics and various types of diseases are present here.

Artificial Neutral Network

Artificial Neural Network (AAN) is a class of learning and a piece of the computing system that is designed to process information of the human brain analyses. It gives by Artificial Intelligence. ANN is connecting with each other by their connecting systems. ANN simulates the functioning of the human brain. Figure 1 shows the various applications of ANN in medicine.

Figure 1. Applications of ANN in medicine

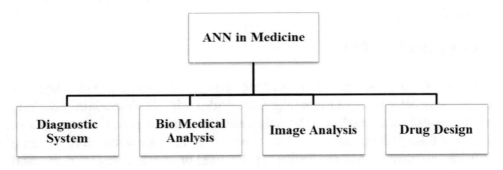

ANN is like the human brain and acts like human brains. The human brain works with hundreds of billions of cells. That cells are called neurons and one neuron is made up of a cell body and that is processing inputs and output which is given by the brain. Artificial Neural Networks are used for multiple medical purposes like signal processing that is used for biometric signal filtering and evaluations, interpretation of instrumental and physical findings to archive more accurate diseases, and also it provides prognostic information that is given by retrospective parameter analysis.

Basically, ANN (Artificial Neural Network) has been applied in the complete area of operations (Cortesm, 1995). It is also usually called neural network (NNs) and it is inspired by the biological neural networks. A huge amount of information is available in present to various types of biomedical data and each type of data provides information related to a particular pathology during the diseases process.

Support Vector Machine (SVM)

It is a kind of mechanism which works on the machine learning procedure, and it is used for arrangement problems as well as regression problems. SVM is developed by Cortes and Vapnik in the year 1990s. SVM solves cases by separating boundaries i.e., hyper lane. The main advantage of SVM is to consist of a constrained quadratic optimization problem, so it is avoiding the drawback of neural network (Dix, 2003).

Support Vector Machine is detecting common diseases such as pre-diabetes and diabetes in persons. Awarding to some optimality criterion approach has its roots in SLT which is stands for statistical learning theory and built "optimum classifiers". To measure the complexity of any model, SLT develops the Vapnik Chervonenkis (VC) dimensions. Some strengths of SVM are: no local optimal unlike in neural network, training is relatively easy, non-traditional data like string and tress can be controlled explicitly. Solving a quadratic programming problem and training, an SVM is equivalent. SVM basically identifies two different classes in the multidimensional environment by working as the liner separator between two data points (Emilio & Javier, 2020).

Deep Learning (DL)

It is a part of Artificial Intelligence that consisting present research and technology innovations that give us much more algorithms to deal with big scale data in healthcare, medicine, games, biomedical information, robotics, neuroscience, computer vision, learning theory, drug discovery, etc. these are some area where deep learning provides efficient algorithms. Various applications of deep learning are mentioned in figure 2. In the past few years, deep learning and many technologies related to artificial intelligence or computational intelligence are changing the shape of the healthcare and medical sector. Each of these technologies connected and provided something different to the industry and completely change the medical industries as well as healthcare. Deep learning to analyze data at extraordinary speed without any compromising on reality or purity. There is multiple application of deep learning in the healthcare sector like imaging solutions, catboats that can identify patterns in patient symptoms, imaging solution that use deep learning to identify diseases or any type of pathology, and deep learning algorithms that can identify types of cancer (Huang, 2011).

Figure 2. Applications of deep learning

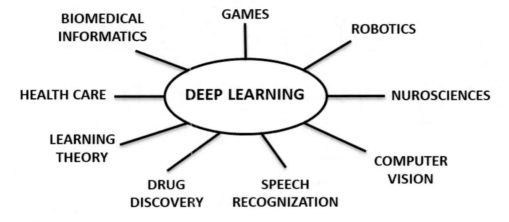

Genetic Algorithm

The genetic algorithm is based on machine learning and inspired by the laws of genetics and follows the lead of reproduction, evolution, and the survival for the fittest theory by Darwin. To produce the second generation there are the laws of genetics, cross-over and mutations occur in chromosomes. Figure 3 shows the two most useful methods for diversifying individuals. These methods basically induce diversity in the population of individuals. In figure 3 (a), during cross-over, one part of the chromosomes is exchanged by another fragment of another chromosome; and in figure 3 (b) during mutations, one or more databases on a chromosome are converted to different ones. These alterations will generate new individuals whose fittest will survive (Kohler, 2019).

Figure 3. Methods to induce diversity in the population of individuals

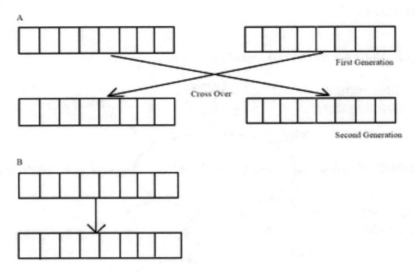

There is multiple application of the genetic algorithm in the medical field like oncology, radiology, cardiology, endocrinology, obstetrics, surgery, gynecology, pediatrics, pulmonary, infectious infections, radiotherapy, rehabilitation drug, orthopedics, neurology, pharmacotherapy and healthcare management.

DNA Computing

DNA (Deoxyribose Nucleic Acid) computing is natural computing using biological molecules apart from traditional. In 1994 Leonard Adelman has proposed the first theory of DNA computing. DNA computing is also known as computing. Instead of the conventional digital components, DNA computing uses the processing power of molecule information. The reaction of DNA is slower than the DNA of computer-based on silicon and the DNA strands to compute has led to high parallel computation that made the processing of the chip is slower. It serves the alternative technology and solves complex problems. It has the biggest processing capabilities. That's why DNA- based computers are mostly used to solve complex problems (Kan, 2019).

ARTIFICIAL INTELLIGENCE IN HEALTHCARE SYSTEM AND MEDICAL EDUCATION

In digital healthcare, AI helps to save millions of lives by their technologies. Artificial intelligence is a new and revolutionary technology for the medical and healthcare system. Artificial intelligence expands its technology in every sector like medical, industrial, economic, societal sector, deface, transport, manufacturing, space, remote sensing, security, vehicles, and many more. The artificial intelligence term is associated with cognitive function by computers. Artificial intelligence in various fields of industries, there is an endless range of possibilities. The main area of artificial intelligence is the medical and healthcare system where we can monitor the health of patients and also manage the data of patients, surgery, drug development medical statistics and imaging.

Radiology is one of the main areas of artificial intelligence application. To make a perfect diagnosis and treatment planning and quick analysis of reading image training by self of machines for MRI, CT and ultrasound increase their efficiency of medical operation capacities. Artificial intelligence can help radiologists with image acquisition and also can help with reconstruction (Kolodner, 1993).

After radiology, artificial intelligence can be extremely used. It consists of the application of artificial intelligence for improving diseases, diagnostics, education of primary care professions, clinical decision making, practice management, etc. To improve and optimize demonstrate an ability to do this. Based on the study of patients older times, at present, diagnostics of heart failure is the main disease; and also their physical examination can be done through ultrasound, CT, and MRI.

Classification of the Applications of Artificial Intelligence in the Field of Medical and Healthcare

In medical and healthcare, according to their detrimental and beneficial character, we propose an important classification of AI and AI applications. Here, we discuss some important applications, their inculcated level of availability in research centers. In this classification of the application of AI in medicine and healthcare, we propose the uses and the outcome of the uses.

Here, some exclusive examples of AI applications in healthcare are –

Table 1.

Application – Genomics *Aim*- It is the application based on deep neural networks (NN) that validate the ability of a computational state in single cells. *Outcome* – Deep Neural Network is predicting more accurately than previous or old methods. This application provides the model parameter that can be interpreted, so they provide how arrangement composition affects methylation changeability.
Application – Drug Development *Aim* – This application is similar to statistical language processing like recurrent neural network (NN) can be skilled as reproductive models for molecular structure. *Outcome* – This recurrent neural network (NN) is centered on the long short time memory (LSTM) and this can be functional to learn the statistical chemical language ideal.
Application – MRI *Aim* – In order to detect spontaneous and localized intracranial aneurysms during flight MR angiography developed an in-depth learning algorithm. *Outcome* – A DL algorithm explore intracranial aneurysm with a high diagnostic performance.
Application – Ultrasound Imaging *Aim* - Ultrasound Imaging detect expansion of deep learning for real-time recognition of breast cancer. *Outcome* – This is the method to realize the real-time assist for detection of breast lessons was developed.

Specific implementations of various some other applications are reported here Loshmi and Indumathi (2016).

- *AI* – mediated technology – IOT, Wearable, mHealth
  Specific Implementation – Automatic clinical/health surveillance in any environment/ Institutions/automated drug delivery.
- *AI*- mediated technology – Gene Editing
  Specific Implementation – Self experimentation medicine, bio-hacking, gene enhanced 'superhuman'. Disease treatment, prevention.
- *AI* – mediated technology – CT Imaging
  Specific Implementation – Deep learning image reconstruction improved CT abdominal examination in the venous portal section. It should be chosen to estimate the death rate you want.
- *AI* – mediated technology – Algorithm for computer aided diagnosis.
  Specific Implementation – Software for decision support in clinical area.
- *AI* – mediated technology – Human animal embryos.
  Specific Implementation – Organs for transplant
- *AI* – mediated technology – Digital pathology
  Specific Implementation – Software for automated, extensive analysis
- *AI* – mediated technology – Big data collection and analysis
  Specific Implementation – Prevention and monitoring of disease outbreaks.

DATA MINING

Various sectors or various fields use data mining like retail sectors to display customer response and banking sectors to predict customer profitability and uses in many sectors. Data mining is a combination of machine learning and data science. It is the procedure of education and structures from data using computerized systems (Maskut & Timur, 2020). So, data mining is knowledge to automotive industries, education, healthcare, manufacturing, telecom, and many more.

In the medical sector, data mining is going to be more famous, and necessary. Before doctors are write patient record information in the paper where the data was hard to collect. As technology and innovations are increasing so efforts by the human being is reduced such as computers that hold millions of records of patients with accuracy and also give us quality. But, healthcare services is the one where the major challenges came and this is the area where data mining has proven most useful.

Data mining applications in healthcare services are the treatment of breast cancer diagnosis and prognosis. Taking data mining beyond the academic research we follow three systems and these three systems are as shown in figure 4.

Figure 4. Three systems of health care

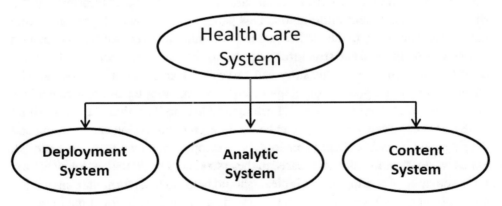

The Analytics System: The analytics system is the system where we collect all the information comprehend it and standardize measurement (Michael & Sonoo, 2001). All the data like aggregating clinical patient satisfaction, financial and all other data are collected into an enterprise data warehouse (EDW). This is the foundation of the system.

The Content System: The content system consists of standardizing knowledge about clinical best practices and the content system applies evidence-based best practices to care delivery.

The Deployment System: Over the new hierarchical structure the deployment system involves driving changes mechanism. It consists of implementing group structures. Throughout an organization, it requires a real hierarchical change.

Data mining is used in healthcare and among all the applications are as follows: Neural Networks, SVM, K-means, decision trees, logical reversion, KNN (K-nearest neighbors), and naive Bayes classification. Today, healthcare organizations seek similar befits from data mining and forecasting. In healthcare, data mining has proven to be effective in the area such as forecasting, customer relationship management the effectiveness of certain treatments.

Ontology and Semantic Reasoning

One of the most challenging problems in the field of health care is to ensure communication between healthcare programs. Ontology promotes communication in the healthcare system is over delays than other areas such as finance their ontology is better. Ontology can help build robust as well interactive information systems. They can maintain the need for a health care system to be reused, transmitting and sharing personal patient information. This paper will introduce the semantic role network and ontology in the medical area. It is committed to the role of information technology in this area and structures that need to be taken into account for technical solutions. Information on this story can serve as a starting point for anyone who wishes to study and practice ontology again web semantics technology. Sematic is the process of conveying enough information to lead to its action (Mirza & Mittal 2018). The sequence of symbols can be used for communication and meaning and their connection can it affect behaviors. For example, when we read this material, which we do combine ideas expressed in these sentences by all that we know before. If the semantic of writing in that is clear, should help students formulate an opinion about ontology and web semantics to serve as a starting point for something else great works, if semantics is not achieved, then the students will not gain much from the study. Therefore semantics is very important and it is the most important thing to do consider for any type of work. We summarize three important issues that provide semantic web support: model building, considering defining the world in an incomprehensible way, to allow for a simple understanding of complex truth. Knowledge-based information, trying to build consulting machines that can logical conclusions from the encrypted information. For details of the exchange, pass on a complex source of information between computers that allows us to disseminate and integrate information at the international level. Figure 5 shows an example of an ontology for the healthcare domain.

Figure 5. An example-of-an-ontology-for-the-healthcare-domain

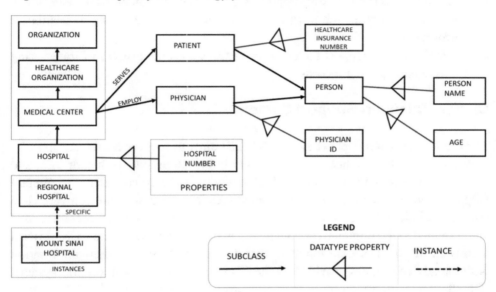

Semantic technology has the power to provide multi-border solutions, offer advanced features access to information based on metadata usage processed by machines. Through semantics, we can improve the way information is presented. Basically for all web applications that are essential for ontology use (Moher & Liberati, 2009). They simplify information sharing and reuse between agents, either personal or artificial. The name "ontology" comes from logos and is a science of being. In computer science, ontology is an organized representation of information from different perspectives within the domain and the relationship between concepts.

The use of ontology in medicine focuses on medical representation and planning words. Doctors have settled their own special languages to service them save and communicate effectively with general practitioners patient information and knowledge. That right terminology, made for man processing, appears in a certain number of information that is not clearly indicated. Meanwhile, medical information systems should be able to link with complex and detailed medical ideas. This is a difficult task and needs an in-depth analysis of the structure and concepts of medical terms. It can be detected by building a medical ontology field to introduce medical terminology programs. Benefits of ontology in this area:

- Ontology can help built strong and more powerful systems of information communication in healthcare. Interaction in healthcare is a skill of various technologies information systems and software applications to swap data and use this information namely changed.
- Ontology has the ability to support the addition of information and data, which can be regarded as the most important benefit they can bring to healthcare programs.
- Ontology may support the need for healthcare in the process of transferring and reusing patient records.

Clinical Decision Support System

The clinical decision support system (CDSS) aims to recover health transport by improving targeted medical results clinical information, patient health info, and other health information. Modern CDSS contains software considered to directly help in medical decision making, where features for each patient are compared to a computer clinic database and patient-specific tests or approvals are recommended and provided to the clinician for conclusion making is provided. The CDSS is used mainly in the field of care today so that doctors can combine their information with the advice or ideas provided by the CDSS. Clinical decision support systems (CDSSs) were suggested more than 50 years ago with the aim of helping health care providers make better decisions and improve patient care. This aid influences diagnosis and treatment. According to several courses, if used properly, it can help to increase the quality, safety, and performance of healthcare. A cornerstone of CDSS's achievement is well described as "The aim of CDSS is to provide relevant information, in the appropriate format, in the appropriate channel, to the appropriate person, at a positive point in the work process, to improve health care decisions and outcomes (Paun, 1999).

Standard CDSS can be divided into two parts-

- Knowledge-based
- Non-knowledge-based

In knowledge-based systems, laws (IF-THEN statements) are formed along with law enforcement data recovery systems to produce an output; Law can be made using document-based, practical or patient-based witness. Naive CDSS still requires data sources but uses artificial intelligence (AI), machine reading (ML), or mathematical pattern acknowledgment, rather than being designed to track decision technical information. Providing more experience and with precise design, the authors have used a number of information-complex features inclination, ontology thinking, and a complex analysis process (FAHP) in their framework. Figure 6 shows the key connections in a knowledge-based and Non-knowledge-based CDSS. The proposed system offers many distinct and significant enhancements to fair use, a powerful, intelligent and rendering CDSS.

Figure 6. A figure of key connections in a knowledge-based and Non-knowledge-based CDSS

KNOWLEDGE BASED SINGLE SYSTEM CDSS

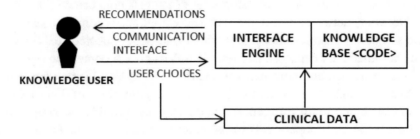

NON-KNOWLEDGE BASED SINGLE SYSTEM CDSS

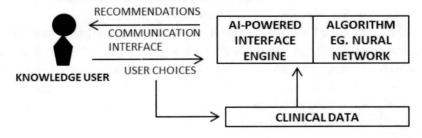

They are built on (1) foundation: proper laws organized into a system (based on information), an algorithm used to simulate a decision (based on information), and data available, (2) communication method: website, uses, or EHR frontend boundary, where the end operator encounters the system (3) input engine: takes the rules designed or determined by the AI, and the data constructions, and put them to the clinic data on the manufacture of the product or action, provided through the end-user (e.g. physician).

The CDSS is approved through the United States Government's Health as well Medicare operates, financially encouraging the implementation of CDS in EHRs. In 2013, an expected 41% of US hospitals have EHR, had CDSS, and in 2017, 40.3% of US hospitals have improved CDS Strength (HIMSS Stage 6). By remainder programs of another medical event, not just those of medicine-related CDSS improve patient safety. Among the multiple examples, CDSS blood glucose rate in ICU can reduce hypoglycemia events. This CDSS automatically motivates nurses to take according to the local glucose monitoring process, glucose measurement specifying how often to measure it should be done according to particular patient statistics as well previous glucose level / trends (Pawlak, 1991).

Smart Homes

A smart home is a living space using a set of gadgets connected to a LAN (Local Area Network) network, or the Internet. These appliances comprise sensors, RFID (radio frequency identification), and added Internet-connected (IoT) devices that can be automatically censored and retrieved. Visualize a home where your shower provides an immediate, non-invasive health check as soon as you get inside, and your bed is furnished with arteries that can identify any signs of illness. Composed data is distributed to all different home devices and provides warnings to ensure your health does not cooperate. These situations are now the truth. In the near future, we will be able to live in affordable housing. Smart houses become the structures of smart cities where resources can be efficiently and efficiently distributed, while the individual facilities delivered to each person do not live up to their different customs and needs (Pramanik & Mukhopadhyay, 2019).

From smartphones to smart households, most of the present established and emerging republics depend on it especially in assistive technology in everyday life. As technology brings new prospects to improve the well-being and worth of lifecycle for its operators, but far from being a good thing, technology becomes a requirement particularly in the field of health care. By the World Health Organization (WHO), the population of the world is growing at an alarming rate due to age-linked diseases like Parkinson's disease and dementia. Its significance raised concerns for health care and medical resources and increased reliance on families, caregivers, and the community. Contrary to this, the focus should be on supporting technological independence, especially at home. Where the main resolution of a smart home is to help caution for the people who live in it, Earth can continue to improve. Focus on how Smart Home (SH) can help its citizens through ADL (Activities of Daily Living), given that observing, forecasting, and indexing support independent living. Smart home becomes an addition of traditional services and includes not only cure but also security. This sector-based healthcare system has been created with technologically advanced advances and a more open environment in technology in general. Smart homes can prove to be economical to help the elderly and disabled stay home longer. This can allow for larger independence and quality of life while reducing the risk of segregation. The use of smart home components such as sensors, characters, controls, and tools allows citizens to monitor and interact and, when equipped with biomedical devices, add personal information to the data collection of objects. This technology can create 24 /7 days a week for the most vulnerable healthcare solutions. In Digital Health Care: Day One, Is It a Well-Managed Home Have you been in a hospital? Experts agree that numerous health circumstances, particularly chronic diseases, can be diagnosed and treated in a home-prepared with the necessary smart home products. However, there will nearly always be a need for hospital and direct health interventions. Still, associated home life is an idea that should be cheered. It provides many occasions to empower and control patients as well as reduce health costs in most cases. Intelligent connected homes may not yet be able to fully reinstate existing health care services, but they can add worth to the field of health care, improve the excellence of care, and enhance the health care system. There are several ways to reduce the pressure. It's important to note that smart homes deal with big details. If you use data mining and ML (machine learning) which is interesting in predicting, finding, and helping smart home situations.

Smart homes are suitable increasingly popular within the technical community as well as five obstacles the end user faces:

1. Balancing the current and changing lifestyles of users
2. Easy access to smart home technology
3. Interaction between systems
4. Honesty
5. Privacy and security

Other blocks to their acquisition are high charge, poor utilization, consistency, and shortage of complete user participation. Without advances within the scientific community in the search for new results for smart homes, their acquisition still falls short of the needs of end-users, leading to the search for new strategies. Smart homes and healthcare depend on the capability to collect data from a diversity of sources, with the environment, the home, and the patient himself. Hardware compatible with software can form an environment-wise environment and independent power that is most interesting to those who depend on supportive care. Sensors are the pillar of any smart home and as well as the main input to data-driven methods and information-driven processes, their selection and their overall value is an important decision point for any solutions engineer. Combining smart home technology with the goal of helping you find more research from years ago. Others, such as MavHome, combine several techniques together to provide a more consistent solution while others focus on a single aspect such as the patient's needs between night-time or living daily activity activities.

Medical Big Data

Big data has opened a new door for health care. Due to the great profits and limited chances, it has involved a lot of care from all the shareholders of the healthcare developed. The purpose of this review is to deliver a complete understanding of the great health care data. The chapter uses 10 'V' of comprehensive health care data and analyses various health data including forecast and set statistics. The clear benefits of using high-tech information technology in health care are carefully described. The application field with a decent amount of active use cases is too deliberated. Managing Big Data leftovers is the main task. The review outlines the challenges of all the possibilities in accessing health care benefits big data. This review also provides a brief overview of equipment and stages, buildings, and viable infrastructure for big health care data (Reed & Baumgart, 2020).

The Uses of 'V's in Healthcare Big Data

Volume: The word 'Big' in health care Big Data ensures that the capacity of health care data generated and accumulated is very large. Over the ages, it is predictable to rise slowly. Experimental data and clinical notes, laboratory results, medical histories, claim details, FDA proposals, medical device information, human genetics and personal information, genomics, radiology photography, 3D imaging, and biometric sensory studies are not provided they do not produce important data about importance. growth of health care data.

Variety: Health care data comes from a variety of sources and, therefore, from a variety of factors (e.g. formal, informal) (e.g. basic text, text blocks, images, video, health image, etc.) and dimensions.

Velocity: Details of health care can be made by people or nerves. Traditional health care management systems are often filled with man-made (man-made) data. In that situation, the amount at which information enters the structure can be controlled. But the extensive uses of IoT and smart health plans have led to the creation of real-time health information.

Veracity: Veracity represents data quality. Here, data quality includes aggregation, reliability, full completeness, selectivity, and sound. Keeping these abilities in health information is a big dare because the diversity of sources and channels. Clearly, authenticity is, perhaps, the most complex issue in between all 'V's in health care Big Data.

Validity: Performance signifies the correctness and precision of the data. The validity of the data is also dignified by how high it is to date and developed by standard conventions and technical methods.

Viability: From the sea of health care data, it is essential to identify appropriate information for individual cases. Data compatibility is necessary to preserve the desired result and accuracy using methods of analysis and prediction.

Volatility: As stated above, health care data is produced and modified at a quick rate. Therefore, see they live shorter lives. But the problem is how short is it? How fast is the data changing? It is essential to find out how long the data is worth, how lengthy to keep it, and how lengthy the data should be considered for analysis.

Vulnerability: Needless to say, privacy and security are important to health care data especially as information is stored in the cloud and goes to different sides of the information.

Visualization: Healthcare information not only needs to be precise, but it must also be existing anonymously, attractive too to the operator. Huge and difficult clinical reports want to be offered in a descriptive and time-consuming way. Proper visual cues help to obtain important information such as showing details in a clear and concise manner.

Value: The main purpose of health analysis with Big Data is to analyze profits in the form of improved health services. Improved governance, improved statistics, and wise decisions are the key to building high value without health care data. In health care organizations, Big Data brings worth by converting profit ponds has been positive by reducing total costs.

Big data shows the efficiency of the public health sector in everything. This capability evolved from "monitoring people's health in real-time" to "add-ons and information sources where multiple diseases are found". Data mining is widely used in big data environments, which can mean they are highly linked. We know that data mining procedures are most effective when the amount of data is very big.

The use of big data analytics in the medical field is capable. Therefore, it is important to identify some of the challenges facing the use of big data in health care:

1. Data of practical profits of a large amount of information is rare.
2. There are numerous procedural problems, such as information value, data conflict and variability, limits of observational studies, authentication, analysis glitches and legal issues.

RADIOLOGY

Radiology is one of the main areas of use of artificial intelligence in health care. By training imaging machines and rapid analysis, increase the effectiveness of medical practice skills. This is based on learning algorithms that can integrate and interact with MRI machines to enhance image resilience without interruption. Some of the

Artificial Intelligence applications will be discussed in this chapter Ultrasound imaging (Rucker, 2020). Radiology, also termed imaging analytic, is a sequence of numerous trials that take images of numerous body parts. The variety of these tests is unique because they allow doctors to see inside the body. Many different tests can be used to provide this impression, including X-ray, MRI, ultrasound scan, CT scan, mammography, nuclear medicine, fluoroscopy, bone mineral densitometry, and PET scan. (Sayani, 2019).

With the wide selection of equipment and techniques available, along with staging and treatment, the role of radiology lies in the management of the disease. Analytic imaging delivers complete data about physical or pathological changes (Salem, 2020). Initial analysis protects lives. Without analysis, there will be no cure for CT imaging.

CT Imaging

Computerized Tomography (CT) scans include a sequence of X-ray pictures taken of different parts of your body and practice computerized processing to form images (slices) of the bones, blood vessels, and soft tissues within your body. CT scans deliver more detailed information than blank X-rays.

Use of CT scans has many uses, but it is best to promptly investigate people who have been injured in car accidents or other types of trauma. CT scans can be used to visualize almost every part of the body and are used to diagnose diseases or injuries, as well as to plan treatment, surgery, or radiation therapy. CT scans can be used to classify diseases or harms in different parts of the body. For example, CT has become a valuable diagnostic apparatus for genital warts or cysts. Cardiac CT scans can be administered when a variety of heart syndrome or irregularities are suspected. CT can be used to diagnose head trauma, tissue clots that lead to hitting, hemorrhage, and other circumstances. It can show lungs to specify the presence of tumors, pneumonia (fluid clots), fluid, and other conditions such as emphysema or pneumonia. CT scans are very helpful when considering complex bone breaks, harshly damaged connections, or bone tissue because they often produce additional information than standard X-rays.

Cancer Diagnosis

Use one or extra procedures to detect cancer by your doctor:

Physical Examination: The doctor may sense body parts with swellings that could show cancer. Throughout a physical inspection, the doctor may go for irregularities, like skin bruising or development, which may point out cancer.

Laboratory Testing: Laboratory assessments test like blood tests and urine tests, can advantage doctors classify irregularities that may outcome from cancer. e.g., in a person with leukemia, a normal blood test named a blood count can expose an irregular amount or type of white blood cell.

Testing: Inspection of the images allows doctors to observe bones and inner tissues in a non-invasive method. Imaging trials used to identify cancer can contain computerized tomography (CT) scanning, scan, etc.

Biopsy: Throughout a biopsy, the doctor gathers a sample of cells to be tested in a research workshop. There are numerous ways to collect a sample. Which biopsy method is correct for you depends on your type of cancer and your location. In numerous cases, a biopsy is the only way to openly identify cancer.

In the lab, doctors look at cell examples in a microscope. Regular cells look similar, with the same size and order (Turing, 2009). Cancer cells look less organized, of changing sizes, and without visible construction.

Drug Development

New drugs are revealed through drug discovery. In history, drugs were broadly available by classifying the active materials in traditional medicine or by accident. Later, ancient pharmacology was used to examine chemical libraries including small molecules, natural products, or extruded plants, as well as to find those with therapeutic effects. Based on the sequence of human DNA, retrospective pharmacology has found solutions to current diseases by experimentation. Disease procedures, chemical tests, existing usages with no side special effects, and new technologies sponsor drug availability in the cycle below. Today drug discovery includes advanced testing, medical chemistry, and development kits to minimize the side effects of drugs (increasing solidarity and choice). Performance or strength, physical constancy (half-life), and oral availability are also enhanced at this stage of the drug development procedure. Drug development is a process that needs input and research from a wide range of studies from diagnostic research, through animal metabolism and toxicology, to clinical development, and end-user legal issues (market, health systems, and control systems). In addition, drug development requires regular data review collected from development strategies and strategies in line with the conclusions from this review. Thus, drug development exceeds the capacity of individual investigators and does not borrow from the 'interest book' - review - research proposal - review - the decision-making process (Steele, 2004).

Genomics

The genome is known as the complete set of DNA. Nearly all cell in the body contains approximately three billion copies of the basic pairs, or strands of DNA, that make up the human genome. DNA consists of the data needed to form the complete human body. Genetics usually refers to a DNA chapter that consists of the commands for creating a particular group of proteins. The total estimated 20,000 to 25,000 genes in the human genomic code is an average of proteins. 23 pairs of chromosomes are found which are filled into a human cell, the genes adjust the construction of proteins with the help of enzyme and messenger particles. Especially, an enzyme duplicates data from genetic DNA to a particle named messenger ribonucleic acid (mRNA). MRNA spreads from the nucleus to the cytoplasm of the cell, where mRNA is declaimed by a small molecular device named the ribosome, and the data are used to assemble minor molecules named amino acids to form a particular protein. Proteins form body structures such as organs and tissues, as well as regulate chemical reactions and regulate signs between cells. When the DNA of a cell is changed, it can produce abnormal protein, which can disrupt normal body procedures and lead to cancer-like illness.

Big Data and E-Health

Over the past few years, big data analysis has expanded and improved and increased management, analysis, and forecasting in health care. The procedure of the big data method has the prospective to expand value, reduce the charge of the care and the number of medical mistakes, and efficiency of the service. There is a worldwide trend as a platform the use of big data that accelerates and facilitates biomedical research and offers many opportunities to discover new results in biology, medicine, genetics and can help reduce the growing numbers of medical information.

The term **Digital Healthcare or E-Health** encompasses a wide range of ideas, ideas, methods and skills like big data, genomics, AI, smart devices, telemedicine, wearable and many other mobile health systems. Over the past few decades, digital health technologies have become widely used in the health care system and they learn about it and use biomedicine, research, and medical education. Through and improving the treatment and diagnosis of various diseases, including the use of digital health concepts. The covid-19 epidemic in all countries has created the need for quick and effective solutions and Artificial Intelligence, Computational Intelligence and many other digital health care systems are helping to get out of this epidemic. New technologies in digital health care systems help medical professionals and assistants with these technologies and reduce the burden on physicians and national health care systems. These stages can simplify the diagnosis, appointment, and action of patients and digital medical technology has already had such a profound effect on the present digital health care system. E.g., the use of telemedicine has facilitated to decrease in hospital admittances and death rates of cardiovascular disease and diabetes.

The study concludes that computer technology is revolutionizing technology in the healthcare sector because of its cost-effectiveness, low cost, and significant risk-based decision-making capabilities.

CONCLUSION

Robust development of intelligent health care system is a very complex process which is highly recommended technical and research experiments that need to be addressed in a different way. This paper examines major paradigms and the use of Computational Intelligence (CI) in health care from the perspective of Artificial Intelligence. There is much work to be done in artificial intelligence, but there is a lack of testing and actual clinical information used by clinicians. This is because, among further things, to the shortage of contact to this clinic information. In addition, the shortage of learning data on data mining procedures, and the general update of this information, has a major effect on the guesses made by these procedures. The range of AI applications and limited AI technology in medicine and health care is vast and growing rapidly, with many powerful effects (good and bad), affecting the individual and community at all levels. Yet, there is a list of queries that want to be replied to before the widespread execution of digital health stages. This includes medical demonstration and validation of these projected technologies. Another problem is the consistency and security of this new digital health system. Because of the lack of legal guidelines and references, participants consisting private and government agencies are facing the difficulty of adequate verification and acceptance of the novel technology's digital life. In this respect, relevant systematic research is needed before the digital invention can be sent to the healthcare sector.

REFERENCES

Azzi, S., Gagnon, S., Ramirez, A., & Richards, G. (2020). Healthcare Applications of Artificial Intelligence and Analytics: A Review and Proposed Framework. *MDPI*, 21.

Bennett, J., & Chen, O. R. (2017). Healthcare in the Smart Home: A Study of Past, Present and Future. *MDPI*, 23.

Buchanan, B. (2005). A (very) brief history of artificial intelligence. *AI Magazine*, *26*, 53.

Cook, D. (2006). Health monitoring and assistance to support aging in place. *JUCS*, *12*(1), 15–29.

Cortes, C. V., & Vapnik, V. (1995). Support vector networks. *Machine Learning*, *20*(3), 273–297. doi:10.1007/BF00994018

Dix, A. F. (2003). *Human–Computer Interaction* (3rd ed.). Prentice Hall.

Emilio, G. G., Emilia, G., Javier, M. R., Manuel, G. C., Isabel, F. L., & María Isabel, R. L. (2020). Artificial intelligence in medicine and healthcare: a review and classification of current and near-future applications and their ethical and social Impact. *arXiv*, 20.

Huang, Y. H. (2011). DNA computing research progress and application. *The 6th International Conference on Computer Science & Education*, 232-235. 10.1109/ICCSE.2011.6028624

Kan, M. M. (2019). Digital technology and the future of health systems," Health Systems & Reform. *Reform*, *5*(2), 113–120.

Kohler, J. E., Falcone, R. A. Jr, & Fallat, M. E. (2019). Rural health, telemedicine and access for pediatric surgery. *Current Opinion in Pediatrics*, *31*(3), 391–398. doi:10.1097/MOP.0000000000000763 PMID:31090582

Kolodner, J. (1993). *Case-Based Reasoning*. Morgan Kaufmann. doi:10.1016/B978-1-55860-237-3.50005-4

Lakshmi, B., Indumathi, T., & Ravi, N. A. (2016). 5 decision tree classification algorithm for risk predictions during pregnancy. *Procedia Technol.*, *24*, 1542–1549. doi:10.1016/j.protcy.2016.05.128

Maskut, S., Timur, S., Zhanar, B., Aigul, A., Marina, Z., & Nazym, A. (2020). *The Recent Progress and Applications of Digital Technologies in Healthcare: A Review*. *International Journal of Telemedicine and Applications*.

Michael, M., Sonoo, T. I., Andrew, A., Andrew, B., Paul, B., & Wendy, C. (2001). *Artificial Intelligence in Health Care:The Hope, the Hype*. National Academy of Medicine.

Mirza, S., Mittal, S., & Zaman, M. (2018). Decision Support Predictive model for prognosis of diabetes using SMOTE and Decision tree. *International Journal of Applied Engineering Research: IJAER*, *13*, 9277–9282.

Moher, D., Liberati, A., Tetzlaff, J., & Altman, D. (2009). Preferred Reporting Items for Systematic Reviews and Meta-Analyses: The PRISMA Statement. *PLoS Med.*

Paun, G. H. R. G. (1999). DNA Computing: New Computing Paradigms. Springer.

Pawlak, Z. R. (1991). *Theoretical Aspects of Reasoning about Data.* Kluwer Academic Publishers.

Pramanik, P. K., Pal, S., & Mukhopadhyay, M. (2019). Healthcare Big Data:A Comprehensive Overview. In P. K. Pramanik, S. Pal, & M. Mukhopadhyay (Eds.), *Healthcare Big Data:A Comprehensive Overview* (pp. 72–100). IGI Global.

Reed, T. S., David, P., Baumgart, D. C., Sadowski, D. C., Fedorak, R. N., & Kroeker, K. I. (2020). An overview of clinical decision support systems: Benefits,risks, and strategies for success. *Digital Medicine*, 10. PMID:32047862

Rucker, M. (2020). The Smart Home: Can It Replace Traditional Health Care? *Verywell Health*, 8.

Russell, S. J. (2003). *Artificial Intelligence: A Modern Approach* (2nd ed.). Prentice Hall.

Salem, A.-B. M. (2020). Computational Intelligence for Digital Healthcare. *CEUR*, 15.

Steele, G. S. (2004). oriented approach to DNA computing. *Proc. of Computational Systems Bioinformatics Conference*, 546-551.

Compilation of References

Abdollahzadeh, S., & Navimipour, N. J. (2016). Deployment strategies in the wireless sensor network: A comprehensive review. *Computer Communications*, *91*, 1–16. doi:10.1016/j.comcom.2016.06.003

Adawe, A., & Oberg, C. (2013). Skin-lightening practices and mercury exposure in the Somali community. *Minnesota Medicine*, *96*(7), 48–49. PMID:24133891

Adegun, A. A., Viriri, S., & Yousaf, M. H. A. (2021). Probabilistic-Based Deep Learning Model for Skin Lesion Segmentation. *Applied Sciences (Basel, Switzerland)*, *11*(7), 3025–3038.

Agarwal, A., Nagi, N., Chatterjee, P., Sarkar, S., Mourya, D., Sahay, R. R., & Bhatia, R. (2020). Guidance for building a dedicated health facility to contain the spread of the 2019 novel coronavirus outbreak. *The Indian Journal of Medical Research*, *151*(2), 177–183. doi:10.4103/ijmr.IJMR_518_20 PMID:32362643

Aghdam, Z. N., Rahmani, A. M., Hosseinzadeh, M. J. C. M., & Biomedicine, P. I. (2020). *The Role of the Internet of Things in Healthcare: Future Trends and Challenges*. Academic Press.

AHA. (2020). *Leading during COVID-19: Lessons Learned from Clinical and Administrative Teams*. Available online at: https://www.aha.org/podcasts/2020-05-28-leading-during-covid-19-lessons-learned-clinical-and-administrative-teams

Ahmad, M. J., & Alam, M. S. (2003). A rapid spectrometric method for the determination of mercury in environmental biological, soil and plant samples using diphenylthiocarbazone. *Spectroscopy (Springfield, Or.)*, *17*, 45–52.

Ahmed, F., Ahmed, N., Pissarides, C., & Stiglitz, J. (2020). Why inequality could spread COVID-19. *The Lancet. Public Health*, *5*(5), e240. doi:10.1016/S2468-2667(20)30085-2 PMID:32247329

Ahmed, I., Jeon, G., & Chehri, A. (2022). An IoT-enabled smart health care system for screening of COVID-19 with multi layers features fusion and selection. *Computing*, 1–18. doi:10.100700607-021-00992-0

Ahsan, M. M. E., Alam, T., Trafalis, T., & Huebner, P. (2020). Deep MLP-CNN model using mixed-data to distinguish between COVID-19 and non-COVID-19 patients. *Symmetry*, *12*(9), 1526. doi:10.3390ym12091526

AlAfandy, K. A., Omara, H., Lazaar, M., & Al Achhab, M. (Eds.). (2019). Artificial Neural Networks Optimization and Convolution Neural Networks to Classifying Images in Remote Sensing: A Review. *Proceeding of The 4th International Conference on Big Data and Internet of Things (BDIoT'19).* 10.1145/3372938.3372945

AlAfandy, K. A., Omara, H., Lazaar, M., & Al Achhab, M. (2020a). Investment of Classic Deep CNNs and SVM for Classifying Remote Sensing Images. *Advances in Science Technology and Engineering Systems Journal, 5*(5), 652–659. doi:10.25046/aj050580

AlAfandy, K. A., Omara, H., Lazaar, M., & Al Achhab, M. (2020b). Using Classic Networks for Classifying Remote Sensing Images: Comparative Study. *Advances in Science Technology and Engineering Systems Journal, 5*(5), 770–780. doi:10.25046/aj050594

Alam, M. Tavakolian, MacKinnon, & Fazel-Rezai. (2016). Automatic Detection and Severity Measurement of Eczema Using Image Processing. *38th IEEE Engineering in Medicine and Biology Society Conference,* 1365-1368.

AlamT. (2021). *Blockchain-Enabled Mobile Healthcare System Architecture for the Real-Time Monitoring of the COVID-19 Patients.* doi:10.2139/ssrn.3772643

Albawi, S., Mohammed, T. A., & Al-Zawi, S. (2017, August). Understanding of a convolutional neural network. In *2017 International Conference on Engineering and Technology (ICET)* (pp. 1-6). IEEE.

AlBeladi, A. A., & Muqaibel, A. H. (2018). Evaluating Compressive Sensing Algorithms in Through-the-wall Radar via F1-score. *International Journal of Signal and Imaging Systems Engineering, 11*(3), 164–171. doi:10.1504/IJSISE.2018.093268

Al-Fuqaha, A., Guizani, M., Mohammadi, M., Aledhari, M., & Ayyash, M. (2015). Internet of things: A survey on enabling technologies, protocols, and applications. *IEEE Communications Surveys and Tutorials, 17*(4), 2347–2376. doi:10.1109/COMST.2015.2444095

Ali, H., & Khan, E. (2018). Bioaccumulation of non-essential hazardous heavy metals and metalloids in freshwater fish. Risk to human health. *Environmental Chemistry Letters, 16*(3), 903–917. doi:10.100710311-018-0734-7

Ali, H., Khan, E., & Sajad, M. A. (2013). Phytoremediation of heavy metals-concepts and applications. *Chemosphere, 91*(7), 869–881. doi:10.1016/j.chemosphere.2013.01.075 PMID:23466085

Allcorn, S. (1990). Using matrix organization to manage health care delivery organizations. *Hospital & Health Services Administration, 35,* 575–590. PMID:10107388

Alloghani, M., Al-Jumeily, D., Mustafina, J., Hussain, A., & Aljaaf, A. J. (2020). A Systematic Review on Supervised and Unsupervised Machine Learning Algorithms for Data Science. In M. Berry, A. Mohamed, & B. Yap (Eds.), *Supervised and Unsupervised Learning for Data Science. Unsupervised and Semi-Supervised Learning.* Springer. doi:10.1007/978-3-030-22475-2_1

Alpaydin, E. (2020). *Introduction to Machine Learning.* MIT Press.

Amarathunga, A. A., Ellawala, E. P., Abeysekar, G. N., & Amalraj, C. R. (2015). Expert System for Diagnosis of Skin Diseases. *International Journal of Scientific and Technology Research*, *4*(1), 174–178.

Angus, K., Cairns, G., Purves, R., Bryce, S., MacDonald, L., & Gordon, R. (2013). *Systematic literature Review to Examine the Evidence for The Effectiveness of interventions that use Theories and Models of Behaviour Change: Towards the Prevention and Control of Communicable Diseases.* Stockholm European Centre for Disease Prevention and Control.

Anzai, Y. (2012). *Pattern Recognition and Machine Learning*. Elsevier Science.

Apostolopoulos, I. D., & Mpesiana, T. A. (2020). Covid-19: Automatic detection from x-ray images utilizing transfer learning with convolutional neural networks. *Physical and Engineering Sciences in Medicine*, *43*(2), 635–640. doi:10.100713246-020-00865-4 PMID:32524445

Armah, F. A., Quansah, R., & Luginaah, I. (2014). Agency for Toxic Substances and Disease Registry (ATSDR). Toxicological Profile for Arsenic. *International Scholarly Research Notices*, 1–37. doi:10.1155/2014/252148

Ascent of machine learning in medicine. (2019). *Nature Materials*, *18*(5), 407. doi:10.103841563-019-0360-1 PMID:31000807

Asperges, E., Novati, S., Muzzi, A., Biscarini, S., Sciarra, M., Lupi, M., Sambo, M., Gallazzi, I., Peverini, M., Lago, P., Mojoli, F., Perlini, S., & Bruno, R. (2020). Rapid response to COVID-19 outbreak in Northern Italy: How to convert a classic infectious disease ward into a COVID-19responsecentre. *The Journal of Hospital Infection*, *105*(3), 477–479. doi:10.1016/j.jhin.2020.03.020 PMID:32205162

Athaya, T., & Choi, S. (2021). An Estimation method of continuous non-invasive arterial blood pressure waveform using photoplethysmography. A U-Net Architecture-Based Approach. *Sensors (Basel)*, *21*(5), 1867. doi:10.339021051867 PMID:33800106

Athey, S. (2018). The impact of machine learning on economics. In *The economics of artificial intelligence: An agenda* (pp. 507–547). University of Chicago Press.

Atiqur, R., Liton, A., & Wu, G. (2020). Content Caching Strategy at Small Base Station in 5G Networks with Mobile Edge Computing. *International Journal of Science and Business.*, *4*(4), 104–112.

Atrey, K., Singh, B. K., & Bodhey, N. K. (2021). Feature Selection for Classification of Breast Cancer in Histopathology Images: A Comparative Investigation Using Wavelet-Based Color Features. In A. A. Rizvanov, B. K. Singh, & P. Ganasala (Eds.), *Advances in Biomedical Engineering and Technology. Lecture Notes in Bioengineering*. Springer. doi:10.1007/978-981-15-6329-4_30

Atrey, K., Singh, B. K., Roy, A., & Bodhey, N. K. (2021). Real-time automated segmentation of breast lesions using CNN-based deep learning paradigm: Investigation on mammogram and ultrasound. *International Journal of Imaging Systems and Technology*, ima.22690. doi:10.1002/ima.22690

Axak, N. M. K. (2020). Cloud Architecture for Remote Medical Monitoring. *IEEE 15th International Conference on Computer Sciences and Information Technologies (CSIT)*, 1-4.

Aziz, H. B., & S. S. (2019). Cloud Based Remote Healthcare Monitoring System Using IoT. *International Conference on Sustainable Technologies for Industry 4.0 (STI)*, 1-5. 10.1109/STI47673.2019.9068029

Aziz, M. N., & Islam, A. (2020). Reviewing Data Mining as an enabling technology for BI. *International Journal of Science and Business*, 4(7), 46–51.

Azzi, S., Gagnon, S., Ramirez, A., & Richards, G. (2020). Healthcare Applications of Artificial Intelligence and Analytics: A Review and Proposed Framework. *MDPI*, 21.

Babar, M., Khan, F., Iqbal, W., Yahya, A., Arif, F., Tan, Z., & Chuma, J. M. (2018). A secured data management scheme for smart societies in industrial internet of things environment. *IEEE Access: Practical Innovations, Open Solutions*, 6, 43088–43099. doi:10.1109/ACCESS.2018.2861421

Bagul, V. R., Shinde, D. N., Chavan, R. P., Patil, C. L., & Pawar, R. K. (2015). New perspective on heavy metal pollution of water. *Journal of Chemical and Pharmaceutical Research*, 7(12), 700–705.

Baker, S. B., Xiang, W., & Atkinson, I. (2017). Internet of things for smart healthcare: Technologies, challenges, and opportunities. *IEEE Access: Practical Innovations, Open Solutions*, 5, 26521–26544. doi:10.1109/ACCESS.2017.2775180

Banerjee, N., & Das, S. (2020). Prediction Lung Cancer. In *Machine Learning Perspective*. IEEE.

Banko, G. (1998). *A Review of Assessing the Accuracy of Classifications of Remotely Sensed Data and of Methods Including Remote Sensing Data in Forest Inventory. International Institution for Applied Systems Analysis (IIASA)*.

Bannister, B., Puro, V., Fusco, F. M., Heptonstall, J., & Ippolito, G. (2009). Framework for the design and operation of high-level isolation units: Consensus of the European network of infectious diseases. *The Lancet. Infectious Diseases*, 9(1), 45–56. doi:10.1016/S1473-3099(08)70304-9 PMID:19095195

Baraldi, P., Razavi-Far, R., & Zio, E. (2011). Bagged ensemble of Fuzzy C-Means classifiers for nuclear transient identification. *Annals of Nuclear Energy*, 38(5), 1161–1171. doi:10.1016/j.anucene.2010.12.009

Barman, M., Chaudhury, J. P., & Biswas, S. (2019). Automated Skin Disease Detection Using Multiclass PNN. *International Journal of Innovations in Engineering and Technology*, 14(4), 19–24.

Baro, E., Degoul, S., Beuscart, R., & Chazard, E. (2015). Toward a literature-driven definition of big data in healthcare. *BioMed Research International*, 2015, 2015. doi:10.1155/2015/639021 PMID:26137488

Barro, Ursua, & Weng. (2020). The Coronavirus and the Great Influenza Epidemic - Lessons from the 'Spanish Flu' for the Coronavirus's Potential Effects on Mortality and Economic Activity. *SSRN.* doi:10.3386/w26866

Basha, N. (2019). Early Detection of Heart Syndrome Using Machine Learning Technique. *4th International Conference on Electrical, Electronics, Communication, Computer Technologies and Optimization Techniques (ICEECCOT).*

Basu, S., Karmakar, A., Bidhan, V., Kumar, H., Brar, K., Pandit, M., & Latha, N. (2021). *Impact of Lockdown Due to COVID-19 Outbreak: Lifestyle Changes and Public Health Concerns in India.* Academic Press.

Bataille, J., & Brouqui, P. (2017). Building an intelligent hospital to fight contagion. *Clinical Infectious Diseases, 65*(suppl_1), S4–S11. doi:10.1093/cid/cix402 PMID:28859348

Bavel, J. J. V., Baicker, K., Boggio, P. S., Capraro, V., Cichocka, A., Cikara, M., Molly, J., Crockett, A. J., Douglas, K.M., Druckman, J. N., Drury, J., Dube, O., Ellemers, N., Finkel, E.J., Fowler, J. H., Gelfand, M., Han, S., Haslam, S. A., Jetten, J., Kitayama, S., ... Willer, R. (2020). Using Social and Behavioural Science to Support COVID-19 Pandemic Response. *Nature Human Behaviour, 460*(4), 460–471.

Bavel, J. J. V., Baicker, K., Boggio, P. S., Capraro, V., Cichocka, A., Cikara, M., Molly, J., Crum, A. J., Douglas, K.M., Druckman, J. N., Drury, J., Dube, O., Ellemers, N., Finkel, E.J., Fowler, J. H., Gelfand, M., Han, S., Haslam, S. A., Jetten, J., Kitayama, S., ... Willer, R. (2020). Using Social and Behavioural Science to Support COVID-19 Pandemic Response. *Nature Human Behaviour, 460*(4), 460–471.

Bawaskar, H. S., & Bawaskar, P. H. (2010). Chronic renal failure associated with heavy metal contamination of drinking water: A clinical report from a small village in Maharashtra. *Clinical Toxicology (Philadelphia, PA), 48*(7), 768–768. doi:10.3109/15563650.2010.497763 PMID:20615151

Beaumont, J. J., Sedman, R. M., Reynolds, S. D., Sherman, C. D., Li, L. H., Howd, R. A., Sandy, M. S., Zeise, L., & Alexeeff, G. V. (2008). Cancer mortality in a Chinese population exposed to hexavalent chromium in drinking water. *Epidem, 19*(1), 12–23. doi:10.1097/EDE.0b013e31815cea4c PMID:18091413

Becker, K., Kaus, S., Krause, C., Lepom, P., Schulz, C., Seiwert, M., & Seifert, B. (2002). German Environmental Survey (1998) (GerES III): Environmental pollutants in blood of the German population. *International Journal of Hygiene and Environmental Health, 205*(4), 297–308. doi:10.1078/1438-4639-00155 PMID:12068749

Bedford, J., Enria, D., Giesecke, J., Heymann, D. L., Ihekweazu, C., Kobinger, G., Lane, H. C., Memish, Z., Oh, M., Sall, A. A., Schuchat, A., Ungchusak, K., & Wieler, L. H. (2020). COVID-19: Towards controlling of a pandemic. *Lancet, 395*(10229), 1015–1018. doi:10.1016/S0140-6736(20)30673-5 PMID:32197103

Belchior, R., Vasconcelos, A., Correia, M., & Hardjono, T. (2021). *HERMES: Fault-Tolerant Middleware for Blockchain Interoperability.* Academic Press.

Benesty. (2008). Springer handbook of speech processing. Springer.

Bengio, Y., Goodfellow, I., & Courville, A. (2017). *Deep Learning.* MIT press.

Bennett, J., & Chen, O. R. (2017). Healthcare in the Smart Home: A Study of Past, Present and Future. *MDPI, 23.*

Bereksi-Reguig, M. A., & Bereksi-Reguig, F. (2017). Photoplethysmogram Signal Processing and Analysis in Evaluating Arterial Stiffness. *International Journal of Biomedical Engineering and Technology, 23*(2–4), 363–378. doi:10.1504/IJBET.2017.10003507

Berlin, M., Zalups, R. K., & Fowler, B. A. (2007). Mercury. IN Handbook on the Toxicology of Metals. Elsevier. doi:10.1016/B978-012369413-3/50088-4

Berstein, A., & Cohen, A. (1985). Speech processing applied for chest diagnosis. *14'th Conv. of Elect. & Electronics Engg.*

Bhavani, R., Prakash, V., Kumaresh, R. V., & Sundra Srinivasan, R. (2019). Vision-Based Skin Disease Identification Using Deep Learning. *International Journal of Engineering and Advanced Technology, 8*(6), 3784–3788.

Birje, M. N., & Hanji, S. S. (2020). Internet of things based distributed healthcare systems: A review. *J. Data Inf. Manag, 2*(3), 149–165. doi:10.100742488-020-00027-x

Bish, A., & Michie, S. (2011). *Demographic and Attitudinal Determinants of Protective Behaviours during a Pandemic.* Department of Health.

Bote-Curiel, L., Muñoz-Romero, S., Gerrero-Curieses, A., & Rojo-Álvarez. José, L. (2019). Deep Learning and Big Data in Healthcare: A Double Review for Critical Beginners. *Applied Sciences (Basel, Switzerland), 9*(11), 2331. doi:10.3390/app9112331

Boubiche, S., Boubiche, D. E., Bilami, A., & Toral-Cruz, H. (2018). Big data challenges and data aggregation strategies in wireless sensor networks. *IEEE Access: Practical Innovations, Open Solutions, 6,* 20558–20571. doi:10.1109/ACCESS.2018.2821445

Boudreaux, E. D., Waring, M. E., Hayes, R. B., Sadasivam, R. S., Mullen, S., & Pagoto, S. (2014). Evaluating and selecting mobile health apps: Strategies for healthcare providers and healthcare organizations. *Translational Behavioral Medicine, 4*(4), 363–371. doi:10.100713142-014-0293-9 PMID:25584085

Bowling, M., Furnkranz, J., Graepel, T., & Musick, R. (2006). Machine Learning and Games. *Machine Learning, Springer, 63*(3), 211–215. doi:10.100710994-006-8919-x

Breiman, L. (1996). Bagging predictors. *Machine Learning, 24*(2), 123–140. doi:10.1007/BF00058655

Buchanan, B. (2005). A (very) brief history of artificial intelligence. *AI Magazine, 26,* 53.

Buchhorn, R., Baumann, C., & Willaschek, C. (2020, August). Heart rate variability in a patient with coronavirus disease 2019. *International Cardiovascular Forum Journal, 20*.

Busev, A. I., Tiptsova, V. G., & Ivanov, M. V. (1981). *Analytical Chemistry of Rare Elements*. Rusian Edn.

Cassenti, D., & Weston. (2020). Advances in Human Factors in Simulation and Modeling. *BMC Public Health, 20*.

Cassenti. D., & Weston. (2020). Advances in Human Factors in Simulation and Modeling. Advances in intelligent systems and computing. BMC Public Health, *20*.

Catarinucci, L., De Donno, D., Mainetti, L., Palano, L., Patrono, L., Stefanizzi, M. L., & Tarricone, L. (2015). An IoT-aware architecture for smart HLC systems. *IEEE Internet of Things Journal, 2*(6), 515–526. doi:10.1109/JIOT.2015.2417684

CBHI. (2019). *National Health Profile 2019*. Central Bureau of Health Intelligence. Directorate General of Health Services. Government of India. Available online at: http://www.cbhidghs.nic.in/showfile.php?lid= 1147

CDC. (2003). *CDC Guidelines for Environmental Infection Control in Health-Care Facilities*. Available online at: https://www.cdc.gov/infectioncontrol/ guidelines/environmental/appendix/air.html

Centeno, J. A., Gray, M. A., Mullick, F. G., Tchounwou, P. B., & Tseng, C. (2005). Arsenic in drinking water andhealth issues. In T. A. Moore, A. Black, J. A. Centeno, J. S. Harding, & D. A. Trumm (Eds.), *Metal Contaminants in New Zealand* (pp. 195–219). Resolution Press.

Centeno, J. A., Tchounwou, P. B., Patlolla, A. K., Mullick, F. G., Murakat, L., Meza, E., Gibb, H., Longfellow, D., & Yedjou, C. G. (2005). Environmental pathology and health effects of arsenic poisoning: acritical review. In R. Naidu, E. Smith, J. Smith, & P. Bhattacharya (Eds.), *Managing Arsenic Inthe Environment: From Soil to Human Health* (pp. 311–327). CSIRO Publishing Corp.

Centers for Disease Control. (1991). *Preventing Lead Poisoning in Young children*. Centers for Disease Control.

Chan, J. F. W., Yuan, S., Kok, K. H., To, K. K. W., Chu, H., Yang, J., & Yuen, K. Y. (2020). A familial cluster of pneumonia associated with the 2019 novel coronavirus indicating person-to-person transmission: A study of a family cluster. *Lancet, 395*(10223), 514–523. doi:10.1016/S0140-6736(20)30154-9 PMID:31986261

Chatterjee, K., Shankar, S., Chatterjee, K., & Yadav, A. K. (2020). Corona virus disease 2019 in India: Post-lockdown scenarios and provisioning for health care. *ELSEVIER Medical Journal, Armed Forces India, 76*(4), 387–394. doi:10.1016/j.mjafi.2020.06.004 PMID:32836711

Chauhan, V. K., Dahiya, K., & Sharma, A. (2019). Problem formulations and solvers in linear SVM: A review. *Artificial Intelligence Review, 52*(2), 803–855. doi:10.100710462-018-9614-6

Chen, L., Wang, S., Fan, W., Sun, J., & Naoi, S. (2015, November). Beyond human recognition: A CNN-based framework for handwritten character recognition. In *2015 3rd IAPR Asian Conference on Pattern Recognition (ACPR)* (pp. 695-699). IEEE.

Cheney, C. (2020). *Coronavirus: 5 Lessons Learned from Temporary Hospitals in China.* Available online at: https://www.healthleadersmedia.com/clinical-care/coronavirus-5-lessons-lear-temporary-hospitals-china

Cheng, Y., Liu, D., Chen, J., Namilae, S., Thropp, J., & Seong, Y. (2018). Human Behavior Under Emergency And Its Simulation Modeling. *RE:view.*

Chen, Y., Jiang, H., Li, C., Jia, X., & Ghamisi, P. (2016). Deep feature extraction and classification of hyperspectral images based on convolutional neural networks. *IEEE Transactions on Geoscience and Remote Sensing, 54*(10), 6232–6251. doi:10.1109/TGRS.2016.2584107

Chief Executives Board for Coordination (CEB) Human Resources Network Version 1.0. (2020). *Administrative Guidelines for Offices on the Novel Coronavirus (COVID-19) Outbreak.* Available online at: https://hr.un.org/sites/hr.un.org/files/Administrative%20Guidelines%20-%20Novel%20 Coronavirus %20Final_Version%201.0_13%20February%202020_0.pdf

Chinese Center for Disease Control and Prevention. (2020). *Epidemic Update and Risk Assessment of 2019 Novel Coronavirus 2020.* Available online at: http://www.chinacdc.cn/yyrdgz/202001/P020200128523354919292. pdf

Chopra, S., Ranjan, P., Singh, V., Kumar, S., Arora, M., Hasan, M. S., Kasiraj, R., Suryansh, Kaur, D., Vikram, N. K., Malhotra, A., Kumari, A., Klanidhi, K. B., & Baitha, U. (2020). Impact of COVID-19 on Lifestyle-Related Behaviours- A Cross-Sectional Audit of Responses from Nine Hundred And Ninety-Five Participants From India. *Diabetes & Metabolic Syndrome, 14*(6), 2021–2030. doi:10.1016/j.dsx.2020.09.034 PMID:33099144

Chowdhury, M. H. (2020). Estimating Blood Pressure from the Photoplethysmogram Signal and Demographic Features Using Machine Learning Techniques. Sensors, 20(11). doi:10.339020113127

Chowdhury, M. E. H., Rahman, T., Khandakar, A., Al-Madeed, S., Zughaier, S. M., Doi, S. A. R., Hassen, H., & Islam, M. T. (2021). An Early Warning Tool for Predicting Mortality Risk of COVID-19 Patients Using Machine Learning. *Cognitive Computation.* Advance online publication. doi:10.100712559-020-09812-7 PMID:33897907

Chowell, G., & Mizumoto, K. (2020). The COVID-19 pandemic in the USA: What might we expect? *Lancet, 395*(10230), 1093–1094. doi:10.1016/S0140-6736(20)30743-1 PMID:32247381

Chui, K. T., Alhalabi, W., Pang, S. S. H., Pablos, P. O. D., Liu, R. W., & Zhao, M. (2017). Disease diagnosis in smart healthcare: Innovation, technologies and applications. *Sustainability, 9*(12), 2309. doi:10.3390u9122309

Chung, J., Gulcehre, C., Cho, K., & Bengio, Y. (2014). *Empirical evaluation of gated recurrent neural networks on sequence modeling.* arXiv preprint arXiv:1412.3555.

Cinaree, & Emiroglu. (2019). *Classification of Brain Tumors by Machine Learning Algorithms.* IEEE.

Cohen, J. (1960). A Coefficient of Agreement for Normal Scales. *Educational and Psychological Measurement, 20*(1), 37–46. doi:10.1177/001316446002000104

Cook, D. (2006). Health monitoring and assistance to support aging in place. *JUCS, 12*(1), 15–29.

Cortes, C., & Vapnik, V. (1995). Support-vector networks. *Machine Learning, 20*(3), 23–297. doi:10.1007/BF00994018

Costa, M., & Klein, C. B. (2006). Toxicity and carcinogenicity of chromium compounds in humans. *Critical Reviews in Toxicology, 36*(2), 155–163. doi:10.1080/10408440500534032 PMID:16736941

COVID-19 coronavirus pandemic. (n.d.). Available: https://www.worldometers.info/coronavirus

Crosta, A. D., Ceccato, I., Marchetti, D., Malva, P. L., Maiella, R., Cannito, R., Cip, M., Mammarella, N., Palumbo, N., Verrocchio, M. C., Palumbo, R., & Domenico, A. D. (2020). Psychological Factors and Consumer Behavior during the COVID-19 Pandemic. *PLoS One*, 1–23. PMID:34398916

Cruz, Garcia, Dimaunahan, Labaclado, Reyes, Riomero, Salamatin & Patrisha. (2019). Eczema, Color histogram, Support vector machine, Psoriasis, RGH-HSV color space, Skin disease, Local binary pattern, Hives. *Proceedings of the 2019- 9th International Conference on Biomedical Engineering and Technology*, 160-165.

Cucinotta, D., & Vanelli, M. (2020). WHO declares COVID-19a pandemic. *Acta Biomedica, 91*, 157–160. doi:10.23750/abm.v91i1.9397 PMID:32191675

Cui, L., Yang, S., Chen, F., Ming, Z., Lu, N., & Qin, J. (2018). A survey on application of machine learning for internet of things. *International Journal of Machine Learning and Cybernetics, 9*(8), 1399–1417. doi:10.100713042-018-0834-5

Dağ, Ö. H. N. (2019). Predicting the success of ensemble algorithms in the banking sector. *International Journal of Business Analytics, 6*(4), 12–31. doi:10.4018/IJBAN.2019100102

Dai, L., & Wang, L., Li. (2018). Multivariate geostatistical analysis and source identification of heavy metals in thesediment of Poyang Lake in China. *Science of EeTotalEnvironment, 621*, 1433–1444. PMID:29056381

Dang, L. M., Piran, M. J., Han, D., Min, K., & Moon, H. (2019). A Survey on Internet of Things and Cloud Computing for Healthcare. *MPDI. Electronics (Basel), 8*(7), 768. doi:10.3390/electronics8070768

Dara, S. S. (1997). Environmental Chemistry and Pollution Control. S. Chand & Company Ltd.

Dargan, S., Kumar, M., Ayyagari, M. R., & Kumar, G. (2020). A Survey of Deep Learning and Its Applications: A New Paradigm to Machine Learning. *Archives of Computational Methods in Engineering, 27*(4), 1071–1092. doi:10.100711831-019-09344-w

Das, G., Jain, S. P., Maheswaran, D., Slotegraaf, R. J., & Srinivasan, R. (2021). Pandemics and Marketing: Insights, Impacts, and Research Opportunities. *Journal of the Academy of Marketing Science, 49*(5), 835–854. doi:10.100711747-021-00786-y PMID:33994600

Davis, R., Campbell, R., Hildon, Z., Hobbs, L., & Michie, S. (2015). Theories of Behaviour and Behaviour Change Across the Social and Behavioural Sciences: A Scoping Review. *Health Psychology Review, 9*(3), 323–344. doi:10.1080/17437199.2014.941722 PMID:25104107

Dayanand, J., & Neethi, P. (2020). Thyroid Disease Prediction Using Feature Selection And Machine Learning Classifiers. *The International Journal of Analytical and Experimental Modal Analysis.*

Debels, P., Ricardofigueroaoberto, U. R. B., & Niel, X. (2005). Evaluation of Water Quality in the Chillán River (Central Chile) Using Physicochemical Parameters and a Modified Water Quality Index. *Environmental Monitoring and Assessment, 110*(1-3), 301–322. doi:10.100710661-005-8064-1 PMID:16308794

Dehkordi, S. A., Farajzadeh, K., Rezazadeh, J., Farahbakhsh, R., Sandrasegaran, K., & Dehkordi, M. A. (2020). A survey on data aggregation techniques in IoT sensor networks. *Wireless Networks, 26*(2), 1243–1263. doi:10.100711276-019-02142-z

J. Deng, W. Dong, R. Socher, L. Li, K. Li, & L. Fei-Fei (Eds.). (2009). ImageNet: A Large-Scale Hierarchical Image Database. In *Proceeding of the 2009 IEEE Conference on Computer Vision and Pattern Recognition.* IEEE. 10.1109/CVPR.2009.5206848

Deng, X., & Huangfu, F. (2019). Collaborative variational deep learning for healthcare recommendation. *IEEE Access: Practical Innovations, Open Solutions, 7*, 55679–55688. doi:10.1109/ACCESS.2019.2913468

Deng, X., Liu, Q., Deng, Y., & Mahadevan, S. (2016). An Improved Method to Construct Basic Probability Assignment Based on the Confusion Matrix for Classification Problem. *Information Sciences, Elsevier, 340-341*, 250–261. doi:10.1016/j.ins.2016.01.033

Deshpande, N., Thakur, K., & Zadgaonkar, A. S. (2014, May). Assessment of heart rate variability from speech analysis. In *Proceedings of Meetings on Acoustics 167ASA* (Vol. 21, No. 1, p. 055004). Acoustical Society of America.

Deshpande, A., Thakur, K., & Zadgaonkar, A. S. (2014, April). Assessment of heart rate variability from speech analysis. *The Journal of the Acoustical Society of America, 135*(4), 2427. doi:10.1121/1.4878075

Devani, U. D. (2016). Implementation of E-health care system using web services and cloud computing. *International Conference on Communication and Signal Processing (ICCSP)*, 1034-1036.

Devi, R., Alemayehu, E., Singh, V., Kumar, A., & Mengistie, E. (2008). Removal of fluoride, arsenic and coli form bacteria by modified homemade filter media from drinking water. *Bioresource Technology*, *99*, 2269–2274.

Dev, K., Khowaja, S. A., Bist, A. S., Saini, V., & Bhatia, S. (2021). Triage of potential COVID-19 patients from chest X-ray images using hierarchical convolutional networks. *Neural Computing & Applications*. Advance online publication. doi:10.100700521-020-05641-9 PMID:33649695

Dhillon, A., Singh, A. J., & World, T. (2019). *Machine learning in healthcare data analysis: a survey.* Academic Press.

Dilip., R. (2020). Development of Graphical System for Patient Monitoring using Cloud Computing. *International Journal of Advanced Science and Technology*, 29.

DiMeglio, J. L., & Rosenthal, J. (2013). Selective conversion of CO2 to CO with high efficiency using an bismuth-based electrocatalyst. *Journal of the American Chemical Society*, *135*(24), 8798–8801.

Dix, A. F. (2003). *Human–Computer Interaction* (3rd ed.). Prentice Hall.

Drury, R. L., Jarczok, M., Owens, A., & Thayer, J. F. (2021). Wireless Heart Rate Variability in Assessing Community COVID-19. *Frontiers in Neuroscience*, 15.

Duffus, J. H. (2002). Heavy metals-a meaningless term? *Pure and Applied Chemistry*, *74*(5), 793–807. doi:10.1351/pac200274050793

Ebdon, L., Foulkes, M. E., Roux, S. L., & Munoz-Olivas, R. (2002). Cold vapour atomic fluorescence spectrometry and gas chromatography-pyrolysis-atomic fluorescence for routine determination of total and organometallic mercury in food samples. *Analyst (London)*, *127*(8), 1108–1114. doi:10.1039/B202927H PMID:12195954

Edel, J., & Sabbioni, E. (1985). Pathways of Cr (III) and Cr (VI) in the rat after intra tracheal administration. *Human Toxicology*, *4*(4), 409–416. doi:10.1177/096032718500400407 PMID:4018821

Edelstein, M., & Ben-Hur, M. (2018). Heavy metals and metalloids:sources, risks and strategies to reduce their accumulation inhorticultural crops. *Scientia Horticulturae*, *234*, 431–444. doi:10.1016/j.scienta.2017.12.039

ElNaqa, I., & Murphy, M. J. (2015). What is Machine Learning? In I. Issam ElNaqa & M. J. Murphy (Eds.), *Machine Learning in Radiation Oncology* (pp. 3–11). Springer. doi:10.1007/978-3-319-18305-3_1

Elngar, A. A., Kumar, R., Hayat, A., & Churi, P. (2020). Intelligent System for Skin Disease Prediction using Machine Learning. *6th International Conference on Advanced Computing and Communication Systems (ICACCS)*, 599-605.

Emilio, G. G., Emilia, G., Javier, M. R., Manuel, G. C., Isabel, F. L., & María Isabel, R. L. (2020). Artificial intelligence in medicine and healthcare: a review and classification of current and near-future applications and their ethical and social Impact. *arXiv*, 20.

Emu, M. (2020). *Assisting the Non-invasive Diagnosis of Liver Fibrosis Stages using Machine Learning Methods*. IEEE.

Engel, B. T., & Chism, R. A. (1967). Effect of increases and decreases in breathing rate on heart rate and finger pulse volume. *Psychophysiology*, *4*(1), 83–89.

Engler, R. (1985). Technology out of control. *Nation (New York, N.Y.)*, *240*(16), 488–500.

Ensafi Ali, A., Katiraei Far, A., & Meghdadi, S. (2009). Highly selective optical-sensing film for lead(II) determination in water samples. *Journal of Hazardous Materials*, *172*(2-3), 1069–1075. doi:10.1016/j.jhazmat.2009.07.112 PMID:19709813

Erkol, B., Moss, R. H., Stanley, R. J., Stoecker, W. V., & Hvatum, E. (2005). Automatic Lesion Boundary Detection in Dermoscopy Images Using Gradient Vector Flow Snakes. *Skin Research and Technology*, *11*(1), 17–26. doi:10.1111/j.1600-0846.2005.00092.x PMID:15691255

Esmaili, A., Kachuee, M., & Shabany, M. (2017). Nonlinear Cuffless Blood Pressure Estimation of Healthy Subjects Using Pulse Transit Time and Arrival Time. *IEEE Transactions on Instrumentation and Measurement*, *66*(12), 3299–3308. doi:10.1109/TIM.2017.2745081

Evtodieva, T. E., Chernova, D. V., Ivanova, N. V., & Wirth, J. (2020). The internet of things: possibilities of application in intelligent supply chain management. In *Digital Transformation of the Economy: Challenges, Trends and New Opportunities* (pp. 395–403). Springer. doi:10.1007/978-3-030-11367-4_38

Fan, P., Peiyu, H., Shangwen, L., & Wenfeng, D. (2015). *Feature extraction of photoplethysmography signal using wavelet approach*. doi:10.1109/ICDSP.2015.7251876

Fant, G. (1960). *Acoustic theory of speech production*. Mouton.

Farid, D. M., Zhang, L., Rahman, C. M., Hossain, M. A., & Strachan, R. (2014). Hybrid Decision Tree and Naive Bayes Classifiers for Multi-class Classification Tasks. *Expert Systems with Applications, Elsevier*, *41*(4), 1937–1946. doi:10.1016/j.eswa.2013.08.089

Fathi-Hafshejani, P., Azam, N., Wang, L., Kuroda, M. A., Hamilton, M. C., Hasim, S., & Mahjouri-Samani, M. (2021). Two-dimensional-material-based field-effect transistor biosensor for detecting COVID-19 Virus (SARS-CoV-2). *ACS Nano*, *15*(7), 11461–11469. doi:10.1021/acsnano.1c01188 PMID:34181385

Fathollahi-Fard, A. M., Abbas, A., & Behrooz, K. (2021). Multi-Objective Optimization of Home Healthcare with Working-Time Balancing and Care Continuity. *Sustainability*, *13*(22), 12431. doi:10.3390u132212431

Feldman & Martin. (2012). *Big Data in Healthcare Hype and Hope*. Academic Press.

Firouzi, F., Rahmani, A. M., Mankodiya, K., Badaroglu, M., Merrett, G. V., Wong, P., & Farahani, B. (2018). Internet-of-Things and big data for smarter healthcare: From device to architecture, applications and analytics. *Future Generation Computer Systems*, *78*, 583–586. doi:10.1016/j.future.2017.09.016

Fizi, F., & Askar, S. (2016). A novel load balancing algorithm for software defined network based datacenters. *International Conference on Broadband Communications for Next Generation Networks and Multimedia Applications (CoBCom)*, 1-6. 10.1109/COBCOM.2016.7593506

Francisco, R., Pedro, M., Delvecchio, E., Espada, J. P., Morales, A., Mazzeschi, C., & Orgiles, M. (2020). Psychological Symptoms and Behavioral Changes in Children and Adolescents during the Early Phase of COVID-19 Quarantine in Three European Countries. *Frontiers in Psychiatry*, *11*, 1–14. doi:10.3389/fpsyt.2020.570164 PMID:33343415

Frederick, W. O. (1979). *Toxicity of heavy metals in the environment*. Part I & II Marcel Dekker, Inc.

Frias, M. E., Williamson, G., & Frias, M. V. (2011). Agent-Based Modeling of Epidemic Spreading Using Social Networks and Human Mobility Patterns. *Proceedings Third International Conference on Privacy, Security, Risk and Trust and IEEE third international conference on social computing*, 57–64.

Friedberg Charles, K. (1966). *Diseases of the Heart*. Saunders Pub.

Fukushima, K., Miyake, S., & Ito, T. (1983). Neocognitron: A Neural Network Model for a Mechanism of Visual Pattern Recognition. *IEEE Transactions on Systems, Man, and Cybernetics*, *SMC-13*(5), 826–834. doi:10.1109/TSMC.1983.6313076

Funk, S., Bansal, S., Bauch, C. T., Eames, K. T., Edmunds, W. J., & Galvani, A. P. (2015). Nine challenges in Incorporating the Dynamics of Behaviour in Infectious Diseases Models. *Epidemics, 10*, 21–5.

Funk, S., Bansal, S., Bauch, C. T., Eames, K. T., Edmunds, W. J., & Galvani. (2015). Nine challenges in Incorporating the Dynamics of Behaviour in Infectious Diseases Models. *Epidemics, 10*, 21–5.

Gabby, P. N. (2003). Lead. In *Environmental Defense "Alternatives to Lead-Acid Starter Batteries."* Pollution Prevention Fact Sheet. Available at http://www.cleancarcampaign.org/FactSheet_BatteryAlts.pdf

Gabby, P. N. (2006). Lead. In *Mineral Commodity Summaries* (pp. 92–93). U.S. Geological Survey. Available https://minerals.usgs.gov/minerals/pubs/commodity/lead/lead_mcs05.pdf

Gad, A. F. (2018). Practical Computer Vision Applications Using Deep Learning with CNNs. Apress. doi:10.1007/978-1-4842-4167-7

Gang, Y., & Malik, M. (2009). Non-invasive risk stratification for implantable cardioverter-defibrillator placement—heart rate variability. *The American Heart Hospital Journal*, *7*(1), 39–44. https://doi.org/10.15420/ahhj.2009.7.1.39

Gao, K., Mei, G., Piccialli, F., Cuomo, S., Tu, J., & Huo, Z. (2020). Julia language in machine learning: Algorithms, applications, and open issues. *Computer Science Review*, *37*, 100254. doi:10.1016/j.cosrev.2020.100254

Gay & Proop. (1993). *Aspects of river pollution*. Butterworth's Scientific Publication.

Ge, M., Bangui, H., & Buhnova, B. (2018). Big data for internet of things: A survey. *Future Generation Computer Systems*, *87*, 601–614. doi:10.1016/j.future.2018.04.053

Gemignani, V., Bianchini, E., Faita, F., Giannoni, M., Pasanisi, E., Picano, E., & Bombardini, T. (2008, September). *Assessment of cardiologic systole and diastole duration in exercise stress tests with a transcutaneous accelerometer sensor. In 2008 Computers in Cardiology*. IEEE.

Ghate, V. V., & Vijayakumar, V. (2018). Machine learning for data aggregation in wsn: A survey. *International Journal of Pure and Applied Mathematics*, *118*(24), 1–12.

Ghose, A., Pal, A., Choudhury, A. D., Chattopadhyay, T., Bhowmick, P. K., & Chattopadhyay, D. (2014). *Internet of things application development*. U.S. Patent Application 14/286,068.

Ghosh, A. M., Halder, D., & Hossain, S. A. (2016, May). Remote health monitoring system through IoT. In *2016 5th International Conference on Informatics, Electronics and Vision (ICIEV)* (pp. 921-926). IEEE. 10.1109/ICIEV.2016.7760135

Ginsberg, J., Mohebbi, M. H., Patel, R. S., Brammer, L., Smolinski, M. S., & Brilliant, L. (2009). Detecting influenza epidemics using search engine query data. *Nature*, *457*(7232), 1012–1014. doi:10.1038/nature07634 PMID:19020500

Glanz, K., & Bishop, D. B. (2010). The Role of Behavioral Science Theory in Development and Implementation of Public Health Interventions. *Annual Review of Public Health*, *31*(1), 399–418. doi:10.1146/annurev.publhealth.012809.103604 PMID:20070207

Gobe, G., & Crane, D. (2010). Mitochondria, reactive oxygen species and cadmium toxicity in the kidney. *Toxicology Letters*, *198*(1), 49–55. doi:10.1016/j.toxlet.2010.04.013 PMID:20417263

Goh, K. J., Wong, J., Tien, J. C., Ng, S. Y., Duu Wen, S., Phua, G. C., & Leong, C. K.-L. (2020). Preparing your intensive care unit for the COVID-19 pandemic: Practical considerations and strategies. *Critical Care (London, England)*, *24*(1), 215. doi:10.118613054-020-02916-4 PMID:32393325

Gopal, K. V. (2003). Neurotoxic effect of mercury on auditory cortex networks growing on microelectrode arrays: A preliminary analysis. *Neurotoxicology and Teratology*, *25*(1), 69–76. doi:10.1016/S0892-0362(02)00321-5 PMID:12633738

Guo, H., & Wang, W. (2019). Granular Support Vector Machine: A Review. *Artificial Intelligence Review, Springer*, *51*(1), 19–32. doi:10.100710462-017-9555-5

Gupta, A., Singla, R., Caminero, J. A., Singla, N., Mrigpuri, P., & Mohan, A. (2020). Impact of COVID-19 on tuberculosis services in India. *The International Journal of Tuberculosis and Lung Disease*, *24*(6), 637–639. doi:10.5588/ijtld.20.0212 PMID:32553014

Gutenbrunner, C., Jureckova, J., Koenker, R., & Portnoy, S. (1993). Tests of Linear Hypotheses Based on Regression Rank Score. *Journal of Nonparametric Statistics*, *2*(4), 307–331. doi:10.1080/10485259308832561

Halgurd, S., Maghdid, A. T., Asaad, K. Z., Ali Safaa, S., & Khurram Khan, M. (2020). *Diagnosing COVID-19 Pneumonia from X-Ray and CT Images using Deep Learning and Transfer Learning Algorithms*. arXiv preprint arXiv:2004.00038.

Hamann, C.R., Boonchai, W., Wen, L., Sakanashi, E.N., Chu, C.Y. & Hamann, K. (2014). *Spectrometric analysis of mercury content in 549 skin-lightening products: Is mercury toxicity a hidden global health hazard?* Academic Press.

Hameed, K., Bajwa, I. S., Ramzan, S., Anwar, W., & Khan, A. (2020). An intelligent IoT based healthcare system using fuzzy neural networks. *Scientific Programming*, *2020*, 2020. doi:10.1155/2020/8836927

Harfiya, L. N., Chang, C., & Li, Y. H. (2021). Continuous blood pressur estimation using exclusively photopletysmography by LSTM based signal-to-signal translation. *Sensors (Basel)*, *21*(9), 2952. doi:10.339021092952 PMID:33922447

Hasanzadeh, N., Ahmadi, M. M., & Mohammadzade, H. (2020). Blood Pressure Estimation Using Photoplethysmogram Signal and Its Morphological Features. *IEEE Sensors Journal*, *20*(8), 4300–4310. doi:10.1109/JSEN.2019.2961411

Hasty, F., García, G., Dávila, H., Wittels, S. H., Hendricks, S., & Chong, S. (2021). Heart rate variability as a possible predictive marker for acute inflammatory response in COVID-19 patients. *Military Medicine*, *186*(1-2), e34–e38.

Hawkes, S. J. (1997). What is a heavy metal? *Journal of Chemical Education*, *74*(11), 1374. doi:10.1021/ed074p1374

Hawkins, D. M. (2004). The Problem of Overfitting. *Journal of Chemical Information and Computer Sciences, ACM*, *44*(1), 1–12. doi:10.1021/ci0342472 PMID:14741005

Hay, R. J., Johns, N. E., & Williams, H. C. (2014). The global burden of skin disease in 2010: An analysis of the prevalence and impact of skin conditions. *The Journal of Investigative Dermatology*, *134*, 1527–1534. doi:10.1038/jid.2013.446 PMID:24166134

Heart rate variability: standards of measurement, physiological interpretation and clinical use. Task Force of the European Society of Cardiology and the North American Society of Pacing and Electrophysiology. (1996). *Circulation, 93*(5), 1043–1065.

Hemdan, E. E. D., Shouman, M. A., & Karar, M. E. (2020). *Covidx-net: A framework of deep learning classifiers to diagnose covid-19 in x-ray images*. arXiv preprint arXiv:2003.11055.

He, X., Goubran, R. A., & Liu, X. P. (2014). Secondary Peak Detection of PPG Signal for Continuous Cuffless Arterial Blood Pressure Measurement. *IEEE Transactions on Instrumentation and Measurement*, *63*(6), 1431–1439. doi:10.1109/TIM.2014.2299524

Heymann, D.L., & Shindom N. (2020). COVID-19: what is next for public health? *Lancet, 395,* 542-50. . doi:10.1016/S0140-6736(20)30374-3

Hill, S. J. (1997). Speciation of trace metals in the environment. *Chemical Society Reviews*, *26*(4), 291–298. doi:10.1039/cs9972600291

Hjemdahl, P. (2000). Cardiovascular system and stress. Encyclopedia of Stress, 1, 389-403.

Hochreiter, S. (1998). The vanishing gradient problem during learning recurrent neural nets and problem solutions. *International Journal of Uncertainty, Fuzziness and Knowledge-based Systems*, *6*(02), 107–116. doi:10.1142/S0218488598000094

Hochreiter, S., & Schmidhuber, J. (1997). Long short-term memory. *Neural Computation*, *9*(8), 1735–1780. doi:10.1162/neco.1997.9.8.1735 PMID:9377276

Holmes, P., James, K A F., & Levy, L. S. (2009). Is low-level environmental mercury exposure of concern to human health? *The Science of the Total Environment*, *408*(2), 171–182. doi:10.1016/j.scitotenv.2009.09.043 PMID:19850321

Horry, M. J., Chakraborty, S., Paul, M., Ulhaq, A., Pradhan, B., Saha, M., & Shukla, N. (2020). *X-ray image based COVID-19 detection using pre-trained deep learning models*. Academic Press.

Hosseinifard, M., Naghdi, T., Morales-Narváez, E., & Golmohammadi, H. (2021). Toward Smart Diagnostics in a Pandemic Scenario: COVID-19. *Frontiers in Bioengineering and Biotechnology*, *9*, 510. doi:10.3389/fbioe.2021.637203 PMID:34222208

Huang, Y. H. (2011). DNA computing research progress and application. *The 6th International Conference on Computer Science & Education*, 232-235. 10.1109/ICCSE.2011.6028624

Huang, C., Wang, Y., Li, X., Ren, L., Zhao, J., Hu, Y., & Cao, B. (2020). Clinical features of patients infected with 2019 novel coronavirus in Wuhan, China. *Lancet*, *395*(10223), 497–506. doi:10.1016/S0140-6736(20)30183-5 PMID:31986264

Hunter, D., Bomford, R.R., & Russell, D.S. (1940). *Poisoning by methylmercury compounds*. Academic Press.

Hunter, D. J. (2020). Covid-19 and the Stiff Upper Lip— The Pandemic Response in the United Kingdom. *The New England Journal of Medicine*, *382*(16), e31. doi:10.1056/NEJMp2005755 PMID:32197002

Hussain, W., Hussain, F. K., Hussain, O. K., & Chang, E. (2016). Provider-Based Optimized Personalized Viable SLA (OPV-SLA) Framework to Prevent SLA Violation. *The Computer Journal*, *59*(12), 1760–1783. doi:10.1093/comjnl/bxw026

Hussain, W., Hussain, F. K., Hussain, O., Bagia, R., & Chang, E. (2018). Risk-based framework for SLA violation abatement from the cloud service provider's perspective. *The Computer Journal*, *61*(9), 1306–1322. doi:10.1093/comjnl/bxx118

Hutson, J. C. (2005). Effects of Bismuth Citrate on the Viability and Function of Leydig Cells and Testicular Macrophages. *Journal of Applied Toxicology*, *25*(3), 234–238. doi:10.1002/jat.1060 PMID:15856528

International Agency for Research on Cancer (IARC). (2003). Monographs – Cadmium. Its toxicopathologic implications for public health. *Environmental Toxicology*, *18*, 149–175. PMID:12740802

Ishaq, E. A.-A. (2020). Online Monitoring Health Station Using Arduino Mobile Connected to Cloud service: "Heart Monitor" System. *International Conference on Promising Electronic Technologies (ICPET)*, 38-43.

Ivakhnenko, A. G., & Lapa, V. G. (1966). Cybernetic Predicting Devices. Technical Report, DTIC Document, Purdue University.

Jabbar, H. K., & Khan, R. Z. (2015). Methods to Avoid Over-fitting and Under-fitting in Supervised Machine Learning (Comparative Study). *Computer Science, Communication and Instrumentation Devices*, *2015*, 163–172. doi:10.3850/978-981-09-5247-1_017

Jafari, A., Mirhossaini, H., Kamareii, B., & Dehestani, S. (2008). Physicochemical Analysis of Drinking Water in Kohdasht City Lorestan, Iran. *Asian Journal of Applied Sciences*, *1*(1), 87–92. doi:10.3923/ajaps.2008.87.92

Jana, E., Subban, R., & Saraswathi, S. (2017). Research on Skin Cancer Cell Detection using Image Processing. *IEEE International Conference on Computational Intelligence and Computing Research (ICCIC)*, 1-8.

Jijesh, J. J., & S. L. (2018). Design and Development of Intuitive Environment with Health Monitoring System Using Internet of Things. *IEEE International Conference on Recent Trends in Electronics,Information Technology & Communication Technology (RTEICT)*, 1351-1355. 10.1109/RTEICT42901.2018.9012157

Jog, S., Kelkar, D., Bhat, M., Patwardhan, S., Godavarthy, P., & Dhundi, U. (2020). Preparedness of Acute Care Facility and a Hospital for COVID-19 Pandemic: What We Did! *Indian Journal of Critical Care Medicine: Peer-Reviewed, Official Publication of Indian Society of Critical Care Medicine*, *24*(6), 385–392. doi:10.5005/jp-journals-10071-23416 PMID:32863628

Jones, L. (n.d.). *The Big Ones: How Natural Disasters Have Shaped Humanity*. New York, NY: Anchor Books Press.

Joshi, S. J. (2019). A Sensor based Secured Health Monitoring and Alert Technique using IoMT. *International Conference on Intelligent Communication and Computational Techniques (ICCT)*, 152-156. 10.1109/ICCT46177.2019.8969047

Kaiser, J. (2000). Toxicology-mercury report backs strict rules. *Science*, *289*(5478), 371–372. doi:10.1126cience.289.5478.371a PMID:10939938

Kaliyaperumal, D., Karthikeyan, R. K., Alagesan, M., & Ramalingam, S. (2021). Characterization of cardiac autonomic function in COVID-19 using heart rate variability: A hospital based preliminary observational study. *Journal of Basic and Clinical Physiology and Pharmacology*, *32*(3), 247–253.

Kamaleswaran, R., Sadan, O., Kandiah, P., Li, Q., Thomas, T., Blum, J., ... Buchman, T. (2021). 227: Altered Heart Rate Variability Predicts Mortality Early Among Critically Ill COVID-19 Patients. *Critical Care Medicine*, *49*(1), 99.

Kan, M. M. (2019). Digital technology and the future of health systems," Health Systems & Reform. *Reform*, *5*(2), 113–120.

Kanne, J. P., Little, B. P., Chung, J. H., Elicker, B. M., & Ketai, L. H. (2020). *Essentials for radiologists on COVID-19: An update—radiology scientific expert panel*. Academic Press.

Karimkhani, C., Dellavalle, R. P., Coffeng, L. E., Flohr, C., Hay, R. J., Langan, S. M., Nsoesie, E. O., Ferrari, A. J., Erskine, H. E., Silverberg, J. I., Vos, T., & Naghavi, M. (2017). Global skin disease morbidity and mortality: An update from the Global Burden of Disease Study. *JAMA Dermatology*, *153*(5), 406–412. doi:10.1001/jamadermatol.2016.5538 PMID:28249066

Kaur, G., & Oberoi, A. (2020). Novel Approach for Brain Tumor Detection Based on Naïve Bayes Classification. In Data Management, Analytics and Innovation. Springer. doi:10.1007/978-981-32-9949-8_31

Kean & Sam. (2011). *The Disappearing Spoon (and other true tales of madness, love, and the history of the world from the Periodic Table of Elements)*. Back Bay Books.

Keti, F., & Askar, S. (2015). Emulation of Software Defined Networks Using Mininet in Different Simulation Environments. *6th International Conference on Intelligent Systems, Modelling and Simulation*, 205-210. 10.1109/ISMS.2015.46

Khalid, S. G., Zhang, J., Chen, F., & Zheng, D. (2018). Blood Pressure Estimation Using Photoplethysmography Only: Comparison between Different Machine Learning Approaches. *Journal of Healthcare Engineering*, *2018*, 2018. doi:10.1155/2018/1548647 PMID:30425819

Khanum, M., Mahboob, T., Imtiaz, W., Abdul Ghafoor, H., & Sehar, R. (2015). A Survey on Unsupervised Machine Learning Algorithms for Automation, Classification and Maintenance. *International Journal of Computers and Applications*, *119*(13), 34–39. doi:10.5120/21131-4058

Kim, H. G., Cheon, E. J., Bai, D. S., Lee, Y. H., & Koo, B. H. (2018). Stress and Heart Rate Variability: A Meta-Analysis and Review of the Literature. *Psychiatry Investigation*, *15*(3), 235–245. https://doi.org/10.30773/pi.2017.08.17

Kittler, J., Hatef, M., Duin, R. P. W., & Matas, J. (1998). On combining classifiers. *IEEE Transactions on Pattern Analysis and Machine Intelligence*, *20*(3), 226–239. doi:10.1109/34.667881

Koda, S., Zeggada, A., Melgani, F., & Nishii, R. (2018). Spatial and Structured SVM for Multilabel Image Classification. *IEEE Transactions on Geoscience and Remote Sensing*, *56*(10), 5948–5960. doi:10.1109/TGRS.2018.2828862

Kohler, J. E., Falcone, R. A. Jr, & Fallat, M. E. (2019). Rural health, telemedicine and access for pediatric surgery. *Current Opinion in Pediatrics*, *31*(3), 391–398. doi:10.1097/MOP.0000000000000763 PMID:31090582

Kollamparambil, U., & Oyenubi, A. (2021). Behavioural Response to the COVID-19 2021 Pandemic in South Africa. *PLoS One*, 1–19. PMID:33861811

Kollamparambil, U., & Oyenubi, A. (2021). Behavioural Response to the COVID-19. Pandemic in South Africa. *PLoS One*, 1–19. PMID:33861811

Kolodner, J. (1993). *Case-Based Reasoning*. Morgan Kaufmann. doi:10.1016/B978-1-55860-237-3.50005-4

Komal Kumar, N. (2020). Analysis and Prediction of Cardio Vascular Disease using Machine Learning Classifiers. *6th International Conference on Advanced Computing & Communication Systems*.

Kononenko, I. (2001). Machine Learning for Medical Diagnosis: History, State of the Art and Perspective. *Journal of Artificial Intelligence in Medicine*, *1*(1), 89–109. doi:10.1016/S0933-3657(01)00077-X PMID:11470218

Kotsiantis, S. B., Kanellopoulos, D., & Zaharakis, I. D. (2006). Bagged averaging of regression models. *IFIP Int. Fed. Inf. Process.*, *204*, 53–60. doi:10.1007/0-387-34224-9_7

Kruk, M.E., Myers, M., Varpilah, S.T., & Dahn, B.T. (2015). What is a resilient health system? Lessons from Ebola. *Lancet, 385*, 1910-2. . doi:10.1016/S0140-6736(15)60755-3

La Marca, A., Capuzzo, M., Paglia, T., Roli, L., Trenti, T., & Nelson, S. M. (2020, September). Testing for SARS-CoV-2 (COVID-19): A systematic review and clinical guide to molecular and serological in-vitro diagnostic assays. *Reproductive Biomedicine Online*, *41*(3), 483–499. doi:10.1016/j.rbmo.2020.06.001 PMID:32651106

Lakshmi, B., Indumathi, T., & Ravi, N. A. (2016). 5 decision tree classification algorithm for risk predictions during pregnancy. *Procedia Technol.*, *24*, 1542–1549. doi:10.1016/j.protcy.2016.05.128

Lakshmi, L., & A. N. (2021). The preeminence of Fog Computing and IoT enabled Cloud Systems in Health care. *International Conference on Intelligent Communication Technologies and Virtual Mobile Network (ICICV)*, 365-375. 10.1109/ICICV50876.2021.9388408

Lancet Infectious Diseases. (2020). Challenges of coronavirus disease 2019. *The Lancet. Infectious Diseases*, *20*(3), 261. doi:10.1016/S1473-3099(20)30072-4 PMID:32078810

Lashkari, B., Rezazadeh, J., Farahbakhsh, R., & Sandrasegaran, K. (2018). Crowdsourcing and sensing for indoor localization in IoT: A review. *IEEE Sensors Journal*, *19*(7), 2408–2434. doi:10.1109/JSEN.2018.2880180

Latif, S., Afzaal, H., & Zafar, N. A. (2018). Intelligent traffic monitoring and guidance system for smart city. In *International Conference on Computing, Mathematics and Engineering Technologies (iCoMET)*. IEEE. 10.1109/ICOMET.2018.8346327

Compilation of References

Lee, I., & Lee, K. (2015). The internet of things (IoT): Applications, investments, and challenges for enterprises. *Business Horizons, 58*(4), 431–440. doi:10.1016/j.bushor.2015.03.008

Leermakers, M., Baeyens, W., Quevauviller, P., & Horvat, M. (2005). Mercury in environmental samples: Speciation, artifacts and validation. *Trac-Trend. Analytical Chemistry, 24*, 383–393.

Lee, S. I., Celik, S., Logsdon, B. A., Lundberg, S. M., Martins, T. J., Oehler, V. G., Estey, E. H., Miller, C. P., Chien, S., Dai, J., Saxena, A., Blau, C. A., & Becker, P. S. (2018). A machine learning approach to integrate big data for precision medicine in acute myeloid leukemia. *Nature Communications, 9*(1), 4. doi:10.103841467-017-02465-5 PMID:29298978

Legido-Quigley, H., Asgari, N., Teo, Y.Y., Leung, G.M., Oshitani, H., & Fukuda, K. (2020). Are high-performing health systems resilient against the COVID-19 epidemic? *Lancet, 395*, 848-50. . doi:10.1016/S0140-6736(20)30551-1

Lide, D. (1992). *'CRC Handbook of Chemistry and Physics* (73rd ed.). CRC Press.

Listed, N. A. (2020). *Michigan National Guard Building Temporary Medical Station in Detroit to Support Coronavirus Patients*. Available online at: https://www.mlive.com/public-interest/2020/04/michigan-national-guard-building-temporary-medical-station-in-detroit-to-support-coronavirus-patients.html

Liu, C., Cao, Y., Alcantara, M., Liu, B., Brunette, M., Peinado, J., & Curioso, W. (2017, September). TX-CNN: Detecting tuberculosis in chest X-ray images using convolutional neural network. In *2017 IEEE international conference on image processing (ICIP)* (pp. 2314-2318). IEEE.

Liu, J., Shen, H., Narman, H.S., Chung, W., & Lin, Z. (2018). A survey of mobile crowd sensing techniques: A critical component for the internet of things. *ACM Transactions on Cyber-Physical Systems, 2*(3), 1–26.

Liu, C., Frazier, P., & Kumar, L. (2007). Comparative Assessment of the Measures of Thematic Classification Accuracy. *Remote Sensing of Environment, Elsevier, 107*(4), 606–616. doi:10.1016/j.rse.2006.10.010

Liu, H., Li, L., Yin, C., & Shan, B. (2008). Fraction distribution and risk assessment of heavy metals in sediments of Moshui Lake. *Journal of Environmental Sciences (China), 20*(4), 390–397. doi:10.1016/S1001-0742(08)62069-0 PMID:18575121

Liu, J., Li, W., Zhao, N., Cao, K., Yin, Y., Song, Q., & Gong, X. (2018, September). Integrate domain knowledge in training CNN for ultrasonography breast cancer diagnosis. In *International Conference on Medical Image Computing and Computer-Assisted Intervention* (pp. 868-875). Springer. 10.1007/978-3-030-00934-2_96

Liu, M., Po, L.-M., & Fu, H. (2017). Cuffless Blood Pressure Estimation Based on Photoplethysmography Signal and Its Second Derivative. *International Journal of Computer Theory and Engineering, 9*(3), 202–206. doi:10.7763/IJCTE.2017.V9.1138

Liu, Q., Zhou, F., Hang, R., & Yuan, X. (2017). Bidirectional-convolutional LSTM based spectral-spatial feature learning for hyperspectral image classification. *Remote Sensing, 9*(12), 1330. doi:10.3390/rs9121330

Li, W., Fu, H., Yu, L., & Cracknell, A. (2017). Deep Learning Based Oil Palm Tree Detection and Counting for High-Resolution Remote Sensing Images. *Remote Sensing, 9*(1), 22–34. doi:10.3390/rs9010022

Li, Y., & Xia, L. (2020). Coronavirus disease 2019 (COVID-19): Role of chest CT in diagnosis and management. *AJR. American Journal of Roentgenology, 214*(6), 1280–1286. doi:10.2214/AJR.20.22954 PMID:32130038

Loiseau, P., Henry, P., Jallon, P., & Legroux, M. (1976). Iatro- genic Myoclonic Encephalopathies Caused by Bismuth Salts. *Journal of the Neurological Sciences, 27*(2), 133–143. doi:10.1016/0022-510X(76)90056-3 PMID:1249582

Lokeshwari, H., & Chandrappa, G. T. (2006). Impact of heavy metal contamination of Bellandur Lake on soil and cultivated vegetation. *Current Science, 91*(5), 584.

Lubis, A. R., Lubis, M., & Khowarizmi, A. (2020). Optimization of Distance Formula in K-Nearest Neighbor Method. *Bulletin of Electrical Engineering and Informatics, 9*(1), 326–338. doi:10.11591/eei.v9i1.1464

F. F. Lubis, Y. Rosmansyah, & S. H. Supangkat (Eds.). (2014). Gradient Descent and Normal Equations on Cost Function Minimization for Online Predictive Using Linear Regression with Multiple Variables. In *Proceeding of the 2014 International Conference on ICT For Smart Society (ICISS)*. IEEE. 10.1109/ICTSS.2014.7013173

Ma, X., Wang, Z., Zhou, S., Wen, H., & Zhang, Y. (2018, June). Intelligent HLC systems assisted by data analytics and mobile computing. In 2018 14th International Wireless Communications & Mobile Computing Conference (IWCMC) (pp. 1317-1322). IEEE.

MacLean, O. A., Orton, R. J., Singer, J. B., & Robertson, D. L. (2020). No evidence for distinct types in the evolution of SARS-CoV-2. *Virus Evolution, 6*(1).

Magoulas, G. D., & Prentza, A. (1999, July). Machine learning in medical applications. In *Advanced course on artificial intelligence* (pp. 300–307). Springer.

Mahaffey, K. R. (1990). Environmental lead toxicity: Nutrition as a component of intervention. *Environmental Health Perspectives, 89*, 75–78. doi:10.1289/ehp.908975 PMID:2088758

Mahananda, H. B., Mahanand, M. R., & Mohanty, B. P. (2005). Studies on the physicochemical and biological parameters of fresh water pond water ecosystem as an indicator of water pollution. *Ecol. Env. And Cons., 11*(3-4), 537–541.

Mahdavinejad, M. S., Rezvan, M., Barekatain, M., Adibi, P., Barnaghi, P., & Sheth, A. P. (2018). Machine learning for internet of things data analysis: A survey. *Digital Communications and Networks, 4*(3), 161–175. doi:10.1016/j.dcan.2017.10.002

Mandal, S., Singh, B. K., & Thakur, K. (2021). Majority voting-based hybrid feature selection in machine learning paradigm for epilepsy detection using EEG. *International Journal of Computational Vision and Robotics*, *11*(4), 85–400. doi:10.1504/IJCVR.2021.116558

Mannino, D.M., Holguin, F., Greves, H.M., Savage-Brown, A., Stock, A.L. & Jones, R.L. (2004). *Urinary cadmium levels predict lower lung function in current and former smokers: Data from the Third National Health and Nutrition Examination Survey*. Academic Press.

Marcel, S. (2020). COVID-19 epidemic in Switzerland: On the importance of testing, contact tracing and isolation. *Swiss Medical Weekly*, *150*(11–12), 4–6. doi:10.4414mw.2020.20225 PMID:32191813

Martinis, E. M., Bertón, P., Olsina, R. A., Altamirano, J. C., & Wuilloud, R. G. (2009). Trace mercury determination in drinking and natural water samples by room temperature ionic liquid based-preconcentration and flow injection-cold vapor atomic absorption spectrometry. *Journal of Hazardous Materials*, *167*(1-3), 475–481. doi:10.1016/j.jhazmat.2009.01.007 PMID:19233554

Martins, A., & Astudillo, R. (2016, June). From softmax to sparsemax: A sparse model of attention and multi-label classification. In *International conference on machine learning* (pp. 1614-1623). PMLR.

Maskut, S., Timur, S., Zhanar, B., Aigul, A., Marina, Z., & Nazym, A. (2020). *The Recent Progress and Applications of Digital Technologies in Healthcare: A Review*. International Journal of Telemedicine and Applications.

Matos, A. D., Paiva, A. F. D., Cunha, C., & Voss, G. (2021). Precautionary Behaviours of Individuals with Multimorbidity during The COVID-19 Pandemic. *European Journal of Ageing*, 1–9. PMID:35002593

Matsumura, K., Rolfe, P., Toda, S., & Yamakoshi, T. (2018). Cuffless Blood Pressure Estimation Using Only a Smartphone. *Scientific Reports*, *8*(1), 1–9. doi:10.103841598-018-25681-5 PMID:29740088

Mcculloch, W. S., & Pitts, W. (1990). A Logical Calculus of the Ideas Immanent in Nervous Activity. *Bulletin of Mathematical Biology, Springer*, *52*(1-2), 99–115. doi:10.1016/S0092-8240(05)80006-0 PMID:2185863

Med, J. Am., Assoc. (1994). Blood lead levels in the United States. *The National Health and Nutrition Examination Surveys*, *272*, 284–291. PMID:8028141

Mekid, S. (2021). IoT for health and usage monitoring systems: mitigating consequences in manufacturing under CBM. *International Multi-Conference on Systems, Signals & Devices (SSD)*, 569-574.

Michael, M., Sonoo, T. I., Andrew, A., Andrew, B., Paul, B., Wendy, C., & Seth, H. (2001). *Artificial Intelligence in Health Care:The Hope, the Hype*. National Academy of Medicine.

Michie. S., Van. S. M. M., & West. R. (2011). The Behaviour Change Wheel: A New method for Characterising and Designing Behaviour Change Interventions. *SCI Implement, 6*.

Michie, S., West, R., Campbell, R., Brown, J., & Gainforth, H. (2014). *ABC of Behaviour Change Theories*. Silverback Publishing.

Milway, C. P. (1969). Education in large lakes and impoundments. *Proc. Upplasale Symp. DECO*.

Miotto, R., Wang, F., Wang, S., Jiang, X., & Dudley, J. T. (2018). Deep learning for healthcare: Review, opportunities and challenges. *Briefings in Bioinformatics*, *19*(6), 1236–1246. doi:10.1093/bib/bbx044 PMID:28481991

Mirza, S., Mittal, S., & Zaman, M. (2018). Decision Support Predictive model for prognosis of diabetes using SMOTE and Decision tree. *International Journal of Applied Engineering Research: IJAER*, *13*, 9277–9282.

Mitchell, T. M. (2006). *The Discipline of Machine Learning*. Carnegie Mellon University, School of Computer Science, Machine Learning Department.

Mohammadi, M., Al-Fuqaha, A., Sorour, S., & Guizani, M. (2018). Deep learning for iot big data and streaming analytics: A survey. *IEEE Communications Surveys and Tutorials*, *20*(4), 2923–2960. doi:10.1109/COMST.2018.2844341

Mohammed & Al-Tuwaijari. (2020). Skin Disease Classification System Based on Machine Learning Technique: A Survey. *IOP Conference Series: Materials Science and Engineering (ISCES)*, *1076*, 1-13.

Mohd Affandi, A., Khan, I., & Ngah Saaya, N. (2018). Epidemiology and Clinical Features of Adult Patients with Psoriasis in Malaysia: 10-Year Review from the Malaysian Psoriasis Registry (2007-2016). *Dermatology Research and Practice*.

Moher, D., Liberati, A., Tetzlaff, J., & Altman, D. (2009). Preferred Reporting Items for Systematic Reviews and Meta-Analyses: The PRISMA Statement. *PLoS Med*.

Moher, D., Liberati, A., Tetzlaff, J., Altman, D., & The, P. (2009). Preferred Reporting Items for Systematic Reviews and Meta-Analyses: The PRISMA Statement. *PLoS Medicine*, *6*(7), e1000097. doi:10.1371/journal.pmed.1000097 PMID:19621072

MOHFW. (2020a). *Guidance Document on Appropriate Management of Suspect/ Confirmed Cases of COVID-19*. Available online at: https://www.mohfw.gov.in/pdf/FinalGuidanceonMangaementofCovidcases version2.pdf

MOHFW. (2020b). *Government of India. Ministry of Health and Family Welfare. Directorate General of Health Services (EMR Division). COVID-19: Guidelines on Dead Body Management*. Available online at: https://www.mohfw.gov.in/pdf/1584423700568_COVID19GuidelinesonDeadbodymanagement.pdf

Mol, M. B., Strous, M. T., van Osch, F. H., Vogelaar, F. J., Barten, D. G., Farchi, M., ... Gidron, Y. (2021). Heart-rate-variability (HRV), predicts outcomes in COVID-19. *PLoS One*, *16*(10), e0258841.

Monteiro, K., É. R. (2018). Developing an e-Health System Based on IoT, Fog and Cloud Computing. *IEEE/ACM International Conference on Utility and Cloud Computing Companion (UCC Companion)*, 17-18. 10.1109/UCC-Companion.2018.00024

Muñana, C., Hamel, L., Kates, J., & Michaud, J. (2020). *The Public's Awareness of Concerns About Coronavirus. Global Health Policy.* Henry J. Kaiser Family Foundation, KFF Health Tracking Poll. Available online at: https://www.kff.org/global-health-policy/issue-brief/the-publicsawareness-of-and-concerns-about-coronavirus/

Mustafat, S., & Kimura, A. (2018). A SVM-Based Diagnosis of Melanoma Using Only Useful Image Features. *International Workshop on Advanced Image Technology (IWAIT)*, 1-4.

Nagarathna, R., Anand, A., Rain, M., Srivastava, V., Sivapuram, M. S., Kulkarni, R., Ilavarasu, J., Sharma, M. N. K., Singh, A., & Nagendra, H. R. (2021). Yoga Practice Is Beneficial for Maintaining Healthy Lifestyle and Endurance Under Restrictions and Stress Imposed by Lockdown During COVID-19 Pandemic. *Frontiers in Psychiatry*, *12*, 1–20. doi:10.3389/fpsyt.2021.613762 PMID:34239456

Narin, A., Kaya, C., & Pamuk, Z. (2020). *Automatic Detection of Coronavirus Disease (COVID-19) Using X-ray Images and Deep Convolutional Neural Networks.* arXiv preprint arXiv:2003.10849.

Naser, W. N., Ingrassia, P. L., Aladhrae, S., & Abdulraheem, W. A. (2018l). A study of hospital disaster preparedness in South Yemen. *Prehospital and Disaster Medicine*, *33*(2), 133–138. doi:10.1017/S1049023X18000158 PMID:29455694

National Institute of Health. (2020). *News Release: NIH Clinical Trial Shows Remdesivir Accelerates Recovery From Advanced COVID-19.* Available online at: https://www.nih.gov/news-events/news-releases/nih-clinical-trialshows-remdesivir-accelerates-recovery-advanced-covid-19

Naudé, W. (2020). Artificial intelligence vs COVID-19: Limitations, constraints and pitfalls. *AI & Society*, *35*(3), 761–765. doi:10.100700146-020-00978-0 PMID:32346223

Neloy, A., S. A. (2019). Machine Learning based Health Prediction System using IBM Cloud as PaaS. *International Conference on Trends in Electronics and Informatics (ICOEI)*, 444-450. 10.1109/ICOEI.2019.8862754

Nevondo, T.S., & Cloete, T.E. (1999). *Bacterial and chemical quality of water in Dertig village settlement water SA.* Academic Press.

Nidhal, K. (2010). Psoriasis Detection Using Skin Colour and Texture Features. *Journal of Computational Science*, *6*(6), 648–652. doi:10.3844/jcssp.2010.648.652

Noble, W. S. (2006). What is a support vector machine? *Nature Biotechnology*, *24*(12), 1565–1567. doi:10.1038/nbt1206-1565 PMID:17160063

NTP. (2007). Technical Report on the Toxicity Study of Sodium Dichromate Dihydrate Administered in Drinking Water to Male and Female F344/N Rats and B6C3F1 Mice and Male BALB/c and am3 - C57BL/6 Mice. National Toxicology Program Toxicity Report Series.

Nunes, E., Cavaco, A., & Carvalho, C. (2014). Children's health risk and benefits of fish consumption: Risk indices based on a diet diary follow-up of two weeks. *Journal of Toxicology and Environmental Health. Part A.*, *77*(1-3), 103–114. doi:10.1080/15287394.2014.866926 PMID:24555651

Olaković, A. Č., & Hadžialić, M. (2018). Internet of things (IoT): A review of enabling technologies, challenges, and open research issues. *Computer Networks*, *144*, 17–39. doi:10.1016/j.comnet.2018.07.017

Orlikoff, R. F., & Baken, R. J. (1989). Fundamental frequency modulation of the human voice by the heartbeat: Preliminary results and possible mechanisms. *The Journal of the Acoustical Society of America*, *85*(2), 888–893.

Oshiro, T. M., Perez, P. S., & Baranauskas, J. A. (2012). How Many Trees in a Random Forest? In *International Workshop on Machine Learning and Data Mining in Pattern Recognition*. Springer. 10.1007/978-3-642-31537-4_13

Otoom, A. F., Abdallah, E. E., Kilani, Y., Kefaye, A., & Ashour, M. (2015). Effective Diagnosis and Monitoring of Heart Disease. *International Journal of Software Engineering and Its Applications*, *9*, 143–156.

Oyewo, O. (2020). Prediction of Prostate Cancer using Ensemble of Machine Learning Techniques. *International Journal of Advanced Computer Science and Applications*, *11*(3).

Ozimek, T. (1975). Field experiment on the effect of municipal sewage on macrophytes and epifauna in the lake littoral. *Bull. Acad. Pol. Sc. Clii*, *23*, 445–447.

Pan, F., Ye, T., Sun, P., Gui, S., Liang, B., Li, L., & Zheng, C. (2020). Time course of lung changes on chest CT during recovery from 2019 novel coronavirus (COVID-19) pneumonia. *Radiology*.

Park, J., Yang, S., Sohn, J., Lee, J., Lee, S., Ku, Y., & Kim, H. C. (2019). Cuffless and Continuous Blood Pressure Monitoring Using a Single Chest-Worn Device. *IEEE Access: Practical Innovations, Open Solutions*, *7*, 135231–135246. doi:10.1109/ACCESS.2019.2942184

Patel, A., D'Alessandro, M. M., Ireland, K. J., Burel, W. G., Wencil, E. B., & Rasmussen, S. A. (2017). Personal protective equipment supply chain: Lessons learned from recent public health emergency responses. *Health Security*, *15*(3), 244–252. doi:10.1089/hs.2016.0129 PMID:28636443

Patel, S. C. (2017). Cloud and sensors based obesity monitoring system. *International Conference on Intelligent Sustainable Systems (ICISS)*, 153-156.

Patil, P. R., Badgujar, S. R., & Wark, A. M. (2001). Evolution of groundwater quality in Ganesh Colony area of Jalgaon City, Maharashtra, India. *Oriental Journal of Chemistry*, *17*(2), 283.

Patil, V., & S. S. (2018). Health Monitoring System Using Internet of Things. *International Conference on Intelligent Computing and Control Systems (ICICCS)*, 1523-1525. 10.1109/ICCONS.2018.8662915

Paun, G. H. (1999). DNA Computing: New Computing Paradigms. Springer.

Paun, G. H. R. G. (1999). DNA Computing: New Computing Paradigms. Springer.

Pawlak, Z. R. (1991). *Theoretical Aspects of Reasoning about Data*. Kluwer Academic Publishers.

Pedregosa, F., Varoquaux, G., Gramfort, A., Michel, V., Thirion, B., Grisel, O., Blondel, M., Prettenhofer, P., Weiss, R., Dubourg, V., Vanderplas, J., Passos, A., Cournapeau, D., Brucher, M., Perrot, M., & Duchesnay, É. (2011). Scikit-learn: Machine Learning in Python. *Journal of Machine Learning Research*, *12*, 2825–2830.

Peihao, M., & Kirati, L. (2021). Central blood pressure estimation from distal ppg measurement using semiclassical signal analysis features. *IEEE Access*. doi:10.1109/ACCESS.2021.3065576

Pfeifer, L. S., Heyers, K., Ocklenburg, S., & Wolf, O. T. (2021). Stress research during the COVID-19 pandemic and beyond. *Neuroscience and Biobehavioral Reviews*, *131*, 581–596. https://doi.org/10.1016/j.neubiorev.2021.09.045

Pharmaceuticals, R. (2020). *News Release: Regeneron and Sanofi Provide Update on US Phase 2/3 Adaptive-Designed Trial of Kevzara R (Sarilumab) in Hospitalized COVID-19 Patients*. Available online at: https://investor. regeneron.com/news-releases/news-release-details/regeneron-and-sanofiprovide-update-us-phase-23-adaptive

Piccialli, F., & Jung, J. E. (2017). Understanding customer experience diffusion on social networking services by big data analytics. *Mobile Networks and Applications*, *22*(4), 605–612. doi:10.100711036-016-0803-8

Piecznska, E., Usikorna, & Olimak, T. (1975). The influence of domestic sewage on the littoral of lakes. *Polskie Archiwum Hydrobiologii*, *22*, 141–146.

Pistofidis, N., Vourlias, G., Konidaris, S., Pavlidou, E., Stergiou, A., & Stergioudis, G. (2007, February). The effect of bismuth on the structure of zinc hot-dip galvanized coating. *Materials Letters*, *61*(4-5), 994–997. doi:10.1016/j.matlet.2006.06.029

Pourghebleh, B., & Navimipour, N. J. (2017). Data aggregation mechanisms in the internet of things: A systematic review of the literature and recommendations for future research. *Journal of Network and Computer Applications*, *97*, 23–34. doi:10.1016/j.jnca.2017.08.006

Pouryazdan, M., Fiandrino, C., Kantarci, B., Soyata, T., Kliazovich, D., & Bouvry, P. (2017). Intelligent gaming for mobile crowd-sensing participants to acquire trustworthy big data in the internet of things. *IEEE Access: Practical Innovations, Open Solutions*, *5*, 22209–22223. doi:10.1109/ACCESS.2017.2762238

Pramanik, P. K., Pal, S., & Mukhopadhyay, M. (2019). Healthcare Big Data: A Comprehensive Overview. In P. K. Pramanik, S. Pal, & M. Mukhopadhyay (Eds.), *Healthcare Big Data: A Comprehensive Overview* (pp. 72–100). IGI Global.

Prathamesh, Somnathe, & Gumaste. (2015). A Review of Existing Hair Removal Methods in Dermoscopic Images. *IOSR Journal of Electronics and Communication Engineering*, 73-76.

Qi, J., Yang, P., Min, G., Amft, O., Dong, F., & Xu, L. (2017). Advanced internet of things for personalised healthcare systems: A survey. *Pervasive and Mobile Computing*, *41*, 132–149. doi:10.1016/j.pmcj.2017.06.018

Qiu, H.-J. (2020). Using the internet search data to investigate symptom characteristics of COVID-19: A big data study. *World J. Otorhinolaryngology-Head and Neck Surgery*, *6*, S40–S48. doi:10.1016/j.wjorl.2020.05.003 PMID:32837757

Rabiner, L. R. (1978). *Digital processing of speech signal*. Academic Press.

Rahat Yasir, R., Rahman, M. A., & Ahmed, N. (2014). Dermatological Disease Detection Using Image Processing and Artificial Neural Network. *8th International Conference on Electrical and Computer Engineering*, 687-690. 10.1109/ICECE.2014.7026918

Rahman, S., Irfan, M., Raza, M., Ghori, K. M., Yaqoob, S., & Awais, M. (2020). Performance analysis of boosting classifiers in recognizing activities of daily living. *International Journal of Environmental Research and Public Health*, *17*(3), 1082. Advance online publication. doi:10.3390/ijerph17031082 PMID:32046302

Rajabi Shishvan, O., Zois, D.-S., & Soyata, T. (2018). Machine Intelligence in Healthcare and Medical Cyber Physical Systems: A Survey. *IEEE Access : Practical Innovations, Open Solutions*, *6*, 46419–46494. doi:10.1109/ACCESS.2018.2866049

Rawat, D., Dixit, V., Gulati, S., Gulati, S., & Gulati, A. (2021). Impact of COVID-19 Outbreak on Lifestyle Behaviour: A Review of Studies Published in India. *Diabetes & metabolic Syndrome*, *15*(1), 331–336.

Rawat, D., Dixit, V., Gulati, S., Gulati, S., & Gulati, A. (2021). Impact of COVID-19 Outbreak on Lifestyle Behaviour: A Review of Studies Published in India. *Diabetes & Metabolic Syndrome, 15*(1), 331–336.

Reddy, S., Fox, J., & Purohit, M. P. (2019). Artificial intelligence-enabled healthcare delivery. *Journal of the Royal Society of Medicine*, *112*(1), 22–28. doi:10.1177/0141076818815510 PMID:30507284

Reed, T. S., David, P., Baumgart, D. C., Sadowski, D. C., Fedorak, R. N., & Kroeker, K. I. (2020). An overview of clinical decision support systems: Benefits,risks, and strategies for success. *Digital Medicine*, 10. PMID:32047862

Rodríguez Martín-Doimeadios, R. C., Berzas Nevado, J. J., Guzmán Bernardo, F. J., Jiménez Moreno, M., Arrifano, G. P. F., Herculano, A. M., do Nascimento, J. L. M., & Crespo-López, M. E. (2014, March 5). Comparative study of mercury speciation in commercial fishes of the Brazilian Amazon. *Environmental Science and Pollution Research International*. Advance online publication. doi:10.100711356-014-2680-7 PMID:24590602

Rodríguez-Mazahua, L., Rodríguez-Enríquez, C.-A., Sánchez-Cervantes, J. L., Cervantes, J., García-Alcaraz, J. L., & Alor-Hernández, G. (2016). A general perspective of big data: Applications, tools, challenges and trends. *The Journal of Supercomputing, 72*(8), 3073–3113. doi:10.100711227-015-1501-1

Roslan, Razly, Sabri, & Ibrahim. (2020). Evaluation of Psoriasis Skin Disease Classification using Convolutional Neural Network. *IAES International Journal of Artificial Intelligence, 9*(2), 349-355.

Roy, A., Singh, B. K., Banchhor, S.K., & Verma, K. (2021). *Segmentation of malignant tumours in mammogram images: A hybrid approach using convolutional neural networks and connected component analysis.* doi:10.1111/exsy.12826

Roy. (2020). *Prediction and Spread Visualization of Covid-19 Pandemic using Machine Learning.* doi: . doi:10.20944/preprints202005.0147.v1

Rubin, R., & Strayer, D. S. (Eds.). (2008). *Environmental and Nutritional pathology. Rubins pathology; Clinico pathologic Foundations of Medicine* (5th ed.). LippincotWilliams & Wilkins.

Rucker, M. (2020). The Smart Home: Can It Replace Traditional Health Care? *Verywell Health*, 8.

Ruder, S. (2016). *An Overview of Gradient Descent Optimization Algorithms.* arXiv preprint arXiv:1609.04747.

Ruman, M. R., & A. B. (2020). IoT Based Emergency Health Monitoring System. *International Conference on Industry 4.0 Technology (I4Tech)*, 159-162.

Ruman, M. R., Barua, A., Rahman, W., Jahan, K. R., Roni, M. J., & Rahman, M. F. (2020, February). IoT based emergency health monitoring system. In *2020 International Conference on Industry 4.0 Technology (I4Tech)* (pp. 159-162). IEEE. 10.1109/I4Tech48345.2020.9102647

Rumelhart, D. E., Hinton, G. E., & Williams, R. J. (1986). Learning representations by back-propagating errors. *Nature, 323*(6088), 533-536.

Russell, S. J. (2003). *Artificial Intelligence: A Modern Approach* (2nd ed.). Prentice Hall.

Sagirova, Z., Kuznetsova, N., Gogiberidze, N., Gognieva, D., Suvorov, A., Chomakhidze, P., Omboni, S., Saner, H., & Kopylov, P. (2021). Cuffless blood pressure measurement using a smartphone-case based ecg monitor with photoplethysmography in hypertensive patients. *Sensors, 21*, 3525. doi:10.3390/s21103525

Saha, H. N., Auddy, S., Pal, S., Kumar, S., Pandey, S., Singh, R., Singh, A. K., Sharan, P., Ghosh, D., & Saha, S. (2017, August). Health monitoring using internet of things (IoT). In *2017 8th Annual Industrial Automation and Electromechanical Engineering Conference (IEMECON)* (pp. 69-73). IEEE.

Sahu, S. P., Londhe, N. D., Verma, S., Singh, B. K., & Banchhor, S. K. (2020). Improved pulmonary lung nodules risk stratification in computed tomography images by fusing shape and texture features in a machine-learning paradigm. *International Journal of Imaging Systems and Technology, 31*(3), 1503–1518. doi:10.1002/ima.22539

Salari, N., Hosseinian-Far, A., Jalali, R., Vaisi-Raygani, A., Rasoulpoor, S., Mohammadi, M., ... Khaledi-Paveh, B. (2020). Prevalence of stress, anxiety, depression among the general population during the COVID-19 pandemic: A systematic review and meta-analysis. *Globalization and Health*, *16*(1), 1–11.

Salem, A.-B. M. (2020). Computational Intelligence for Digital Healthcare. *CEUR*, 15.

Sangeetha, D., & Deepa, P. (2016). An Efficient Hardware Implementation of Canny Edge Detection Algorithm. *29th International Conference on VLSI Design and 2016 15th International Conference on Embedded Systems (VLSID)*, 457-462.

Sanuki, H., Rui Fukui, T., & Warisawa, S. (2017). Cuffless calibration free blood pressure estimation under ambulatory environment using pulse wave velocity and photoplethysmogram signal. *Proceedings of 10ᵗʰ International conference on biomedical engineering system and technology and application (BIOESTEC 2017)*. 10.5220/0006112500420048

Sapna Singh kshatri Verified reviews. (2020). Academic Press.

Saritha, B., Giri, A., & Reddy, T. S. (2014). Direct spectrophotometric determination of Pb (II) in alloy, biological and water samples using 5-bromo-2-hydroxyl -3-methoxybenzaldehyde-4-hydroxy benzoichydrazone. *Journal of Chemical and Pharmaceutical Research*, *6*(7), 1571–1576.

Sarkar, B. K. (2017). Big data for secure healthcare system: A conceptual design. *Complex & Intelligent Systems*, *3*(2), 133–151. doi:10.100740747-017-0040-1

Scarpone, C., Brinkmann, S. T., Große, T., Sonnenwald, D., Fuchs, M., & Walker, B. B. (2020). A multimethod approach for county-scale geospatial analysis of emerging infectious diseases: A cross-sectional case study of COVID-19 incidence in Germany. *International Journal of Health Geographics*, *19*(1), 1–17. doi:10.118612942-020-00225-1 PMID:32791994

Schubert, C., Lambertz, M., Nelesen, R. A., Bardwell, W., Choi, J. B., & Dimsdale, J. E. (2009). Effects of stress on heart rate complexity—A comparison between short-term and chronic stress. *Biological Psychology*, *80*(3), 325–332.

Schuller, B., Friedmann, F., & Eyben, F. (2013, May). Automatic recognition of physiological parameters in the human voice: Heart rate and skin conductance. In *2013 IEEE International Conference on Acoustics, Speech and Signal Processing* (pp. 7219-7223). IEEE.

Sengupta, M., Roy, A., Ganguly, A., Baishya, K., Chakrabarti, S., & Mukhopadhyay, I. (2021, June 1). Challenges Encountered by Healthcare Providers in COVID-19 Times: An Exploratory Study. *Journal of Health Management*, *23*(2), 339–356. doi:10.1177/09720634211011695

Sen, P. C., Hajra, M., & Ghosh, M. (2020). Supervised Classification Algorithms in Machine Learning: A Survey and Review. In J. Mandal & D. Bhattacharya (Eds.), *Emerging Technology in Modelling and Graphics. Advances in Intelligent Systems and Computing* (Vol. 937). Springer. doi:10.1007/978-981-13-7403-6_11

Seshadri, M. S., Seshadri, M. S., & John, T. J. (2020, April 4). Hospital Readiness for COVID-19: The Scenario from India with Suggestions for the world. *Christian Journal for Global Health*, *7*(1), 33–36. doi:10.15566/cjgh.v7i1.375

Sethy, P. K., & Behera, S. K. (2020). *Detection of coronavirus disease (covid-19) based on deep features*. Academic Press.

Shahamiri, S. R., & Thabtah, F. (2020). Autism AI: A new autism screening system based on Artificial Intelligence. *Cognitive Computation*, *12*(4), 766–777. doi:10.100712559-020-09743-3

Shahbazi, Z., & Byun, Y.-C. (2020). Towards a Secure Thermal-Energy Aware Routing Protocol in Wireless Body Area Network Based on Blockchain Technology. *Sensors (Basel)*, *20*(12), 3604. doi:10.339020123604 PMID:32604851

Shahbazi, Z., & Byun, Y.-C. (2021). Improving Transactional Data System Based on an Edge Computing–Blockchain–Machine Learning Integrated Framework. *Processes (Basel, Switzerland)*, *9*(1), 92. doi:10.3390/pr9010092

Shakeel, V. T. (2017). Monitoring Health Care System Using Internet of Things - An Immaculate Pairing. *International Conference on Next Generation Computing and Information Systems (ICNGCIS)*, 153-158.

Shanmuganathan, S. (2016). Artificial Neural Network Modelling: An Introduction. In Series in Artificial Neural Network Modelling (pp. 1-14). Springer. doi:10.1007/978-3-319-28495-8_1

U. S. Shanthamallu, A. Spanias, C. Tepedelenlioglu, & M. Stanley (Eds.). (2017). A Brief Survey of Machine Learning Methods and Their Sensor and IoT Applications. In *Proceeding of the 8th International Conference on Information, Intelligence, Systems & Applications (IISA)*. IEEE. 10.1109/IISA.2017.8316459

Sharma, S., & Yoon, W. (in press). *Multiobjective Reinforcement Learning Based Energy Consumption in C-RAN enabled Massive MIMO*. Academic Press.

Sharma, R. K., Agrawal, M., & Marshall, F. M. (2009). Heavy Metals in Vegetables Collected from Production and Market Sites of a Tropical Urban Area of India. *Food and Chemical Toxicology*, *47*(3), 583–591. doi:10.1016/j.fct.2008.12.016 PMID:19138719

Sharma, S., Srivastava, S., Kumar, A., & Dangi, A. (2018). Multi-Class Sentiment Analysis Comparison Using Support Vector Machine (SVM) and BAGGING Technique-An Ensemble Method. *2018 International Conference on Smart Computing and Electronic Enterprise (ICSCEE)*, 1–6. 10.1109/ICSCEE.2018.8538397

Sharma, S., & Yoon, W. (2018). Multi-objective energy efficient resource allocation for WPCN. *International Journal of Engineering Research & Technology (Ahmedabad)*, *11*, 2035–2043.

Sharma, S., & Yoon, W. (2019). Multiobjective Optimization for Energy Efficiency in Cloud Radio Access Networks. *International Journal of Engineering Research & Technology (Ahmedabad)*, *12*(5), 607–610.

Sharma, S., & Yoon, W. (2021). Multiobjective Optimization for Resource Allocation in Full-duplex Large Distributed MIMO Systems. *Advances in Electrical and Computer Engineering*, *21*(2), 67–74. doi:10.4316/AECE.2021.02008

Sharma, Y., & Singh, B. K. (2022). One-dimensional convolutional neural network and hybrid deep-learning paradigm for classification of specific language impaired children using their speech. *Computer Methods and Programs in Biomedicine*, *213*, 106487. doi:10.1016/j.cmpb.2021.106487 PMID:34763173

Sharmin, M., Ahmed, S., Ahamed, S. I., Haque, M. M., & Khan, A. J. (2006, March). Healthcare aide: towards a virtual assistant for doctors using pervasive middleware. In *Fourth Annual IEEE International Conference on Pervasive Computing and Communications Workshops (PERCOMW'06)*. IEEE. 10.1109/PERCOMW.2006.63

Shekhawat, K., Chatterjee, S., & Joshi, B. (2015). Chromium Toxicity and its Health Hazards. *International Journal of Advanced Research*, *3*(7), 167–172.

Shemirani, F., Baghdadi, M., Ramezani, M., & Jamali, M. R. (2005). Determination of ultra trace amounts of bismuth in biological and water samples by electrothermal atomic absorption spectrometry (ET-AAS) after cloud point extraction. *Analytica Chimica Acta*, *534*(1), 163–169. doi:10.1016/j.aca.2004.06.036

Shi, H., Han, X., Jiang, N., Cao, Y., Alwalid, O., Gu, J., Fan, Y., & Zheng, C. (2020). Radiological findings from 81 patients with COVID-19 pneumonia in Wuhan, China: A descriptive study. *The Lancet. Infectious Diseases*, *20*(4), 425–434. doi:10.1016/S1473-3099(20)30086-4 PMID:32105637

Shi, L. (2013). Learning theory estimates for coefficient-based regularized regression. *Applied and Computational Harmonic Analysis, Elsevier*, *34*(2), 252–265. doi:10.1016/j.acha.2012.05.001

Shimizu, K. (2020). 2019-nCoV, fake news, and racism. *Lancet*, *395*(10225), 685–686. doi:10.1016/S0140-6736(20)30357-3 PMID:32059801

Shinde, P. P., & Shah, S., Dr. (Eds.) (2018). A Review of Machine Learning and Deep Learning Applications. In *Proceeding of the 2018 Fourth International Conference on Computing Communication Control and Automation (ICCUBEA)*. IEEE. 10.1109/ICCUBEA.2018.8697857

Shirvanimoghaddam, M., Dohler, M., & Johnson, S. J. (2017). Massive non-orthogonal multiple access for cellular IoT: Potentials and limitations. *IEEE Communications Magazine*, *55*(9), 55–61. doi:10.1109/MCOM.2017.1600618

Shorten, C., & Khoshgoftaar, T. M. (2019). A Survey on Image Data Augmentation for Deep Learning. *Journal of Big Data*, *6*(1), 1–48. doi:10.118640537-019-0197-0

Singh, A., Thakur, N., & Sharma, A. (2016). A review of supervised machine learning algorithms. *Proceedings of the 2016 3rd International Conference on Computing for Sustainable Global Development*, 1310–1315.

Compilation of References

Singhal, Y., Jain, A., Batra, S., Varshney, Y., & Rathi, M. (2018). Review of Bagging and Boosting Classification Performance on Unbalanced Binary Classification. *2018 IEEE 8th International Advance Computing Conference (IACC)*, 338–343. 10.1109/IADCC.2018.8692138

Singhal, T. (2020). A review of coronavirus disease-2019 (COVID-19). *Indian Journal of Pediatrics*, *87*(4), 281–286. doi:10.100712098-020-03263-6 PMID:32166607

Singh, B. K., Verma, K., & Thoke, A. S. (2015). Investigations on impact of feature normalization techniques on classifier's performance in breast tumor classification. *International Journal of Computers and Applications*, *116*(19).

G. Singh, B. Kumar, L. Gaur, & A. Tyagi (Eds.). (2019). Comparison between multinomial and Bernoulli naïve Bayes for text classification. In *Proceeding of the 2019 International Conference on Automation, Computational and Technology Management (ICACTM)*. IEEE. 10.1109/ICACTM.2019.8776800

Singh, K., Raghav, P., Singh, G., Pritish Baskaran, T. B., Bishnoi, A., Gautam, V., Chaudhary, A. K., Kumar, A., Kumar, S., & Sahu, S. (2021). Lifestyle and Behavioral Changes During Nationwide Lockdown in India-A Cross-Sectional Analysis. *Journal of Family Medicine and Primary Care*, *10*(7), 2661–2667. doi:10.4103/jfmpc.jfmpc_2464_20 PMID:34568152

Skopin, D., & Baglikov, S. (2009, June). Heartbeat feature extraction from vowel speech signal using 2D spectrum representation. *Proc. the 4th Int. Conf. Information Technology*.

Skowronski, D. M. (2005). Article. *Annual Review of Medicine*, *56*(1), 357–381. doi:10.1146/annurev.med.56.091103.134135 PMID:15660517

Smith, A., Goycolea, M., Haque, R., & Bigs, M. L. (1998). Marked increase in bladder and lung cancer mortality in a region of northern Chile due to arsenic in drinking water. *American Journal of Epidemiology*, *147*(7), 660–669. doi:10.1093/oxfordjournals.aje.a009507 PMID:9554605

Sokol, R. Z., & Berman, N. (1991). The effect of age of exposure on lead-inducedtesticular toxicity. *Toxicology*, *69*(3), 269–278. doi:10.1016/0300-483X(91)90186-5 PMID:1949051

Soliman, N. (2019). A Method of Skin Disease Detection Using Image Processing and Machine Learning. *Procedia Computer Science*, *163*, 85–92.

Srinivasu, SivaSai, Ijaz, Bhoi, Kim, & Kang. (2021). Classification of Skin Disease Using Deep Learning Neural Networks with MobileNet V2 and LSTM. *Sensors (Basel)*, *21*(8), 2852–2879.

Srivastava, P. K., Han, D., Rico-Ramirez, M. A., Bray, M., & Islam, T. (2012). Selection of Classification Techniques for Land Use / Land Cover Change Investigation. *Advances in Space Research*, *50*(9), 1250–1265. doi:10.1016/j.asr.2012.06.032

Steele, G. S. (2004). oriented approach to DNA computing. *Proc. of Computational Systems Bioinformatics Conference*, 546-551.

Steenland, K., & Boffetta, P. (2000). Lead and cancer in humans: Where are we now. *American Journal of Industrial Medicine, 38*(3), 295–299. doi:10.1002/1097-0274(200009)38:3<295::AID-AJIM8>3.0.CO;2-L PMID:10940967

Sultan, N. (2015). Reflective thoughts on the potential and challenges of wearable technology for healthcare provision and medical education. *International Journal of Information Management, 35*(5), 521–526. doi:10.1016/j.ijinfomgt.2015.04.010

Sundaravadivel, P., Kougianos, E., Mohanty, S. P., & Ganapathiraju, M. K. (2017). Everything you wanted to know about smart health care: Evaluating the different technologies and components of the internet of things for better health. *IEEE Consumer Electronics Magazine, 7*(1), 18–28. doi:10.1109/MCE.2017.2755378

Surakratanasakul, K. P. (2017). A study of integration Internet of Things with health level 7 protocol for real-time healthcare monitoring by using cloud computing. *10th Biomedical Engineering International Conference (BMEiCON)*, 1-5.

Swapnarekha, H., Behera, H. S., Nayak, J., & Naik, B. (2020). Role of intelligent computing in COVID-19 prognosis: A state-of-the-art review. *Chaos, Solitons, and Fractals, 138*, 109947. doi:10.1016/j.chaos.2020.109947 PMID:32836916

Taccone, S. F., Gorham, J., & Vincent, J. L. (2020). Hydroxy chloroquine in the management of critically ill patients with COVID-19: The need for an evidence base. *The Lancet. Respiratory Medicine, 8*(6), 539–541. doi:10.1016/S2213-2600(20)30172-7 PMID:32304640

Taheri, S., & Mammadov, M. (2013). Learning the Naïve Bayes Classifier With Optimization Models. *International Journal of Applied Mathematics and Computer Science, 23*(4), 787–795. doi:10.2478/amcs-2013-0059

Tamilselvi, V., & S. S. (2020). IoT Based Health Monitoring System. *International Conference on Advanced Computing and Communication Systems (ICACCS)*, 385-389.

Tayarani, N. M.-H. (2021). Applications of artificial intelligence in battling against covid-19: A literature review. Chaos, Solitons, and Fractals, 142, 110338. doi:10.1016/j.chaos.2020.110338 PubMed doi:10.1016/j.chaos.2020.110338 PMID:33041533

Tchounwou, P. B., Centeno, J. A., & Patlolla, A. K. (2004). Arsenic toxicity, mutagenesis and carcinogenesis – a health risk assessment and management approach. *Molecular and Cellular Biochemistry, 255*(1/2), 47–55. doi:10.1023/B:MCBI.0000007260.32981.b9 PMID:14971645

Tchounwou, P. B., Wilson, B., & Ishaque, A. (1999). Important considerations in the development of public health advisories for arsenic and arsenic-containing compounds in drinking water. *Reviews on Environmental Health, 14*(4), 211–229. doi:10.1515/REVEH.1999.14.4.211 PMID:10746734

Tchounwou, P. B., Wilson, B., & Ishaque, A. (2000). *Important considerations in the development of public TP-92/09. Georgia.* Center for Disease Control.

Thayer, J. F. (2009). *Heart rate variability: A neurovisceral integration model.* Academic Press.

Tian, S., Yang, W., Le Grange, J. M., Wang, P., Huang, W., & Ye, Z. (2019). Smart healthcare: Making medical care more intelligent. *Global Health Journal*, *3*(3), 62–65. doi:10.1016/j. glohj.2019.07.001

Tibor, V., Varga, T. V., Bu, F., Dissin, A. S., Elsenburg, L. K., Bustamante, J. J. H., Matta, J., Zon, S. K. R. V., Brouwer, S., Beultmann, U., Fancourt, D., Hoeyer, K., Goldberg, M., Melchior, M., Larsen, K. S., Zins, M., Clotworthy, A., & Rod, N. H. (2021). Loneliness, worries, anxiety, and precautionary behaviors in response to the COVID-19 pandemic: A longitudinal analysis of 200,000 Western and Northern Europeans. *The Lancet Regional Health - Europe*, *2*, 1–9.

Tikka, S. K., Singh, B. K., Nizamie, S. H., Garg, S., Mandal, S., Thakur, K., & Singh, L. K. (2020). Artificial intelligence-based classification of schizophrenia: A high density electroencephalographic and support vector machine study. *Indian Journal of Psychiatry*, *62*(3), 273. doi:10.4103/psychiatry. IndianJPsychiatry_91_20 PMID:32773870

Tjajjadi, H., & Ramli, K. (2020). Noninvasive blood pressure classification based on photoplethysmography using K-nearest neighbors algorithm: A feasible study. *Information*, *11*(93). . doi:10.3390/info11020093

Trivedi, R. K. (1990). Physicochemical characteristic and Phytoplankton of the river Panchganga near Kolhapur, Maharashtra. In K. Trivedi (Ed.), *River pollution on India* (pp. 159–178). Ashish Publishing House.

Tromberg, B. J., Schwetz, T. A., Pérez-Stable, E. J., Hodes, R. J., Woychik, R. P., Bright, R. A., Fleurence, R. L., & Collins, F. S. (2020). Rapid Scaling Up of Covid-19 Diagnostic Testing in the United States— The NIH RADx Initiative. *The New England Journal of Medicine*, *383*(11), 1071–1077. doi:10.1056/NEJMsr2022263 PMID:32706958

Tsai, C.-W., Lai, C.-F., Chao, H.-C., & Vasilakos, A. (2015). Big data analytics: A survey. *Journal of Big Data*, *2*(1), 21. doi:10.118640537-015-0030-3 PMID:26191487

Uddin, M. S., & J. B. (2017). Real time patient monitoring system based on Internet of Things. *International Conference on Advances in Electrical Engineering (ICAEE)*, 516-521. 10.1109/ ICAEE.2017.8255410

UNDP (United Nations Development Programme). (2006). *Human Development Report 2006. Beyond scarcity Power, Povertyh and the global water crises*. Available at http//hdr.undp.org/ hdr2006/

UNICEF. (2008). *UNICEF Hnad book on Water Quality*. Available at: www.uniceforg/wes/files/ WQ_Handbook_final_signed_16_April_2008.

UNICEF. (2011). *Official Homepage of UNICEF Promotion of household water treatment and safe storage m UNICEF wash programmes 2011*. http.www.unicef.org

Unnithan, P. S. G. (2020). Kerala Reports First Confirmed Coronavirus Case in India. *India Today*. Available online at: https://www.indiatoday.in/india/ story/kerala-reports-first-confirmed-novel-coronavirus-case-in-india1641593-2020-01-30

USFDA Press Announcement. (2020). *Coronavirus (COVID-19) Update: FDA Issues Emergency Use Authorization for Potential COVID-19 Treatment*. Available online at: https://www.fda.gov/news-events/press-announcements/coronavirus-covid-19-update-fda-issues-emergency-use-authorizationpotential-covid-19-treatment

Usman, S. (2019). Second Derivative and Contour Analysis of PPG for Diabetic Patients. *2018 IEEE EMBS Conference on Biomedical Engineering and Sciences, IECBES 2018 – Proceedings*, 59–62.

Vaishya, R., Javaid, M., Khan, I. H., & Haleem, A. (2020). Artificial Intelligence (AI) applications for COVID-19 pandemic. *Diabetes & Metabolic Syndrome*, *14*(4), 337–339. doi:10.1016/j.dsx.2020.04.012 PMID:32305024

Vapnik, V. N. (2000). *The Nature of Statistical Learning Theory*. Springer Science. doi:10.1007/978-1-4757-3264-1

Velasco, Pascion, Alberio, Apuang, Cruz, & Gomez, Molina, Tuala, Thio-ac, & Jorda. (2019). A Smartphone-Based Skin Disease Classification Using MobileNet CNN. *International Journal of Advanced Trends in Computer Science and Engineering*, *8*(5), 2632–2637.

Venugopal, B., & Lucky, T. D. (1978). *Metal Toxicity in Mammals*. Plenum Press.

Verdhan, V. (2020). Supervised Learning with Python. Apress. doi:10.1007/978-1-4842-6156-9

Veslind, P. J. (1993). '·National Geographic Senior Writer. *National Geographic*, *5*, 183.

Vezhnevets, V., Sazonov, V., & Andreeva, A. (2003). A Survey on Pixel-based Skin Colour Detection Techniques. *Proceedings of International Conference Graphicon*, 85-92.

Vick, D. J., Wilsom, A. B., & Fisher, M. (2018). Assessment of community hospital disaster preparedness in New York State. *Journal of Emergency Management (Weston, Mass.)*, *16*, 213–227. doi:10.5055/jem.2018.0371 PMID:30234908

Vidya, M., & Karki, M. V. (2020). *Skin Cancer Detection using Machine Learning Techniques*. IEEE.

Vigneshvar, S., Sudhakumari, C. C., Senthilkumaran, B., & Prakash, H. (2016). Recent advances in biosensor technology for potential applications–an overview. *Frontiers in Bioengineering and Biotechnology*, *4*, 11. doi:10.3389/fbioe.2016.00011 PMID:26909346

Vincent, J. L., & Taccone, F. S. (2020). Understanding pathways to death in patients with COVID-19. *The Lancet. Respiratory Medicine*, *8*(5), 430–432. doi:10.1016/S2213-2600(20)30165-X PMID:32272081

Vollenweidre, R. A. (1986). *Scientific fundamental of the eutrophication of lakes and flowing waters v-rith special reference to nitrogen and phosphorus as factoring eutrophication*. OECD.

Compilation of References

Von Ehrenstein, O. S., GuhaMazumder, D. N., Hira-Smith, M., Ghosh, N., Yuan, Y., Windham, G., Ghosh, A., Haque, R., Lahiri, S., Kalman, D., Das, S., & Smith, A. H. (2006). Pregnancy outcomes, infant mortality, and arsenic in drinking water in west Bengal, India. *American Journal of Epidemiology*, *163*(7), 662–669. doi:10.1093/aje/kwj089 PMID:16524957

Waldron, H. A. (1983). Did the Mad Hatter have mercury poisoning? *British Medical Journal (Clinical Research Ed.)*, *287*(6409), 1961. doi:10.1136/bmj.287.6409.1961 PMID:6418283

Wang, Huang, & Chen. (2016). Preprocessing of PPG and ECG Signal to estimate blood pressure based on noninvasive wearable device. *Proceeding of International conference on engineering technology and application (ICETA 2016)*.

Wang, J. J. Y. (2021). Design of Cloud Computing Platform Based Accurate Measurement for Structure Monitoring Using Fiber Bragg Grating Sensors. *IEEE 2nd International Conference on Big Data, Artificial Intelligence and Internet of Things Engineering (ICBAIE)*, 807-811.

Wang, J., Li, P., Ran, R., Che, Y., & Zhou, Y. (2018). A Short-Term Photovoltaic Power Prediction Model Based on the Gradient Boost Decision Tree. *Applied Sciences (Basel, Switzerland)*, *8*(5), 689. Advance online publication. doi:10.3390/app8050689

Wang, L., Lin, Z. Q., & Wong, A. (2020). Covid-net: A tailored deep convolutional neural network design for detection of covid-19 cases from chest x-ray images. *Scientific Reports*, *10*(1), 1–12. doi:10.103841598-020-76550-z PMID:33177550

T. Wang, & W. H. Li (Eds.). (2010). Naïve Bayes Software Defect Prediction Model. In *Proceeding of 2010 International Conference on Computational Intelligence and Software Engineering*. IEEE. 10.1109/CISE.2010.5677057

Waveform DatabaseMIMICII. (2012). https://physionet.org/mimic2/mimic2_waveform_overview.shtml

Weenink, D. (2014). Speech signal processing with Praat. *Haettu*, *16*.

Wei, H. C., Xiao, M.-X., Chen, H.-Y., Li, Y.-Q., Wu, H.-T., & Sun, C.-K. (2018). Instantaneous Frequency from Hilbert-Huang Transformation of Digital Volume Pulse as Indicator of Diabetes and Arterial Stiffness in Upper-Middle-Aged Subjects. *Scientific Reports*, *8*(1), 1–8. doi:10.103841598-018-34091-6 PMID:30361528

Weston, D. I. A., & Amlot, R. (2020). Examining the Application of Behavior Change Theories in the Context of Infectious Disease Outbreaks and Emergency Response: A Review of Reviews. *BMC Public Health*, *20*(1), 1–19. doi:10.118612889-020-09519-2 PMID:33004011

Weston, D., Hauck, K., & Amlot, R. (2018). Infection Prevention Behaviour and Infectious Disease Modeling: A Review of The Literature and Recommendations For The Future. *BMC Public Health*, *18*(1), 336. doi:10.118612889-018-5223-1 PMID:29523125

Weston, D., Ip, A., & Amlot, R. (2020). Examining the Application of Behavior Change Theories in the Context of Infectious Disease Outbreaks and Emergency Response: A Review of Reviews BMC. *Public Health*, *20*, 1–19. PMID:33004011

West, R., Michie, S., Rubin, G. J., & Amlot, R. (2020). Applying Principles of Behavior Change to Reduce SARS-Cov-2 Transmission. *Nature Human Behaviour, 4*(5), 451–459. doi:10.103841562-020-0887-9 PMID:32377018

WHO. (2004). *Guidelines for Drinking-Water Quality, Recommendations.* WHO.

WHO. (2020a). *WHO Disease Outbreak News. Pneumonia of unknown cause – China.* Available online at: https://www.who.int/csr/don/05-january-2020pneumonia-of-unkown-cause-china/en/

WHO. (2020b). *WHO Director-General's Opening Remarks at the Media Briefing on COVID-19 - 11 March 2020.* Available online at: https://www.who.int/ dg/speeches/detail/who-director-general-s-opening-remarks-at-the-mediabriefing-on-covid-19--11-march-2020

Wikipedia. (2020). *2020 Coronavirus Lockdown in India.* Available online at: https://en.wikipedia.org/wiki/2020_coronavirus_lockdown_in_India

Williams, L., Rasmussen, S., Kleczkowski, A., Maharaj, S., & Cairns, N. (2015). Protection Motivation Theory and Social Distancing Behaviour in Response to a Simulated Infectious Disease Epidemic. *Psychology Health and Medicine, 20*(7), 832–837. doi:10.1080/13548506.2015.1028946 PMID:25835044

Wilson, D. N. (1988). Cadmium - market trends and influences. *Proceedings of the 6th International Cadmium Conference*, 9-16.

World Health Organization. (2020). *Middle East respiratory syndrome corona virus.* MERS-CoV.

World Health Organization. (2020). *Pneumonia of unknown cause-China. Emergencies preparedness, response Web site.* WHO.

World Health Organization. (2020c). *WHO Director-General's Opening Remarks at the Media Briefing on COVID-19.* Available online at: https://www.who. int/dg/speeches/detail/who-director-general-s-opening-remarks-at-themedia-briefing-on-covid-19---11-march-2020

World Health Organization. (2020d). *Coronavirus Disease 2019 (COVID-19) Situation Report-51.* Available online at: https://www.who.int/docs/defaultsource/coronaviruse/situation-reports/20200311-sitrep-51-covid-19.pdf? sfvrsn=1ba62e57_10

World Health Organization. (2020e). *Modes of Transmission of Virus Causing COVID19: Implications for IPC Precaution Recommendations: Scientific Brief.* World Health Organization. Available online at: WHO/2019-nCoV/ Sci_Brief/Transmission_modes/2020.2

World Health Organization. (2020f). *Coronavirus Disease 2019 (COVID-19) Situation Report-43.* Available online at: https://www.who.int/docs/defaultsource/coronaviruse/situation-reports/20200303-sitrep-43-covid-19.pdf? sfvrsn=76e425ed_2

World Health Organization. (2020g). *Coronavirus Disease 2019 (COVID-19) Situation Report-47.* Available online at: https://www.who.int/docs/defaultsource/coronaviruse/situation-reports/20200307-sitrep-47-covid-19.pdf? sfvrsn=27c364a4_4

World Health Organization. (2020h). *Coronavirus Disease 2019 (COVID-19) Situation Report−53*. Available online at: https://www.who.int/docs/defaultsource/coronaviruse/situation-reports/20200313-sitrep-53-covid-19.pdf? sfvrsn=adb3f72_2

World Health Organization. (2020i). *Coronavirus Disease (COVID-19) Advice for the Public*. Available online at: https://www.who.int/emergencies/diseases/ novel-coronavirus-2019/advice-for-public

World Health Organization. (2020j). *Q & A on Coronaviruses (COVID-19)*. Available online at: https://www.who.int/news-room/q-a-detail/q-acoronaviruses

World Health organization. (2020k). *Coronavirus Disease 2019 (COVID-19) Situation Report-153*. Available online at: https://www.who.int/docs/defaultsource/coronaviruse/situation-reports/20200621-covid-19-sitrep-153.pdf? sfvrsn=c896464d_2

World Health Organization. (2021). *Medical doctors (per 10,000)*. Retrieved from https://www.who.int/data/gho/data/indicators/indicator-details/GHO/medical-doctors-(per-10-000-population)

Wu, F., Zhao, S., Yu, B., Chen, Y. M., Wang, W., Song, Z. G., & Zhang, Y. Z. (2020). A new coronavirus associated with human respiratory disease in China. *Nature*, *579*(7798), 265–269. doi:10.103841586-020-2008-3 PMID:32015508

Wu, H., Huangc, J., Casper, J. P. Z., Zonglin, H., & Ming, W. K. (2020). Facemask shortage and the novel coronavirus disease (COVID-19) outbreak: Reflections on public health measures. *EClinicalMedicine*, *21*, 100329. doi:10.1016/j.eclinm.2020.100329 PMID:32292898

Wu, J., Wang, J., Nicholas, S., Maitland, E., & Fan, Q. (2020). Application of big data technology for COVID-19 prevention and control in China: Lessons and recommendations. *Journal of Medical Internet Research*, *22*(10), e21980. Advance online publication. doi:10.2196/21980 PMID:33001836

Wu, Y., Ianakiev, K., & Govindaraju, V. (2002). Improved K-Nearest Neighbor Classification. *Pattern Recognition, Elsevier*, *35*(10), 2311–2318. doi:10.1016/S0031-3203(01)00132-7

Xie, X., Zhong, Z., Zhao, W., Zheng, C., Wang, F., & Liu, J. (2020). Chest CT for Typical Coronavirus Disease 2019 (COVID-19) Pneumonia: Relationship to Negative RT-PCR Testing. *Radiology*, *296*(2), E41–E45. doi:10.1148/radiol.2020200343 PMID:32049601

Xiong, Y., & Z. J. (2019). Research on Health Condition Assessment Method for Spacecraft Power Control System Based on SVM and Cloud Model. *Prognostics and System Health Management Conference (PHM-Paris)*, 143-149. 10.1109/PHM-Paris.2019.00032

Xu, B., & L. X. (2014). Architecture of M-Health Monitoring System Based on Cloud Computing for Elderly Homes Application. *Enterprise Systems Conference*, 45-50. 10.1109/ES.2014.11

Yadav, S., & Jadhav, S. (2019). Machine Learning Algorithms for Disease Prediction Using IoT Environment. *International Journal of Engineering and Advanced Technology*, *8*(6), 8. doi:10.35940/ijeat.F8914.088619

Yamaguchi, S., Sano, K., & Shimojo, N. (1983). On the biological half-time of hexavalent chromium in rats. *Industrial Health*, *21*(1), 25–34. doi:10.2486/indhealth.21.25 PMID:6841147

Yaman, E., & Subasi, A. (2019). Comparison of Bagging and Boosting Ensemble Machine Learning Methods for Automated EMG Signal Classification. *BioMed Research International*, *2019*, 9152506. doi:10.1155/2019/9152506 PMID:31828145

Yang, Z., Zhou, Q., Lei, L., Zheng, K., & Xiang, W. (2016). An IoT-cloud based wearable ECG monitoring system for smart healthcare. *Journal of Medical Systems*, *40*(12), 1–11. doi:10.100710916-016-0644-9 PMID:27796840

Ye, J., Chow, J.-H., Chen, J., & Zheng, Z. (2009). Stochastic gradient boosted distributed decision trees. *Proceedings of the 18th ACM conference on Information and knowledge management—CIKM'09*. 10.1145/1645953.1646301

Yu, W., Liu, T., & Valdez, R. (2010). Application of support vector machine modeling for prediction of common diseases: the case of diabetes and pre-diabetes. *BMC Med Inform Decis Mak, 10*, 16. doi:10.1186/1472-6947-10-16

Yuvaraj, N., & SriPreethaa, K. R. (2017). Diabetes prediction in healthcare systems using machine learning algorithms on Hadoop cluster. *Cluster Computing*, *22*(S1), 1–9. doi:10.100710586-017-1532-x

Zabirul Islam, Md., Milon Islam, Md., & Amanullah, A. (2020). *A combined deep CNN-LSTM network for the detection of novel coronavirus (COVID-19) using X-ray images*. Elsevier.

Zaki, A. M., van Boheemen, S., Bestebroer, T. M., Osterhaus, A. D., & Fouchier, R. A. (2012). Isolation of a novel coronavirus from a man with pneumonia in Saudi Arabia. *The New England Journal of Medicine*, *367*(19), 1814–1820. doi:10.1056/NEJMoa1211721 PMID:23075143

Zaman, C.L. (2002). A Nested Case control study of Methanoglobinemia risk factor in children of Transilvania Romania. *Env. Health Perspt., 110*(B).

Zaqout, I. (2019). *Diagnosis of skin lesions based on Dermoscopic Images Using Image Processing Techniques*. In *Pattern Recognition Selected Methods and Applications*. Intech Open.

Zhang, N., Jia, W., Lei, H., Wang, P., Zhao, P., Guo, Y., Dung, C. H., Bu, Z., Xue, P., Xie, J., Zhang, Y., Cheng, R., & Li, Y. (2019). Effects of Human Behavior Changes During the Coronavirus Disease 2019 (COVID-19) Pandemic on Influenza Spread in Hong Kong. Oxford University Press.

Zhang, S., Li, X., Zong, M., Zhu, X., & Cheng, D. (2017). Learning K for KNN Classification. *ACM Transactions on Intelligent Systems and Technology*, *8*(3), 1–19. doi:10.1145/2990508

Zhang, Y., Xin, J., Li, X., & Huang, S. (2020). Overview on routing and resource allocation based machine learning in optical networks. *Optical Fiber Technology*, *60*, 102355. doi:10.1016/j.yofte.2020.102355

Zhang, Z., & Sabuncu, M. R. (2018, January). Generalized cross entropy loss for training deep neural networks with noisy labels. *32nd Conference on Neural Information Processing Systems (NeurIPS).*

L. Zhao, M. Mammadov, & J. Yearwood (Eds.). (2010). From Convex to Nonconvex: A Loss Function Analysis for Binary Classification. In *Proceeding of the 2010 IEEE International Conference on Data Mining Workshops.* IEEE. 10.1109/ICDMW.2010.57

Zhao, S., Xie, B., Li, Y., Zhao, X., Kuang, Y., Su, J., He, X., Wu, X., Fan, W., Huang, K., Su, J., Peng, Y., Navarini, A., Huang, W., & Chen, X. (2020). Smart Identification of Psoriasis by Images Using Convolutional Neural Networks: A case Study in China. *Journal of the European Academy of Dermatology and Venereology, 34*(3), 518–524.

Zhao, W., Zhong, Z., Xie, X., Yu, Q., & Liu, J. (2020). Relation between chest CT findings and clinical conditions of coronavirus disease (COVID-19) pneumonia: A multicentre study. *AJR. American Journal of Roentgenology, 214*(5), 1072–1077. doi:10.2214/AJR.20.22976 PMID:32125873

Zhao, X., Liu, L., Qi, S., Teng, Y., Li, J., & Qian, W. (2018). Agile convolutional neural network for pulmonary nodule classification using CT images. *International Journal of Computer Assisted Radiology and Surgery, 13*(4), 585–595. doi:10.100711548-017-1696-0 PMID:29473129

Zhong, B. L., Luo, W., Li, H. M., Zhang, Q. Q., Liu, X. G., Li, W. T., & Li, Y. (2020). Knowledge, attitudes, and practices towards COVID-19 among Chinese residents during the rapid rise period of the COVID-19 out break: A quick online cross-sectional survey. *International Journal of Biological Sciences, 16*(10), 1745–1752. doi:10.7150/ijbs.45221 PMID:32226294

Zhu, H., Wu, C. K., Koo, C. H., Tsang, Y. T., Liu, Y., Chi, H. R., & Tsang, K. F. (2019). Smart healthcare in the era of internet-of-things. *IEEE Consumer Electronics Magazine, 8*(5), 26–30. doi:10.1109/MCE.2019.2923929

Zhu, N., Zhang, D., Wang, W., Li, X., Yang, B., Song, J., Zhao, X., Huang, B., Shi, W., Lu, R., Niu, P., Zhan, F., Ma, X., Wang, D., Xu, W., Wu, G., Gao, G. F., & Tan, W. (2020). A novel coronavirus from patients with pneumonia in China, 2019. *The New England Journal of Medicine, 382*(8), 727–733. doi:10.1056/NEJMoa2001017 PMID:31978945

Zou, L., Zheng, J., Miao, C., Mckeown, M. J., & Wang, Z. J. (2017). 3D CNN based automatic diagnosis of attention deficit hyperactivity disorder using functional and structural MRI. *IEEE Access: Practical Innovations, Open Solutions, 5*, 23626–23636. doi:10.1109/ACCESS.2017.2762703

About the Contributors

Sapna Singh Kshatri received the Ph.D. degree from MATS University, Raipur. She has completed her M.C.A. from Rungta College of Eng. & Technology Bhilai, India. She was Assistant Professor in Ashoka Institute technology and management. She is Head of Department Of computer science In Bharti University Durg. She has 5 years of teaching and academic experience. She has over 10 research article chapters and national and international conference papers and received Best Paper Awards in 1 International Conferences, reviewer of several journals. She has delivered more than 5 Keynote/Invited Talks and Chaired many Technical Sessions in International/ national Conferences. She has reviewed many papers in reported journals like IEEE, IET, Oxford. Her research interests include Bio-medical, Machine Learning, and Data Science.

Kavita Thakur received her B.E. (Electrical Engineering) in 1989, M.E. (Electronics & Telecommunication Engineering - Control and Guidance) in 1991, Doctoral degree in Electrical Engineering in 1999 at Pt. Ravishankar Shukla University, Raipur, C.G. and is presently working as Professor in School of Studies in Electronics & Photonics, Pt. Ravishankar Shukla University, Raipur, C.G., Chhattisgarh, India. She has published more than 140 research papers in various National / International Journals and Conferences of repute. She has successively supervised 08 students for the award of Ph. D. degree. Her areas of interest are Speech, Image and Biomedical signal processing. She is member of many Professional bodies viz. ISTE, senior member IEEE, ASI, ACM and APSIPA. She has published 02 books with ISBN 978-3-8465-4338-2 and ISBN 978-3-659-17007-2, LAP LAMBERT Academic Publishing GmbH & Co, Germany. She is recipient of Rashtriya Gaurav Award for year 2010-2011 & 2014 from IIFS, New Delhi, India and Best citizen award for the year 2011 from IPS, New Delhi, India.

Maleika Heenaye Mamode Khan is currently working as Associate Professor at the Department of Software and Information Systems, University of Mauritius. She has obtained her PhD in the field of Computer Science and Engineering, University of Mauritius. She has 15 years of experience in academia and research in many areas of Computer Science and Engineering. Her research interest includes Computer Vision, Medical Image Processing, Artificial Intelligence, Biometrics and Data Analytics. She has published some research papers in various International Journals (Elsevier, PLOS One and Emerald etc.) and in Proceedings of the reputed International/ National Conferences as well. She is active reviewer of various reputed International Journals in his research areas. She has been the head of department and acting Dean of the Faculty. She has also served as member of senate at the University of Mauritius. She has one completed PhD student and is currently supervising several students at masters and PhD level.

Deepak Singh has published over 13 SCI indexed journal articles and more than 15 papers in conference proceedings, book chapter etc received Best Paper Awards in 1 International Conferences. Dr. Singh is recipient of travel grant from CENTURI to present the project proposal at Luminy campus Marseille, France in the year 2019. His research interests include Evolutionary Computation, Machine Learning, Domain adaptation, Protein mining and Data Mining.

G. R. Sinha is Adjunct Professor at International Institute of Information Technology (IIIT) Bangalore and currently deputed as Professor at Myanmar Institute of Information Technology (MIIT) Mandalay Myanmar. He obtained his B.E. (Electronics Engineering) and M.Tech. (Computer Technology) with Gold Medal from National Institute of Technology Raipur. He received his Ph.D. in Electronics & Telecommunication Engineering from Chhattisgarh Swami Vivekanand Technical University Bhilai. He has published 227 research papers in various international and national journals and conferences. He has authored 06 Books including Biometrics published by Wiley India, a subsidiary of John Wiley and Medical Image Processing published by Prentice Hall of India. He has also published 05 Edited books as Editor, such as Cognitive Science-Two Volumes (Elsevier), Optimization Theory (IOP) and Biometrics (Springer). He is active reviewer and editorial member of more than 12 Reputed International Journals such IEEE Transactions on Image Processing, Elsevier Computer Methods and Programs in Biomedicine, Springer Journal of Neural Computing and Applications, etc.

* * *

Mohammed Al Achhab received his PhD in December 2006 from the University of Franche-Comté, Besançon, France, in the field of formal verification of reactive systems. He received a Master degree in July 2003 from University of Franche-Comté, in the field of software engineering and artificial intelligence.

He was Temporary Lecturer and Research Assistant, at the University of Franche-Comté. He was an assistant professor at Faculty of Sciences Dhar El mehraz, Fez from 2007 to 2012. Currently, he is a professor at the National School of Applied Sciences of Tetuan. He is a member of the steering committee of the department of computer sciences and member of the National School board. His research focuses on analysis and validation of business process, natural language processing, case of study Arabic and adaptive e-learning. He is the co-author of more than 20 peer-reviewed publications. To his credit also, is being Member in many scientific associations notably IEEE, innove, and mocit. He has been participating in many national and international scientific and organizing committees. He is the mentor of the IEEE UAE Student Branch since 2015. He is the conference chair of the 2014 and 2016 IEEE CiSt editions.

Khalid A. AlAfandy was born in Sharkia, Egypt, in 1975. He received the B.Sc. degree in Electronic Engineering - Department of Computer Science and Engineering from Menoufia University, Menouf, Egypt, in 1997, the M.Sc. degree in Engineering Science - Department of Computer Science and Engineering was received from Menoufia University, Menouf, Egypt, in 2017, and now he is PhD student in National School for applied Science (ENSA) in Tetouan, Abdelmalek Essaadi University, Tetouan, Morocco. Through his Master research, he had Authored 3 conference Papers and 3 journal papers, and after finishing his Master research he had authored another 1 journal paper. Through his PhD research, he had Authored 2 conference papers, 3 journal papers, and 2 book chapters, there is 1 journal paper is under review. So, the total publications are 5 conference papers, 7 journal papers, and 2 book chapters.

Ankita has completed her post graduation from Pandit Ravishankar Shukla University, Raipur in 2019 and also worked as guest faculty in School of Studies in Electronics and Photonics.

Jaspal Bagga is PhD in Electronics & Telecommunication and presently she is Vice Principal in SSTC, Bhilai.

Astha Bhanot is working as an assistant professor in the Business Administration Department, College of Business Administration, Princess Nourah bint Abdulrahman University. She has experience of 14 years in teaching and research.

Devanand Bhonsle completed his B.E in Electronics & Telecommunication in 2004 and M.E in Communication(ETC) in 2008.He received his PhD in Electronics & Telecommunication Engineering in 2019 from CSVTU.

Mukesh Kumar Chandrakar is working as Assistant Professor in Bhilai Institute of Technology Durg, Chhattisgarh, India. He has been pursuing his Doctoral Research in the area of Medical Image Diagnosis. He holds M.Tech. degree from Chhattisgarh Swami Vivekaknand Technical University Bhilai.

Neha Dewangan received her B.Sc. degree with first class in Electronics in 2013 and M.Sc. degree with first class in Electronics in 2015 from Pt. Ravishankar Shukla University, Raipur. She is currently working as a Guest lecturer at the School of Studies in Electronics and Photonics, Pt. Ravishankar Shukla University, Raipur. Her research interests include image processing, pattern recognition and biomedical signal processing.

Thomas George obtained his Bachelor's degree in Electronics from Cochin University of Science and Technology, Kerala in 1999. Then he obtained his Master's of Engineering Degree in Applied Electronics from Bharathiar University, Coimbatore in 2001. He is currently working as an Assistant Professor in the Department of Applied Electronics and Instrumentation at Mount Zion College of Engineering, Kadammanitta, APJ Abdul Kalam Technological University, Kerala and is pursuing a PhD from Sathyabama Institute of Science & Technology, Chennai. His specialization includes Advanced Communication, Space Technology, Control Engineering, Embedded Systems, and Instrumentation. His current research interests are Control Engineering, Instrumentation and Space Technology.

Jerin Geo Jacob received his Master's degree in Instrumentation Engineering from Hindustan University, Chennai, India in 2017 and Bachelor's degree in Instrumentation Engineering from Mahatma Gandhi University, Kerala, India in 2014. He is currently an Assistant Professor in the Department of Applied Electronics and Instrumentation Engineering at Mount Zion College of Engineering, Pathanamthitta, Kerala. He has worked in the field of Automation, Robotics, and the Internet of Things (IoT). His research interests include Robotics and Automation, Medical Image Processing, Smart Farming, Computer Networks, and Video Processing. Deep Learning and Internet of Things (IoT).

Mathew K. received his Ph. D in Computer Science and Engineering from Karpagam University Coimbatore, India in 2016 and a Master's degree in Computer Science and Engineering from Allahabad Agricultural Deemed University, India in 2006. He is currently a Professor in Computer Science and Engineering at Mount Zion College of Engineering Pathanamthitta, Kerala, India. His research interest includes Image processing, Deep learning, and High-performance Computing.

Naila Khan is working as an associate professor in the College of Business Administration, Princess Nourah bint Abdulrahman University. She has experience of 17 years in teaching.

Arun Kumar received B.E. from Pt.RSU raipur in 2003 complete M.Tech from CSVTU Bhilai in 2008 done my Ph.D from CVRU Bilaspur 2016 currently working as professor in the department of Electronics & Telecommunication in bhilai institute of technology Durg, India my field of interests are machine/biomedical signal processing, embedded systems.

Mohamed Lazaar received his PhD in March 2013 from the Faculty of Sciences and Technics, Sidi Mohammed Ben Abdellah university of Fez. He is a Professor of Computer Science and Artificial Intelligence at National School of Computer Sciences and Systems Analysis, Mohammed V University in Rabat. Dr. Mohamed Lazaar is a member in Smart Systems Laboratory and in Rabat IT Center at ENSIAS. His research interests include the performance of Machine Learning Methods and their applications in NLP, Recommender Systems, Multimedia Processing, etc.

Sunandan Mandal received his B. Sc. Degree in Electronics in 2007, M. Sc. Degree in Electronics in 2009 and M. Tech. Degree in 2012 from Pt. R.S.U. Raipur, India. He is currently a Research Scholar at the School of studies in Electronics & Photonics, Pt. R. S. U. Raipur, India. His research interests include biomedical signal processing, pattern recognition and data mining.

Hicham Omara is currently Professor in the Department of Computer Science in the Faculty of Science, Abdelmalek Essaadi University. His current research interests include recommender systems and machine learning.

Roshni Rahangdale is B.E in Electrical Engineering in 2001 and M.E in Power System Engineering in 2010.Recently pursuing PhD in Electrical Engineering from CSVTU Bhilai, Chhattisgarh, India.

Tanu Rizvi is B.E in Electrical & Electronics Engineering in 2008 and M.E in Power System Engineering(Electrical) in 2013.She is pursuing her PhD in Electrical Engineering from CSVTU Chhattisgarh.

Arun S. received his Bachelor's Degree in Applied Electronics and Instrumentation from Mahatma Gandhi University and Master's Degree in Applied Electronics from Anna University. He is currently working as the Assistant Professor in the Department of Applied Electronics and Instrumentation Engineering at Mount Zion

College of Engineering, Pathanamthitta, Kerala, India. His area of interest includes Biomedical Engineering, Occupational Health and Safety, and automation.

Ashima Sharma is a researcher, publishing many research papers in reputed journals, completed PhD from NIT, Raipur in Nano Science and Nano Technology. Reviewer of many national and international journals and research consultant. Field of research area is nuclear chemistry, environmental science, nanoscience, hydrochemistry, etc.

Pramisha Sharma completed PhD from CV Raman University. Working as Professor in MM College of Technology, Raipur, C.G.

Sameer Sharma has completed his MS in Renewable Energy from Carl von Ossietzky University of Oldenburg. Currently he is working as Design Engineer with RWE Renewables.

Shruti Sharma received her M.Sc. degree in Electronics from Pt. Ravishankar Shukla University, Raipur, C.G., and India in 2008. Further, she completed her Diploma in Embedded System Design from C-DAC, Kolkata, India and Post Graduate Diploma in Computer Applications form Guru Ghasidas University, Bilaspur. From 2011 to 2014, she served in GENPACT multinational firm. She also worked as Assistant Professor in CMD College, Bilaspur, and C.G. India from 2014 to 2015. Currently, she is research scholar in Electrical and Computer Engineering from Ajou University, South Korea. Her research interests include embedded design, machine learning, 5G communication, and massive MIMO.

Siji A. Thomas received her Master's degree in Communication Engineering from APJ Abdul Kalam Technological University, India in 2019 and Bachelor's degree in Instrumentation Engineering from Mahatma Gandhi University, Kerala, India in 2016. She is currently an Assistant Professor in Department of Applied Electronics and Instrumentation Engineering, Mount Zion College of Engineering, Pathanamthitta, Kerala, India. She has worked in the field of Instrumentation Maintenance, Medical Image Processing, Internet of Things, and Robotics. Her research interests include Biomedical Image Processing, Neural Networks, Deep Learning, Robotics, Smart Farming and Internet of Things (IoT).

Sini K. Thomas received her Master's degree in Communication Engineering from APJ Abdul Kalam Technological University, India in 2017 and Bachelor's degree in Electronics and Communication Engineering from Mahatma Gandhi University, Kerala, India in 2012. She is currently an Assistant Professor in Department of Electronics and Communication Engineering, VISAT Engineering College, Ernakulam, Kerala, India. She has worked in the field of different Image Processing techniques. Her research interests include Computer Networks, Optical Communication, Advanced Communication System, Biomedical Image Processing and Neural Networks.

Ruhi Uzma is B.E in Electrical & Electronics Engineering in 2005 and M.E in Power System Engineering (Electrical) in 2010. She received her PhD in 2021 in Electrical Engineering.

Gulab Singh Verma received his B.Sc degree from Govt. N P G College of Science, Raipur and M.Sc degree in Electronics & Photonics from Pt. Ravishankar Shukla University, Raipur Chhattisgarh, India. He is awarded by DST Inspire Fellowship, India. Presently is doing project on Wireless Solar Mobile Charger. His research interests include bio medical sensor and cloud computing.

Prafulla Vyas received his M. Sc. degree in Electronics in 1996 and Ph. D. degree in 2014 from Pandit Ravishankar Shukla University Raipur, India. He is currently working as Assistant Professor and Head of Department of Electronics in Disha College Raipur.

Index

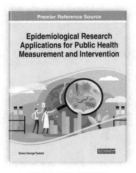
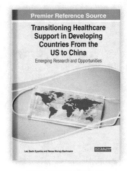
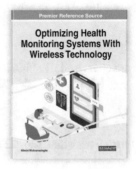
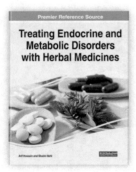
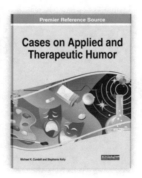
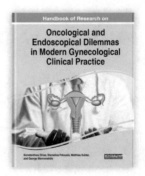
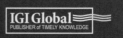

Ensure Quality Research is Introduced to the Academic Community

Become an Evaluator for IGI Global Authored Book Projects

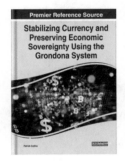

Premier Reference Source

Stabilizing Currency and Preserving Economic Sovereignty Using the Grondona System

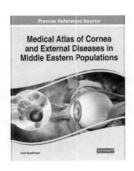

Premier Reference Source

Medical Atlas of Cornea and External Diseases in Middle Eastern Populations

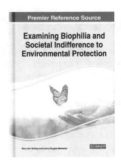

Premier Reference Source

Examining Biophilia and Societal Indifference to Environmental Protection

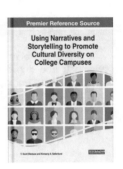

Premier Reference Source

Using Narratives and Storytelling to Promote Cultural Diversity on College Campuses

The overall success of an authored book project is dependent on quality and timely manuscript evaluations.

Applications and Inquiries may be sent to:
development@igi-global.com

Applicants must have a doctorate (or equivalent degree) as well as publishing, research, and reviewing experience. Authored Book Evaluators are appointed for one-year terms and are expected to complete at least three evaluations per term. Upon successful completion of this term, evaluators can be considered for an additional term.

If you have a colleague that may be interested in this opportunity, we encourage you to share this information with them.

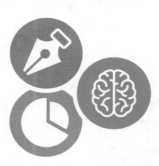
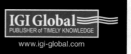

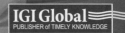

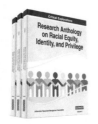
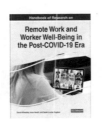
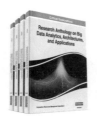
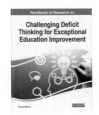

Printed in the United States
by Baker & Taylor Publisher Services